Medical Radiology

Diagnostic Imaging

For further volumes:
http://www.springer.com/series/4354

Mariano Scaglione • Ulrich Linsenmaier
Gerd Schueller

Editors

Emergency Radiology of the Abdomen

Imaging Features and Differential Diagnosis for a Timely Management Approach

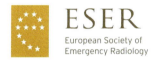

ESER
European Society of
Emergency Radiology

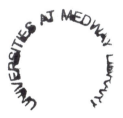

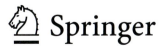

Springer

Mariano Scaglione
Department of Diagnostic Imaging
Pineta Grande Medical Center
Castel Volturno
Italy

Ulrich Linsenmaier
Department of Clinical Radiology
Ludwig-Maximilians-University
Munich
Germany

and

Director Institute of Diagnostic Radiology
    and Interventional Therapy Klinikum
    München Pasing & Perlach (KMPP)
Munich
Germany

Prof. Dr. Gerd Schueller, MBA
Department of Radiology
Medical University of Vienna
General Hospital of Vienna
Vienna
Austria

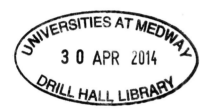
ISSN 0942-5373
ISBN 978-88-470-2512-7   e-ISBN 978-88-470-2513-4
DOI 10.1007/978-88-470-2513-4
Springer Heidelberg New York Dordrecht London

Library of Congress Control Number: 2012932402

Printed on acid-free paper

Springer is part of Springer Science+Business Media (www.springer.com)

To my beloved sons, Pietro e Ruben, for their love, encourage and support

Mariano Scaglione

My thanks go to my family, my beloved children Laura and Lukas, my brother Jörg and all friends for supporting me and encouraging my scientific work

Ulrich Linsenmaier

For Claudia, my wife, whose constant support is a great asset in my life: and to my daughters Nadja, Mona, and Linda, who tried but eventually did not preclude the writing of this book

Gerd Schueller

Foreword

Emergency Radiology of the Abdomen

Imaging Features and Differential Diagnosis for a Timely Management Approach

Things may at the same time become more difficult and easier. This very general remark also applies to the topic of this book "Emergency Radiology of the Abdomen". On one hand state-of-the-art imaging technologies allow for a straight forward diagnosis in many cases of acute abdomen, trauma to the abdomen and other emergency conditions related to diseases of abdominal organs. On the other hand, radiologists have to be more and more aware of clinical entities and pathological conditions in order to fulfil their duty, namely to provide our clinical partners with practically useful information.

It is not so long ago, that surgeons had to perform laparotomy in order to make a definite diagnosis in cases of ambiguous clinical findings concerning the status of the abdominal organs. Nowadays, imaging has become so precise and reliable, that in almost all cases a definitive diagnosis can be established before patients undergo surgery or in order to prevent unnecessary surgical procedures.

Since we talk about potentially life threatening disorders and diseases, the diagnostic imaging is a critical issue. Therefore, radiologists have to be aware of the clinical needs, the great variability of disorders, which may only be categorized correctly in view of the clinical history and clinical findings. Consequently, close cooperation and common understanding with emergency physicians are indispensable.

I would like to thank the editors of this edition of Medical Radiology/ Diagnostic Imaging for their initiative and for bringing together experts in the field. Considering the steadily increasing importance of diagnostic imaging in the management of patients with acute symptoms of the abdomen, this work may become an indispensible guide for many radiologists and clinicians. I would also like to thank all authors of the various chapters of this edition for their contribution and for the willingness to share their expertise with the readers of this book.

Prof. Dr. med. Dr. h.c. Maximilian Reiser
Department of Clinical Radiology
University Hospitals
Ludwig-Maximilians-University of Munich

Foreword

Over the last 25 years Emergency Radiology has evolved into a specialty of Diagnostic Imaging. Several major Emergency Radiology societies have arisen in many countries, there are now specialty journals on the subject, and many radiology departments throughout the world now have dedicated sections of Emergency Radiology often providing full-time coverage to their institutions. Of course, there has been and continues to be a need to organize this distinctive body of knowledge, which has grown so rapidly, and to educate the radiology community at large on this subject. Fortunately, diagnostic imaging technology has advanced over the last two decades to make the rapid and accurate diagnosis of emergent pathology practical. The evolution of multi-row detector CT has, in the most urgent clinical scenarios, provided a near perfect diagnostic modality.

In this text, the emphasis is on emergent imaging in the abdomen. The origin of the word *abdomen* is not known with certainly. It is possibly derived from the Latin *abdere* meaning to hide, thus it might mean a cavity in which odds and ends are hidden away. This definition alludes to the fact that knowing what's in abdomen and retroperitoneum, as regards acute pathology, is quite difficult making accurate diagnosis of pathology highly challenging. Given that failure to identify and quickly treat life-threatening pathology can permit a patient's death and unnecessarily opening the abdomen surgically to directly see what's inside can lead to morbidity and occasionally mortality. The value of imaging to reveal "truth without intervention" has been of inestimable value.

I have known Editors Uli Linsenmaier, MD and Dr. Mariano Scaglione, MD for many years and I know they bring a wealth of experience and knowledge to their subject. You will find this text comprehensive, current, well-written, well illustrated, and reflective of their personal insights and opinions concerning complex and controversial issues relevant to the topic. You may note some variation between the U.S. and European perspective in the early diagnostic approach to assessing emergent abdominal conditions with a stronger emphasis on sonography in initial imaging in Europe, but less so in the U.S. with greater reliance on immediate CT. They deal with the challenging issue of when to bypass imaging in favor of immediate surgery and how to integrate information obtained from the bedside and lab with imaging data in deciding optimal management. Controversies concerning the most appropriate use of diagnostic imaging are elaborated upon and personal opinions supported.

This book will be a standard for trainees and those needing to both refresh their knowledge of the subject and stay current in the field and will be a reference source to resolve "at the moment" diagnostic uncertainty when time for "quiet reflection" is not available. The information contained herein is very "digestible", that is, easy to assimilate. I fully expect that it will help you resolve many problematical acute abdominal imaging cases.

Stuart E. Mirvis
Professor and Director Section of Emergency Radiology
University of Maryland School of Medicine

Preface

We, as radiologists, face a time in which rapid emergency radiology (ER) diagnosis and intervention are mandatory for the proper management of serious abdominal emergencies. Indeed, the demand for diagnostic imaging in ER departments has risen dramatically over the last decade, with an exponential increase in the use of multi-detector computed tomography (MDCT) of up to 25% per year. In the USA, between 1996 and 2007, MDCT use during ER department visits grew by 330%, with the largest increase in older patients and for the diagnosis of abdominal or chest pain. These rates are a direct result of the technical and methodological improvements in the use of MDCT. Moreover, diagnostic imaging has, at least in part, virtually replaced physical examination for many emergency patients. Particularly in severely injured or critically ill patients referred to an emergency unit, immediate cross-sectional imaging is used as an adjunct to the primary patient survey (ATLS) and has proven to be of substantial benefit in establishing an adequate, timely, and individual therapy.

In order to achieve excellent professional co-operation with referring physicians, it is indispensable that radiologists have a concise understanding of the specific pathologies that are seen in the emergency setting, including appropriate clinical knowledge of acute abdominal disorders.

Our aim in writing this book was to provide a comprehensive review of the traumatic as well as the non-traumatic emergency scenarios of the acute abdomen. The style of the presentation reflects the belief that improved time-lines and greater accuracy in diagnostic and interventional imaging lead to improved clinical management and better patient outcomes. Thus, the book focuses on the imaging features that are relevant to a timely management approach.

It is a pleasure for us to offer this book to an international readership, with the support of the new European Society of Emergency Radiology (ESER), which was founded as a subspecialty society under the auspices of the European Society of Radiology (ESR). In our opinion, emergency radiology requires comprehensive specialized training, consistent with the shift in radiologic education from a modality-based approach to organ—and process-specific practices. Dedicated abdominal emergency radiology training is a remarkable endeavor—one that not only has become an integral part of the core curriculum for residents and fellows but which is also very much in demand in postgraduate training.

We truly believe that this book could help fulfilling the unique demands of modern emergency radiology.

Mariano Scaglione, MD
Ulrich Linsenmaier, MD
Gerd Schueller, MD, MBA

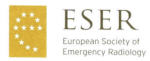

Contents

Contributors

F. E. Avni Department of Radiology, Erasme Hospital, Brussels, Belgium, e-mail: Freddy.Avni@erasme.ulb.ac.be

F. H. Berger Department of Radiology, VU University Medical Center Amsterdam, Amsterdam, The Netherlands

Gianpaolo Carrafiello Department of Radiology, University of Insubria, Varese, Italy, e-mail: gcarraf@gmail.com

M. Cassart Department of Radiology, Medical University of Vienna, General Hospital Vienna, Vienna, Austria

Garry Choy Department of Radiology, Division of Emergency Radiology and Teleradiology, Massachusetts General Hospital, Boston, MA, USA, e-mail: gchoy@partners.org

E. Cotta Department of Radiology, University of Insubria, Varese, Italy

N. Damry Pediatric Imaging, Children's Hospital Queen Fabiola, Brussels, Belgium

V. Di Mizio Radiology Service, Santa Maria della Misericordia Hospital, Rovigo, Italy

M. K. Dighe Department of Radiology, University of Washington, Seattle, WA, USA

C. Fugazzola Department of Radiology, University of Insubria, Varese, Italy

L. L. Geyer Department of Clinical Radiology, University Hospital LMU Munich, Munich, Germany, e-mail: lucas.geyer@med.uni-muenchen.de

R. Grassi Department of Radiology, Second University, Naples, Italy

J. A. Gross Department of Radiology, Harborview Medical Center, University of Washington, Seattle, WA, USA, e-mail: jagross@uw.edu

A. M. Ierardi Department of Radiology, University of Insubria, Varese, Italy

P. N. Khalil Division of General and Visceral Surgery, Department of Surgery, Campus Innenstadt, Ludwig-Maximilians University (LMU), Munich, Germany, e-mail: philipe@me.com

D. R. Kool Department of Radiology, Jeroen Bosch Hospital, S Hertogenbosch, The Netherlands

B. E. Lehnert Department of Radiology, Harborview Medical Center, University of Washington, Seattle, WA, USA

U. Linsenmaier Department of Clinical Radiology, University Hospital LMU Munich, Ludwig-Maximilians-University, Munich, Germany, e-mail: ulrich. linsenmaier@med.lmu.de ; Director Institute of Diagnostic Radiology and Interventional Therapy Klinikum München Pasing & Perlach (KMPP), Munich, Germany, e-mail: ulrich.linsenmaier@kliniken-pasing-perlach.de

M. Mangini Department of Radiology, University of Insubria, Varese, Italy

L. Mannelli Department of Radiology, Harborview Medical Center, University of Washington, Seattle, WA, USA

M. A. Mazzei Department of Radiology, University of Siena, Siena, Italy

V. Miele Department of Emergency Radiology, S. Camillo Hospital, Rome, Italy, e-mail: vittoriomiele@alice.it

R. A. Novelline Department of Radiology, Division of Emergency Radiology and Teleradiology, Massachusetts General Hospital, Boston, MA, USA

F. Piacentino Department of Radiology, University of Insubria, Varese, Italy

A. Pinto Department of Radiology, Cardarelli Hospital, Naples, Italy

C. Recaldini Department of Radiology, University of Insubria, Varese, Italy

L. Romano Department of Radiology, Cardarelli Hospital, Naples, Italy

A. Rotondo Department of Radiology, Second University, Naples, Italy

C. T. Sadro Department of Radiology, Harborview Medical Center, University of Washington, Seattle, WA, USA

M. Scaglione Department of Radiology, Pineta Grande Medical Center, Castel Volturno, Italy, e-mail: mscaglione@tiscali.it

M. K. Scherr Department of Clinical Radiology, University Hospital LMU Munich, Ludwig-Maximilians-University, Munich, Germany, e-mail: michael.scherr@med.uni-muenchen.de

G. Schueller Department of Radiology, Medical University of Vienna, General Hospital of Vienna, Vienna, Austria, e-mail: gerd.schueller@ meduniwien.ac.at

A. K. Singh Department of Radiology, Division of Emergency Radiology and Teleradiology, Massachusetts General Hospital, Boston, MA, USA

J. A. Soto Department of Radiology, Boston Medical Center, Boston University School of Medicine, Boston, MA, USA, e-mail: Jorge.Soto@bmc.org

M. Treitl Department of Clinical Radiology, University Hospital LMU Munich, Munich, Germany, e-mail: marcus.treitl@med.uni-muenchen.de

P. M. Vos Department of Radiology, St. Pauls Hospital Vancouver BC, Vancouver, BC, Canada

S. Wirth Department of Clinical Radiology, University Hospital LMU Munich, Munich, Germany, e-mail: swirth@med.lmu.de

Acute Abdomen: Clinical Context and Indications for Imaging

Philipe N. Khalil

Contents

Abstract

The acute abdomen is characterized by the sudden onset of severe abdominal pain, which requires emergency medical or surgical consultation. It can be caused by diseases of any of the abdominal organs or organ systems, and, as such, the acute abdomen represents a physical condition rather than a disease. However, extra-abdominal disease may also lead cause an acute abdomen. A rapid and accurate diagnosis is essential because various potentially life-threatening processes may be the underlying causes of the physical complaints. Because of the wide spectrum of diseases that may cause an acute abdomen, the use of imaging techniques, in particular, multidetector computed tomography (MDCT) and magnetic resonance imaging (MRI), is often warranted because of their ability to suggest alternative diagnoses if the suspected clinical diagnosis is unconfirmed by ultrasonography (US). Depending on the clinical pattern and basic diagnosis, the treatment of such injuries requires a balance between the quick availability, the possible diagnostic benefit of additional and potential radiation exposures by imaging, possible time delay. These circumstances are particularly relevant for patients with life-threatening illnesses, when MDCT should be immediately be performed, and for pregnant woman when dedicated MRI can be a diagnostic option. Thus, early use of MDCT has been shown to reduce the number of serious diagnoses that are missed. Advanced diagnostics that may be used to guide and treat both trauma and non-trauma patients include such techniques as endoscopy or

P. N. Khalil (✉)
Division of General and Visceral Surgery,
Department of Surgery, Campus Innenstadt,
Ludwig-Maximilians University (LMU),
Nußbaumstraße 20, 80336 Munich, Germany
e-mail: philipe@me.com

M. Scaglione et al. (eds.), *Emergency Radiology of the Abdomen*,
Medical Radiology. Diagnostic Imaging,
DOI: 10.1007/174_2011_464, © Springer-Verlag Berlin Heidelberg 2012

selective angiography, e.g., for the treatment of gastrointestinal or visceral organ hemorrhage. Parenchymateous organ or hollow organ visceral bleeding, including perforations, is representative of classical, life-threatening diagnoses secured by MDCT. However, advanced testing in patients that require surgery for abdominal emergencies will result in a delay in the necessary treatments. The present chapter defines the clinical context of patients presenting with an acute abdomen and provides information's on clinical pattern and diagnostic strategies.

1 Introduction

The acute abdomen is characterized by the sudden onset of severe abdominal pain, which requires emergency medical or surgical consultation. It can be caused by diseases of any of the abdominal organs or organ systems, and, as such, represents a physical condition rather than a disease. However, extra-abdominal disease may also result in an acute abdomen. A rapid and accurate diagnosis is essential because various potentially life-threatening processes may underlie the physical complaints. Given the wide spectrum of diseases that may cause an acute abdomen, the use of imaging techniques, in particular, multi-detector computed tomography (MDCT) and magnetic resonance imaging (MRI), is often warranted based on their ability to suggest alternative diagnoses if the preliminary clinical diagnosis is unconfirmed by ultrasonography (US). Depending on the clinical pattern and the preliminary diagnosis, the treatment of such injuries requires a balance between the rapid availability of a particular treatment, the possible diagnostic benefit of imaging despite additional and potential radiation exposures, and the effects of a possible time delay in treatment. These circumstances are particularly relevant for patients with life-threatening illnesses, in which case MDCT should be immediately performed, and for pregnant woman, in whom dedicated MRI is usually a diagnostic option. This chapter defines the clinical context of patients presenting with an acute abdomen and provides information on the clinical patterns and diagnostic strategies relevant to this condition.

2 General Considerations

The acute abdomen is a common clinical syndrome in patients admitted to the emergency department and can be related to a variety of underlying disease (Stoker et al. 2009; Leschka et al. 2005). Approximately 5–10% of all patients who present to the emergency department are suffering from acute abdominal pain (Laméris et al. 2009). The acute abdomen comprises non-traumatic and traumatic emergencies, and patients come to the attention of physicians in a number of contexts: presenting themselves to the emergency department, transported by ambulance, or while already hospitalized on the ward. The patients may be hemodynamically stable or unstable, conscious or unconscious. An acute abdomen can be caused by diseases of any of the abdominal organs or organ systems, and, as such, the acute abdomen represents a physical condition rather than a disease (Zech and Reiser 2010). These multiple etiologies of the acute abdomen and the challenge of a proper diagnosis led Hugh Dudley to state, "it is as much an intellectual exercise to tackle the problems of belly ache as to work on the human genome" (Schein 2005a). Although the intensity and the time course of the pain often correlate with disease severity, these factors may be masked in immuno-compromised or elderly patients, as well as in children (Spencer et al. 2009; de Dombal 1988; Myren et al. 1988). The acute abdomen is characterized by the sudden onset of severe abdominal pain, which requires emergency medical or surgical consultation (Leschka et al. 2005). Thus, Zachary Cope noted: "the general rule can be laid down that the majority of severe abdominal pains which occur in patients who have been previously fairly well, and which last as long as 6 h, are caused by conditions of surgical import" (Schein 2005a). Physical examination and laboratory tests for this condition are often non-specific, and the clinical presentations may overlap in many diseases (Leschka et al. 2005). A rapid and accurate diagnosis is essential in all patients suffering from an acute abdomen because various potentially life-threatening processes may be the underlying causes of the physical complaints (Schein 2005a). Therefore, Cope's statement holds true, that "all who have had much experience of the group of cases known generally as the acute abdomen will probably agree that in that condition early diagnosis is exceptionally important" (Green 2008). Therefore, an interdisciplinary approach is essential to secure a prompt diagnosis for a patient admitted with an acute abdomen. There is no doubt that, prior to the widespread use of radiological imaging techniques, individuals presenting with abdominal tenderness and rigidity were candidates for surgery; however, with the present availability of diagnostic imaging for the evaluation of an acute abdomen, some of these patients will no longer undergo immediate surgery but, instead, will receive intermittent or definite medical treatment for the underlying disease (Stoker et al. 2009).

2.1 Etiology and Clinical Patterns

There is a long list of diseases that may lead to an acute abdomen. While most of them have their origin in the abdomen, others arise from extra-abdominal regions; for example. an inferior wall myocardial infarction can lead to severe epigastric pain (Schein 2005a). As determined by a multinational OMGE (World Gastroenterology Organization) survey, the vast majority of patients presenting with acute abdominal pain for whom a final diagnosis can be established suffer in particular from appendicitis (28%), cholecystitis (10%), small-bowel obstruction (4%), acute gynecological disease (4%), acute pancreatitis (3%), acute renal colic (3%), perforated peptic ulcer (2.5%), or acute diverticulitis (1.5%), while in approximately one-third of the cases the etiology remains undetermined (de Dombal 1988). A number of attempts have been made to categorize and track the major diseases that cause an acute abdomen. Frequently, these categorizations are based on the anatomic location of the abdominal pain, the decision to treat the disease surgically or non-surgically, and the different medical disciplines involved in treatment. An overview of the categorization of the major diseases according to the anatomic location of the abdominal pain is given in Table 1. However, it is not sufficient in clinical practice to merely consider the most likely causes for the acute abdomen or to rule them out one by one from a long list (Schein 2005a). In the view of Moshe Schein, it is wiser to identify a clinical pattern and to decide upon a course of action from a limited menu of

management options, which in turn will guide the clinician to a specific management option (Schein 2005a). These clinical patterns include: (1) abdominal pain and shock, (2) generalized peritonitis, (3) localized peritonitis, confirmed to one quadrant of the abdomen, (4) intestinal obstruction, and (5) medical illness. The individual management options in such cases are: (1) immediate operation (surgery now), (2) pre-operative preparation and operation (surgery tomorrow morning), (3) conservative treatment (e.g. observations, fluid substitution, and antibiotics), and (4) discharge home (Schein 2005a). Both the clinical pattern and the various management options reflect the larger problem faced by doctors when evaluating patients presenting with an acute abdomen: Since time may affect patient outcome, a timely and priority-based approach in these patients is essential both to minimize the potential for delayed diagnosis and to assure proper further treatment (Khalil et al. 2011a).

2.2 Medical History and Physical Examination

In patients with acute abdomen, past medical history is essential and often path-determining for the later diagnosis of the underlying disease leading. In the case of a critically ill patient, this information is often obtained from relatives or from an observer of the event. In general, the medical history and physical assessment are completed with the help of a standardized questionnaire. The rationale behind this approach is that obtaining a medical history requires time that is often not available for a critically ill patient. Moreover, there is the potential to miss important physical findings (Boffard 2007). A formal medical history generally includes the quality, duration, and localization of the pain prompting admission, as well as previous pain episodes, the presence of nausea or vomiting, and noticeable changes in bowel movements or urination. In addition, medications received, previous abdominal operations, and existing chronic diseases or allergies are essential in this context. However, the assembly of an adequate medical history may be complicated or even impossible in the presence of a language barrier or due to the age or condition of the patient. The latter often applies to a patient with a

Table 1 Categorization of the most common diseases according to the anatomic side of abdominal pain

Right upper quadrant	Epigastrium	Left upper quadrant
	Gastritis	
Cholecystolithiasis	Gastroesophageal reflux	Splenic trauma
Cholecystitis	Peptic ulcer	Splenic infarction
Cholangitis	Myocardial infarction	Nephrolithiasis
Choledocholithiasis	Pancreatitis	Pyelonephritis
Nephrolithiasis		Pleuritis
Pyelonephritis		Pneumothorax
Pleuritis		Subphrenic abscess
Pneumothorax	**Periumbilical**	Diverticulitis
Colitis	Gastroenteritis	Large bowel ischemia
Hepatic tumors	Incisional hernia	Large bowel obstruction
Hepatic trauma	Small bowel obstruction	Large bowel perforation
Subphrenic abscess	Large bowel obstruction	
Subhepatic abscess and bilioma	Pancreatitis	
	Large bowel ischemia	
	Urinary retention	
Right lower quadrant	Intestinal pseudo-obstruction	**Left lower quadrant**
Appendicitis	Mesenterial ischemia	Diverticulitis
Urinary tract infection	Aortic aneurysm incl.	Large bowel obstruction
Renal colic	rupture/dissection	Large bowel perforation
Inguinal hernia	Abdominal hernia	Ischemic colitis
Inflamed Meckel's diverticulum	Inflammatory bowel disease	Urinary tract infection
Large bowel obstruction		Renal colic
Inflammatory bowel disease		Inguinal hernia
Colitis		Inflammatory bowel disease
Cecum ischemia	**Central lower quadrant**	Salpingitis
Large bowel perforation	Cystitis	Ectopic pregnancy
Salpingitis	Salpingitis	Ovary torsion
Ectopic pregnancy	Urinary retention	Ovary cyst rupture
Ovary torsion	Diverticulitis	Volvulus
Ovary cyst rupture	Ovary cyst rupture	
Volvulus	Ectopic pregnancy	
Intestinal invagination	Volvulus	
	Suprapubic herniation	

life-threatening injury as the result of trauma but can also refer to a non-traumatic, unstable patient who is, for instance, suffering from a bleeding event or sepsis. The physical examination is a second important component of the further evaluation and begins with inspection of the patient. For example, patients with abdominal tenderness or rigidity often adduct the lower extremities to reduce the abdominal pain. During visual inspection and later physical examination of the patient and, in particular, of the abdomen, it is worthwhile to search for scars derived from previous celiotomies and to assess the skin color or the volume status by searching for standing wrinkles or peripheral edema. The moisture or dryness of the skin can be determined, and the body temperature estimated. The abdominal wall may be distended or flat. Auscultation of all four quadrants may reveal unsuspicious bowel sounds, hyper- or suspending peristalsis, or complete silence within the abdomen. The bowel sounds can be tympanic or burbling. Palpation may reveal localized or diffuse pain with or without signs of abdominal tenderness. Incisional abdominal wall hernias, intra-abdominal resistances, or tumor formations may be palpable if deeper palpation is tolerated by the patient and not barred by tenderness and rigidity. However, an accurate palpation of the abdomen may be difficult in the adipose patient. Additionally, peripheral perfusion and the pulse should be assessed. When appropriate, a digital rectal examination is performed. In patients with life-threatening illness or abdominal injury, the assessment should be carried out using the primary survey and the ABCDEs (A: airway, B: breathing, C: circulation, D: disability, E: environment) according to the American College of Surgeons and the Advanced Trauma Life Support guidelines (American College of Surgeons—Committee on Trauma 2004; Kool and Blickman 2007). Following completion of the primary survey and depending on the requirement for resuscitative efforts in the patient demonstrating normalization of vital function, the secondary survey should be performed (American College of Surgeons—Committee on Trauma 2004). In this context, it is worthwhile mentioning that, especially in trauma patients, distracting injuries may be present. Thus, patients report those symptoms that they themselves feel most acutely, but not necessarily those that may be of most medical relevance. These symptoms therefore may go initially undetected. On the other hand, many therapeutically relevant conditions can be missed during the primary survey if the focus is only on those that are life-threatening.

3 Basic Diagnostics and Decision-Making

The diagnostics performed on patients evaluated for an acute abdomen will depend, in general, on the observed clinical patterns. In accordance with the Advanced Trauma Life Support protocol, priority is given to resuscitation rather than to an over-extended and time-consuming diagnostic evaluation (Khalil et al. 2011a; Boffard 2007; American College of Surgeons—Committee on Trauma 2004). Measuring and, where necessary, monitoring vital signs, including breathing rate, oxygenation, heart rate, and blood pressure, are imperative in every patient presenting with an acute abdomen. Volume substitution or oxygen should be supplied as needed. Obtaining a venous blood sample after the establishment of a venous access line and performing a focused US of the abdomen constitute the most important diagnostic tools that are rapidly available. In this context, blood tests should include a complete set of the values necessary to assess possible organ dysfunction or damage, as well as those systemic values required to evaluate possible anemia, coagulation or its disturbance, and inflammation. Values for creatinine and thyroid stimulating hormone are required prior to intravenous iodine contrast administration during MDCT; they are however, dispensable in acute emergencies. Additionally, a pregnancy test should be performed for every parous female. It is now well recognized that abdominal US provides a useful and fast tool in the initial physical evaluation that guides the course of decision-making for an acute abdomen, although its accuracy depends on the investigator's level of experience and the available time. A urine test should follow the US where appropriate. An electrocardiogram to detect possible arrhythmias or a myocardial infarction is further recommended. Following a negative or inconclusive US, MDCT yields the highest sensitivity, as with this strategy only 6% of urgent cases are missed, according to one study (Laméris et al. 2009). In that report, 49% of patients required a subsequent MDCT (Laméris et al. 2009). Acute appendicitis, which accounts for approximately 7% of all presentations to the emergency department, is one diagnosis that often requires no further imaging. Instead, the US examination, in conjunction with the clinical presentation, the course of the complaints, and an increase in the markers of inflammation, guides the diagnosis (Howell et al. 2010; Schick et al. 2008; Khalil et al. 2010). The use of MDCT in the evaluation of acute appendicitis is not universally recommended and accepted, especially in young females or during pregnancy. However, remarkable geographic differences are observed in the use of US and MDCT, also depending on the availability and the established clinical and diagnostic pathways (Howell et al. 2010; Khalil et al. 2010). However, the diagnosis of acute appendicitis may be especially challenging in pregnant women. With a frequency of approximately 1 in 1,500 pregnancies, acute appendicitis is the most common reason for non-obstetrical surgical intervention in pregnancy (Khalil et al. 2010; Rosen et al. 2000). US is not useful to visualize the appendix after 34 weeks of gestation (Lim et al. 1992) but a late or missed diagnosis of appendicitis during pregnancy is associated with a fetal loss rate of up to 25% and a maternal mortality of 4% (Kilpatrick and Monga 2007). Therefore, the need for further measures to establish the diagnosis must be carefully balanced. MRI has recently shown great potential in imaging the acute abdomen during pregnancy and after the first trimester the indications are well established (see "The Pelvis"). Uncomplicated cholecystitis is the second most common non-traumatic disease diagnosed solely by US and clinical presentation (Leschka et al. 2005; Grafen et al. 2010). In these patients, MDCT may be reserved for complicated cases, e.g., suspicion of choledocholithiasis or biliary pancreatitis, either of which is considered an endoscopic emergency (Leschka et al. 2005; Cahir et al. 2004; Shakespear et al. 2010; Bortoff et al. 2000). For the treatment of cholecystitis, early (<72 h) or delayed cholecystectomy (>14 days) may be performed by laparoscopy or using an open technique, without any major clinical differences in the postoperative outcome (Johansson et al. 2005; Gurusamy et al. 2010). The timing of the operation depends on the clinical presentation and history of symptoms (Figs. 1 and 2).

3.1 Advanced Diagnostic and Therapeutic Strategies

MDCT is the diagnostic gold standard for evaluating patients presenting with an acute abdomen (Stoker et al. 2009; Federle 2005). The positive effect of imaging on the accuracy of clinical diagnosis of the acute abdomen has been proven, which in turn has led to changes in patient management (Laméris et al. 2009). The early use of MDCT has been shown to reduce the number of serious diagnoses that are missed (Laméris et al. 2009). In contrast, MRI does not play a relevant role in abdominal emergencies except in selected populations and circumstances, including pregnancy (Stoker et al. 2009; Kilpatrick and Monga 2007). Advanced diagnostics that may be

used to guide and treat both trauma and non-trauma patients include endoscopy and selective angiography, e.g., for the treatment of gastrointestinal or visceral organ hemorrhage. Parenchymateous-or hollow-organ visceral bleeding, including perforations, is representative of the classical, life-threatening pathologies secured by MDCT. However, advanced testing in patients who require surgery for abdominal emergencies will result in a delay in the necessary treatments (Rozycki et al. 2002).

Traumatic or non-traumatic hepatic tumor bleeding is one of these conditions. The most comprehensive hepatic injury classification was introduced in 1989 by the Organ Injury Scaling Committee of the American Association for the Surgery of Trauma (AAST) and it includes six grades, from subcapsular hematoma or small capsular tear to a hepatic avulsion (Oniscu et al. 2006). The prevalence of liver injuries among patients who have sustained blunt multiple traumas is reported to be 1–8% (Yoon et al. 2005). Over the past decades, there has been a paradigm shift in the management of blunt liver trauma, with a trend toward non-surgical management in hemodynamically stable patients. This reflects the wide availability of MDCT and the efforts made using interventional radiology (Yoon et al. 2005; Parks et al. 2011). Thus, Pringle's statement from 1908, that "minor liver injuries will heal without operative intervention," still holds true today and the list of injuries may be expanded to include higher-grade hepatic organ lacerations (Yoon et al. 2005; Pringle 1908). In fact, up to 89% of all patients with blunt liver trauma can be treated non-surgically, with success rates of 85–94% (Yoon et al. 2005). This approach is similarly appropriate in up to 65% of patients with blunt spleen injuries and selected stab wounds (Pachter et al. 1998; Madoff et al. 2005). However, unstable patients with grade IV and V lesions, i.e., lacerations involving segmental or hilar vessels and producing major devascularization of >25% of the spleen (IV) as well as a completely shattered spleen or hilar vascular injuries leading to a devascularized spleen (V), require emergency celiotomies to insure hemostasis (Pachter et al. 1998; Moore et al. 1995) (Figs. 3, 4, 5).

The peptic ulcer is a considerable cause of non-traumatic abdominal bleeding and is associated with high morbidity and substantial mortality (Malfertheiner et al. 2009; Wang et al. 2010; Gralnek et al. 2008). In this context, the role of emergency surgery is not to

Fig. 1 Clinical presentation and intraoperative findings in patients admitted with an acute abdomen. **a** Abdominal view, male patient. **b** Umbilical hernia with bowel incarceration. **c** Perineal view, male patient. **d** Perineal hernia with small-bowel incarceration years after abdomino-perineal resection of the rectum for lower rectal cancer. **e** Abdominal view, female patient. **f** Septic multi-organ failure and massive toxic megacolon. **g** Abdominal view, male patient. **h** Keel-shaped distention of the abdomen due to a sigmoid colon volvulus and typical colon twist

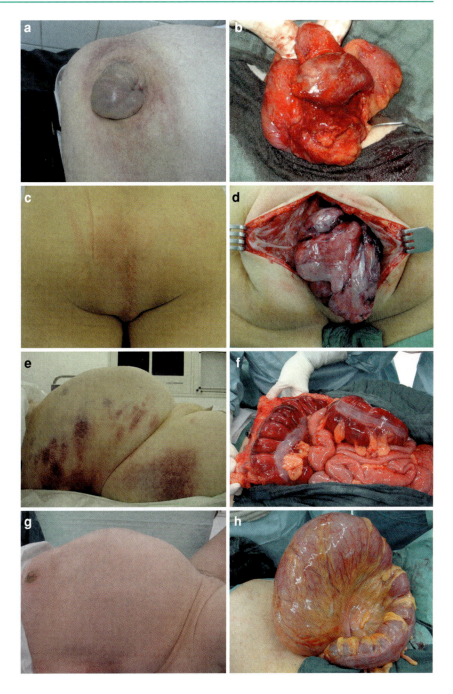

cure the disease but rather to stop a hemorrhage when endoscopic therapy is unavailable or has failed or to treat possible perforations (Malfertheiner et al. 2009). MDCT may be used both to detect the source of upper gastrointestinal bleeding and to confirm a suspected perforation (Jaeckle et al. 2008).

Other common diseases that may cause an acute abdomen and diagnosed primarily by MDCT are inflammatory, vascular-related, or obstructive large- and small-bowel diseases. Inflammatory bowel diseases comprise ulcerative colitis and Crohn's disease, either of which has the potential to cause an acute abdomen with complications of emergent surgical relevance, e.g., toxic megacolon, perforation, severe bleeding, and bowel obstruction (Andersson and Söderholm 2009).

Fig. 2 Clinical presentation and intraoperative findings in patients admitted with an acute abdomen. **a** Abdominal view, male patient. **b** Septic course with four-quadrant peritonitis requiring operative revision. **c** Abdominal view, female insulin-dependent diabetic patient who after sustained cardiopulmonary resuscitation leading to livid skin color was operated on for abdominal compartment syndrome. **d** Generalized mesenteric lymphatic adenopathy (*) with bacteriology-confirmed necrotizing fasciitis originating from the lower extremities. **e** Abdominal view, female patient after coronary artery intervention including coronary stent placement for acute myocardial infarction. **f** Celiotomy showed a gastric perforation (*arrows*). **g** Abdominal view, male patient. **h** Abdominal stab wound following attempted suicide; the small bowel is exposed

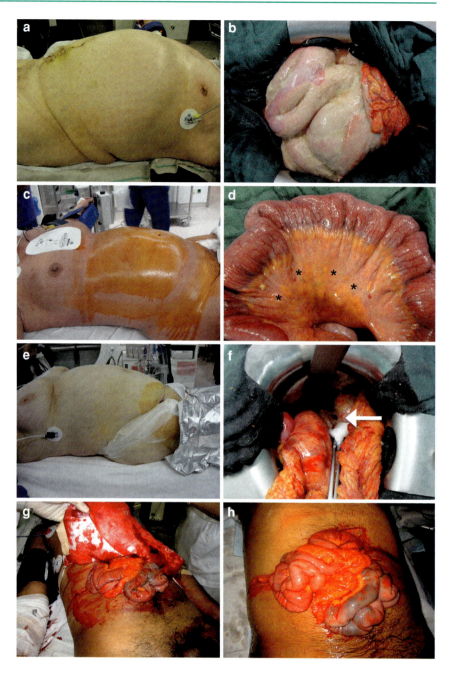

Diverticulitis of the sigmoid colon, also known as left-sided appendicitis, is the classical cause of left lower quadrant pain (Jacobs 2007). The indication for and timing of surgery is determined primarily by disease severity but also includes age and co-existing diseases (Jacobs 2007; Hinchey et al. 1978). Thus, <10% of patients admitted with acute diverticulitis require surgical treatment during the same admission (Jacobs 2007). Among the indications for emergency surgery are generalized peritonitis and sepsis, uncontained visceral perforation, the presence of a large non-draining abscess, and no improvement or worsened course within 3 days (Jacobs 2007). The severity of diverticulitis and the surgical indications are graded according to the Hinchey classification, based on the presence of: localized abscess (I), pelvic abscess (II), purulent peritonitis (III), and feculent peritonitis (IV) (Jacobs 2007; Hinchey et al. 1978;

Fig. 3 Operative features in patients with abdominal hemorrhage who presented with an acute abdomen. **a, b** Unstable male patient after sustained blunt abdominal trauma with massive hemorrhage caused by splenic rupture. Operative field and dorsal view of the spleen compound. **c, d** Unstable male patient after sustained blunt abdominal trauma with massive abdominal hemorrhage caused by hepatic rupture. Intraoperative compression of the liver allows assessment of the extent of the injury after blood evacuation by suction. **e** Young unstable patient with massive abdominal hemorrhage caused by non-traumatic spontaneous rupture of the left hepatic lobe due to focal nodular hyperplasia of the liver. **f** Young male patient who sustained an abdominal stab wound (*arrow*). Emergent laparoscopy verified a small hepatic laceration as the cause for free abdominal fluid (*)

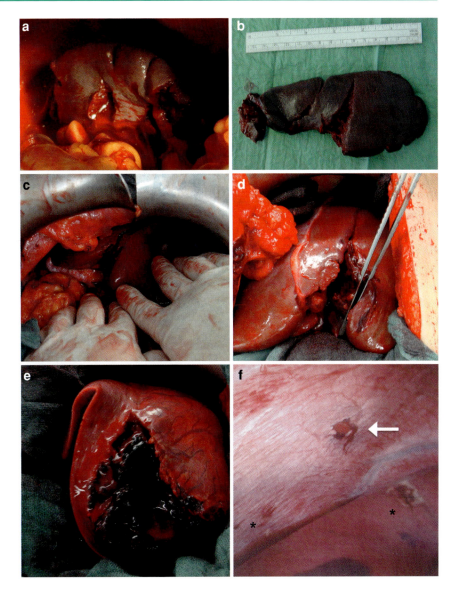

Ambrosetti et al. 2002). Ischemic bowel disease shows a broad spectrum of clinical manifestations. It is commonly due to mesenteric ischemia following embolic arterial occlusion, and less frequently to superior mesenteric vein thrombosis or vasculitis (Shanley and Weinberger 2008; Renner et al. 2011). In selected patients, early reconstructive surgery or interventional procedures can be performed to preserve the mesenteric blood supply; however, these cases often result in poor overall outcome (Renner et al. 2011). In contrast, non-occlusive ischemic colitis can involve every segment of the colon (Khalil et al. 2009) (Figs. 6, 7, 8, 9).

A further common cause of acute abdomen that is regularly diagnosed by MDCT is related to large- and small-bowel obstruction. US cannot detect many adhesions and it likewise often fails due to the presence of gas-filled bowel loops (Silva et al. 2009). While tumors of various types, postoperative adhesions, coprostasis, and volvulus are the most likely reasons for a large-bowel obstruction, 65–75% of small-bowel obstructions are the result of intra-abdominal adhesions, with bowel strangulation, incisional or inner hernias, instussception, peritoneal carcinomatosis, primary or secondary tumors, and gallstones as less frequent causes (Taourel et al. 2003;

Fig. 4 Operative features in patients with an acute abdomen caused by cholecystitis. **a, b** Male patient who presented with local right upper quadrant tenderness. Further diagnostic evaluation showed an acute cholecystitis with choledocholithiasis. After a failed endoscopic stone extraction, open cholecystectomy and stone saving were performed. **c, d** Two examples of the gallbladder after laparoscopic cholecystectomy for cholecystitis. Cholecystitis with the gallbladder completely filled by stones (**c**), an opened ulcerous cholecystitis (**d**). **e** Young pregnant female, 27th week of gestation, who presented with right upper quadrant tenderness. Emergent laparoscopy confirmed purulent cholecystitis. The foreground of the picture shows the uterus (*)

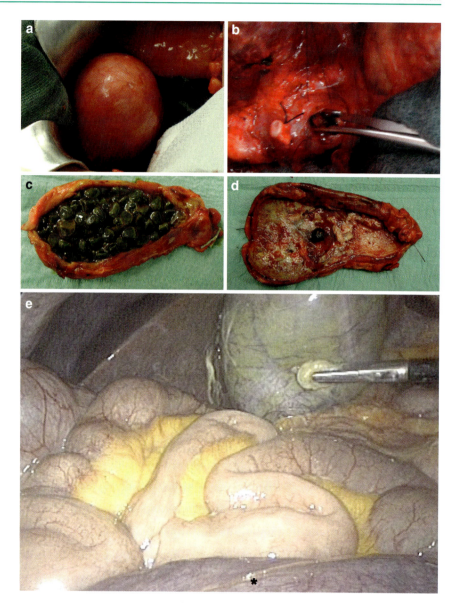

Martin and Steele 2010; Aguirre et al. 2005; Khalil et al. 2011a). In these cases, it is of particular importance to determine the extent of the bowel damage or tumor localization because this information will determine the subsequent medical and surgical strategy. The majority of the cases of acute colonic obstruction are secondary to colorectal cancer, involving 15–20% of all such patients (Trompetas 2008). Simple colostomy, primary resection, the discontinuity resection of Hartmann, or palliative bowel stenting are the prevailing surgical options in this context (Angele et al. 2011). In cases of small- or large-bowel obstruction, MDCT can be used to determine the localization, course, and underlying cause of the obstruction, providing information that guides further surgical approaches, e.g., in cases of singular adhesion bridle, treatment may involve laparoscopy or a minimally fashioned laparotomy (Grafen et al. 2010).

3.2 Demands of Imaging and Interdisciplinary Approach

Given the wide spectrum of diseases that may cause an acute abdomen, the use of imaging techniques, in

Fig. 5 Operative features in patients with bowel obstruction requiring emergent surgery. **a, b** Male patient with mechanical obstruction caused by a bridle adhesion (*arrow*). The obstructed small bowel recovered and no bowel resection was necessary. **c** Male patient with mechanical small bowel obstruction cause by a bridle (*arrow*). **d** The patient presented late and the necrotic segment had to be resected. **e** Male patient presenting with generalized tenderness due to a gangrenous ileum segment due to strangulation and subsequent ischemia. **f** Female patient with a small bowel obstruction caused by abdominal adhesions of small bowel to the abdominal wall (*arrow*), laparoscopic view. **g, h** Patient presenting with a small-bowel obstruction caused by a gallstone. **i** Small-bowel obstruction due to tumor infiltration (*). **j** Patient with large-bowel obstruction caused by a large carcinoma of the sigmoid colon, opened colon after resection (*)

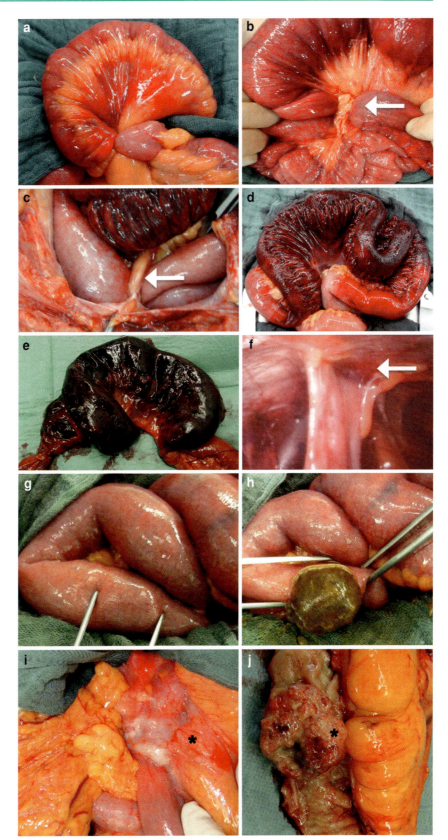

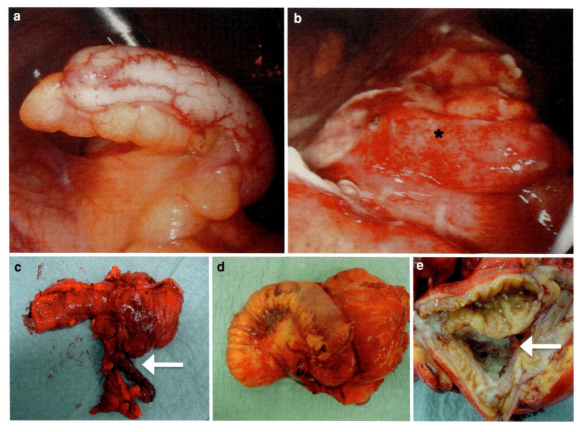

Fig. 6 Operative features in patients with right lower quadrant pain related to the appendix. **a** Acute appendicitis, laparoscopic view. **b** Purulent appendicitis, laparoscopic view (*). **c** Necrotic and perforated appendicitis involving the cecum (*arrow*). **d** Conglomerate of the ileo-cecal segment in a patient with a perforated appendicitis leading to an abscess formation. **e** Retroperitoneal abscess cavity after bowel incision (*arrow*)

particular, MDCT and MRI, is often warranted because of their ability to suggest alternative diagnoses if the suspected clinical diagnosis is unconfirmed by US (Leschka et al. 2005). Acute pancreatitis is representative of pathologies requiring primary, non-surgical management; in an emergent case of acute pancreatitis, the extent is determined using MDCT (Kleespies et al. 2008). However, cholecystectomy and/or endoscopic intervention in cases of biliary pancreatitis, necrosectomy and lavage in progressively infected necrosis and septic course, or emergent celiotomy in case of bleeding or hollow-organ perforation are conditions requiring surgical intervention (Kleespies et al. 2008; Balthazar 2002). In traumatic injuries of the pancreas, the indication for celiotomy depends on whether the lesion is of a grade associated with high morbidity and mortality (Linsenmaier et al. 2008). Depending on the clinical pattern and basic diagnosis, the

treatment of such injuries requires a balance between rapid availability, the possible diagnostic benefit of additional imaging despite further radiation exposures, and the risks of possible time delays (Linsenmaier et al. 2008). These circumstances are particularly relevant for patients with life-threatening illnesses, in which case MDCT should be immediately performed, and for pregnant woman when dedicated MRI can be a diagnostic option. On the other hand, an improper diagnosis, due to an insufficient work-up in which imaging was omitted or improperly executed may have severe or even fatal consequences for the patient. Abdominal surgery begins with surgical access. In many diseases that cause an acute abdomen, e.g., perforated peptic ulcer, acute cholecystitis, appendicitis, pelvic inflammatory disease, or abdominal adhesions, a minimally invasive procedure will usually result in a favorable outcome

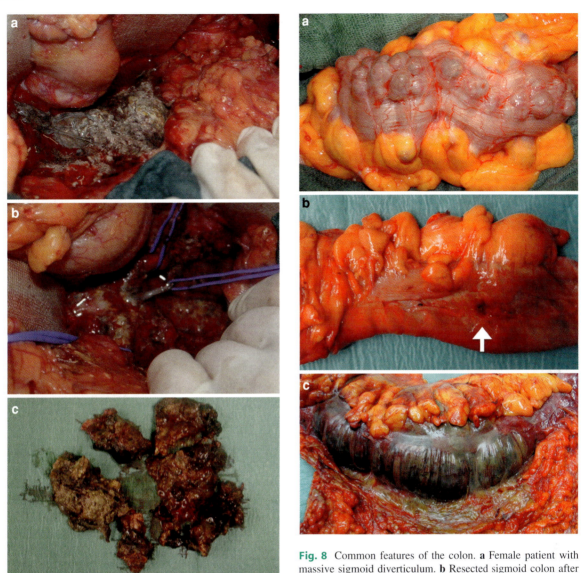

Fig. 8 Common features of the colon. **a** Female patient with massive sigmoid diverticulum. **b** Resected sigmoid colon after perforation and log-sized defect of the muscular layer that occurred during coloscopy (*arrow*). **c** Necrotic colon transversum with gangrenous bowel wall due to mesenterial embolism

Fig. 7 Operative status of a patient with necrotizing infected pancreatitis before (**a**) and after (**b**) necrosectomy; removed pancreatic necrosis (**c**)

(Sauerland et al. 2006). In pregnant woman, abdominal pain should be assessed in an expedient and thorough manner, as surgical intervention is often required (Kilpatrick and Monga 2007). A delay in diagnosis and intervention in a case of an acute abdomen often worsens the outcome for both mother and fetus (Kilpatrick and Monga 2007). A diagnosis made following a complete evaluation determines the

need for further procedures. In case of surgery, the diagnosis determines the surgical approach, e.g., laparoscopic vs. conventional celiotomy of the abdomen. Thus, in experienced hands, a laparoscopic intervention seems to be possible for the majority of patients with acute adhesive small-bowel obstruction (Grafen et al. 2010; Szomstein et al. 2006). A disadvantageous choice based on a deficient or imprecise preoperative diagnosis will often lead to further intraoperative problems and a disastrous outcome.

Fig. 9 Intraoperative vascular features. **a** Male patient with large kinking infrarenal aneurysm. **b** An aortic y-shaped prostheses was implanted; the aneurysmal sac is not yet closed

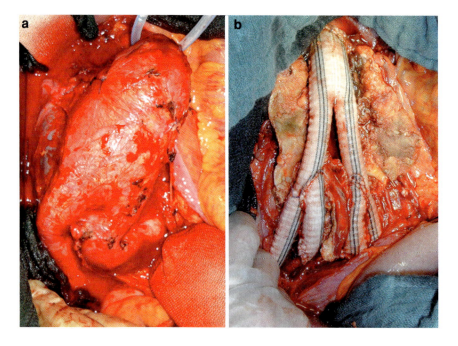

Moreover, it may result in erroneous or inappropriate surgical decision-making. It is well known that changes to a planned procedure made during an operation can be associated with a worse outcome, as, of course, may the wrong diagnosis. Gastrointestinal-tract perforation is a common presentation that requires emergency surgery. MDCT is a sensitive imaging technique for guiding the surgical approach, which differs considerably depending on the site of the lesion (Furukawa et al. 2005). The so-called Valentino appendix should be mentioned as an example of the catastrophic outcome that may occur when a preoperative diagnosis is not carefully re-evaluated intra-operatively. Rudolph Valentino. a glamorous movie actor during the silent-film era, underwent an operation for suspected acute appendicitis. He died at the age of 31 from a perforated peptic ulcer that was hidden from the surgeon, who was misled because fluid secreted from the perforation site likely traveled to the appendix region, where it induced a local inflammatory reaction suggestive of appendicitis (Schein 2005b). Thus, in the clinical routine, it is of particular importance that the radiologist and surgeon work closely together during the work-up of patients presenting with an acute abdomen that requires further imaging. This prerequisite is based on the fact that the clinician may best understand the relevance of the complaints and underlying disease but he or she lacks the skill to interpret every imaging detail, in contrast to radiologists, who are trained to interpret these studies and can most competently do so when fully informed of the patient's major clinical complaints.

In conclusion, this chapter has emphasized the clinical context and imaging indications in patients presenting with an acute abdomen. In recent years, the use of MDCT has increased in this population. The improved diagnostic capability is reflected in the large increase since 1995 in the proportion of patients with acute abdominal pain or flank pain: from 2 to 33% and from 0.4 to 43%, respectively (Larson et al. 2011). These changes highlight the impact and growing importance of modern MDCT in these patients.

References

Aguirre DA, Santosa AC, Casola G, Sirlin CB (2005) Abdominal wall hernias: imaging features, complications, and diagnostic pitfalls at multi-detector row CT. Radiographics 25:1501–1520

Ambrosetti P, Becker C, Terrier F (2002) Colonic diverticulitis: impact of imaging on surgical management–a prospective study of 542 patients. Eur Radiol 12:1145–1149

American College of Surgeons—Committee on Trauma (2004) Initial assessment and management. In: ATLS advanced trauma life support—program for doctors, 7th edn. American College of Surgeons, Chicago, IL, pp 11–29

Andersson P, Söderholm JD (2009) Surgery in ulcerative colitis: indication and timing. Dig Dis 27:335–340

Angele MK, Khalil PN, Spelsberg F, Bruns CJ, Burges A, Jauch KW, Kleespies A (2011) Non-curable tumours of the female genital tract: therapeutic options in bowel stenosis and bleeding. Zentralbl Chir 136:237–243

Balthazar EJ (2002) Complications of acute pancreatitis: clinical and CT evaluation. Radiol Clin North Am 40:1211–1227

Boffard KD (2007) Surgical decision-making. In: Boffard KD (ed) Manual of definitive surgical trauma care, 2nd edn. Hodder Arnold, part of Hachette Livre, London, pp 47–64

Bortoff GA, Chen MY, Ott DJ, Wolfman NT, Routh WD (2000) Gallbladder stones: imaging and intervention. Radiographics 20:751–766

Cahir JG, Freeman AH, Courtney HM (2004) Multislice CT of the abdomen. Br J Radiol 77:64–73

de Dombal FT (1988) The OMGE acute abdominal pain survey. Progress report, 1986. Scand J Gastroenterol Suppl 144:35–42

Federle MP (2005) CT of the acute (emergency) abdomen. Eur Radiol 15(Suppl 4):D100–D104

Furukawa A, Sakoda M, Yamasaki M, Kono N, Tanaka T, Nitta N, Kanasaki S, Imoto K, Takahashi M, Murata K, Sakamoto T, Tani T (2005) Gastrointestinal tract perforation: CT diagnosis of presence, site, and cause. Abdom Imaging 30:524–534

Grafen FC, Neuhaus V, Schöb O, Turina M (2010) Management of acute small bowel obstruction from intestinal adhesions: indications for laparoscopic surgery in a community teaching hospital. Langenbecks Arch Surg 395:57–63

Gralnek IM, Barkun AN, Bardou M (2008) Management of acute bleeding from a peptic ulcer. N Engl J Med 359:928–937

Green JM (2008) When is the faster better? Operative timing in acute care surgery. Curr opin Crit Care 14:423–427

Gurusamy K, Samraj K, Gluud C, Wilson E, Davidson BR (2010) Meta-analysis of randomized controlled trials on the safety and effectiveness of early versus delayed laparoscopic cholecystectomy for acute cholecystitis. Br J Surg 97:141–150

Hinchey EJ, Schaal PG, Richards GK (1978) Treatment of perforated diverticular disease of the colon. Adv Surg 12:85–109

Howell JM, Eddy OL, Lukens TW, Thiessen ME, Weingart SD, Decker WW (2010) Clinical policy: critical issues in the evaluation and manage-ment of emergency department patients with suspected appendicitis. Ann Emerg Med 55:71–116 American College of Emergency Physicians

Jacobs DO (2007) Clinical practice. Diverticulitis. N Engl J Med 357:2057–2066

Jaeckle T, Stuber G, Hoffmann MH, Freund W, Schmitz BL, Aschoff AJ (2008) Acute gastrointestinal bleeding: value of MDCT. Abdom Imaging 33:285–293

Johansson M, Thune A, Nelvin L, Stiernstam M, Westman B, Lundell L (2005) Randomized clinical trial of open versus laparoscopic cholecystectomy in the treatment of acute cholecystitis. Br J Surg 92:44–49

Khalil PN, Huber-Wagner S, Ladurner R, Kleespies A, Siebeck M, Mutschler W, Hallfeldt K, Kanz KG (2009) Natural history,

clinical pattern, and surgical considerations of pneumatosis intestinalis. Eur J Med Res 14:231–239

Khalil PN, Werner JC, Kleespies A (2010) Diagnostic of acute appendicitis in the emergency department. Notfall Rettungsmed 13:249–250

Khalil PN, Kleespies A, Angele MK, Thasler WE, Siebeck M, Bruns CJ, Mutschler W, Kanz KG (2011a) The formal requirements of algorithms and their implications in clinical medicine and quality management. Langenbecks Arch Surg 396:31–40

Khalil PN, Kleespies A, Angele MK, Bruns CJ, Siebeck M (2011b) Small bowel incarceration in recurrent perineal hernia after abdominoperineal resection. Int J Colorectal Dis 26:957–958

Kilpatrick CC, Monga M (2007) Approach to the acute abdomen in pregnancy. Obstet Gynecol Clin North Am 34:389–402

Kleespies A, Thasler WE, Schäfer C, Meimarakis G, Eichhorn ME, Bruns CJ, Jauch KW, Zügel N (2008) Acute pancreatitis: is there a need for surgery? Z Gastroenterol 46:790–798

Kool DR, Blickman JG (2007) Advanced Trauma Life Support. ABCDE from a radiological point of view. Emerg Radiol 14(3):135–141 Jul 2007

Laméris W, van Randen A, van Es HW, van Heesewijk JP, van Ramshorst B, Bouma WH, ten Hove W, van Leeuwen MS, van Keulen EM, Dijkgraaf MG, Bossuyt PM, Boermeester MA, Stoker J, MA OPTI (2009) Imaging strategies for detection of urgent conditions in patients with acute abdominal pain: diagnostic accuracy study. BMJ 338:b2431

Larson DB, Johnson LW, Schnell BM, Salisbury SR, Forman HP (2011) National trends in CT use in the emergency department: 1995–2007. Radiology 258:164–173

Leschka S, Alkadhi H, Wildermuth S, Marincek B (2005) Multi-detector computed tomography of acute abdomen. Eur Radiol 15:2435–2447

Lim HK, Bae SH, Seo GS (1992) Diagnosis of acute appendicitis in pregnant women: value of sonography. AJR Am J Roentgenol 159:539–542

Linsenmaier U, Wirth S, Reiser M, Körner M (2008) Diagnosis and classification of pancreatic and duodenal injuries in emergency radiology. Radiographics 28:1591–1602

Madoff DC, Denys A, Wallace MJ, Murthy R, Gupta S, Pillsbury EP, Ahrar K, Bessoud B, Hicks ME (2005) Splenic arterial interventions: anatomy, indications, technical considerations, and potential complications. Radiographics 25(Suppl 1):S191–S211

Malfertheiner P, Chan FK, McColl KE (2009) Peptic ulcer disease. Lancet 374(9699):1449–1461

Martin MJ, Steele SR (2010) Twists and turns: a practical approach to volvulus and intussusception. Scand J Surg 99:93–102

Moore EE, Cogbill TH, Malangoni MA, Jurkovich GJ, Shackford SR, Champion HR, McAninch JW (1995) Organ injury scaling. Surg Clin North Am 75:293–303

Myren J, Bouchier IA, Watkinson G, Softley A, Clamp SE, de Dombal FT (1988) The OMGE multinational inflammatory bowel disease survey 1976–1986. A further report on 3175 cases. Scand J Gastroenterol 144:11–19

Oniscu GC, Parks RW, Garden OJ (2006) Classification of liver and pancreatic trauma. HPB (Oxford) 8:4–9

Pachter HL, Guth AA, Hofstetter SR, Spencer FC (1998) Changing patterns in the management of splenic trauma: the impact of nonoperative management. Ann Surg 227:708–717

Parks NA, Davis JW, Forman D, Lemaster D (2011) Observation for nonoperative management of blunt liver injuries: how long is long enough? J Trauma 70:626–629

Pringle JH (1908) Notes on the arrest of hepatic heorrhage due to trauma. Ann Surg 48:541–548

Renner P, Kienle K, Dahlke MH, Heiss P, Pfister K, Stroszczynski C, Piso P, Schlitt HJ (2011) Intestinal ischemia: current treatment concepts. Langenbecks Arch Surg 396:3–11

Rosen MP, Sands DZ, Longmaid HE 3rd, Reynolds KF, Wagner M, Raptopoulos V (2000) Impact of abdominal CT on the management of patients presenting to the emergency department with acute abdominal pain. AJR Am J Roentgenol 174:1391–1396

Rozycki GS, Tremblay L, Feliciano DV, Joseph R, DeDelva P, Salomone JP, Nicholas JM, Cava RA, Ansley JD, Ingram WL (2002) Three hundred consecutive emergent celiotomies in general surgery patients: influence of advanced diagnostic imaging techniques and procedures on diagnosis. Ann Surg 235:681–688

Sauerland S, Agresta F, Bergamaschi R, Borzellino G, Budzynski A, Champault G, Fingerhut A, Isla A, Johansson M, Lundorff P, Navez B, Saad S, Neugebauer EA (2006) Laparoscopy for abdominal emergencies: evidence-based guidelines of the European Association for Endoscopic Surgery. Surg Endosc 20:14–29

Schein M (2005a) The acute abdomen. In: Schein M, Rogers PN (eds) Schein's common sense emergency abdominal surgery, 2nd edn. Springer, Berlin, pp 17–25

Schein M (2005b) Acute appendicitis. In: Schein M, Rogers PN (eds) Schein's common sense emergency abdominal surgery, 2nd edn. Springer, Berlin, pp 245–254

Schick KS, Hüttl TP, Fertmann JM, Hornung HM, Jauch KW, Hoffmann JN (2008) A critical analysis of laparoscopic appendectomy: how experience with 1400 appendectomies allowed innovative treatment to become standard in a university hospital. World J Surg 32(7):1406–1413

Shakespear JS, Shaaban AM, Rezvani M (2010) CT findings of acute cholecystitis and its complications. AJR Am J Roentgenol 194:1523–1529

Shanley CJ, Weinberger JB (2008) Acute abdominal vascular emergencies. Med Clin North Am 92:627–647 ix

Silva AC, Pimenta M, Guimarães LS (2009) Small bowel obstruction: what to look for. Radiographics 29:423–439

Spencer SP, Power N, Reznek RH (2009) Multidetector computed tomography of the acute abdomen in the immunocompromised host: a pictorial review. Curr Probl Diagn Radiol 38:145–155

Stoker J, van Randen A, Laméris W, Boermeester MA (2009) Imaging patients with acute abdominal pain. Radiology 253:31–46

Szomstein S, Lo Menzo E, Simpfendorfer C, Zundel N, Rosenthal RJ (2006) Laparoscopic lysis of adhesions. World J Surg 30:535–540

Taourel P, Kessler N, Lesnik A, Pujol J, Morcos L, Bruel JM (2003) Helical CT of large bowel obstruction. Abdom Imaging 28:267–275

Trompetas V (2008) Emergency management of malignant acute left-sided colonic obstruction. Ann R Coll Surg Engl 90:181–186

Wang YR, Richter JE, Dempsey DT (2010) Trends and outcomes of hospitalizations for peptic ulcer disease in the United States, 1993 to 2006. Ann Surg 251:51–58

Yoon W, Jeong YY, Kim JK, Seo JJ, Lim HS, Shin SS, Kim JC, Jeong SW, Park JG, Kang HK (2005) CT in blunt liver trauma. Radiographics 25:87–104

Zech CJ, Reiser MF (2010) Acute abdomen: an interdisciplinary challenge. Radiologe 50:208

Acute Abdomen: Rational Use of us, MDCT, and MRI

Vittorio Miele, Antonio Pinto, and Antonio Rotondo

Contents

V. Miele (✉)
Department of Emergency Radiology,
S. Camillo Hospital,
C.ne Gianicolense, 87,
00151 Rome, Italy
e-mail: vittoriomiele@alice.it

A. Pinto
Department of Radiology,
Cardarelli Hospital,
V. Antonio Cardarelli, 9,
80131 Naples, Italy

A. Rotondo
Department of Radiology,
Second University,
P.za Miraglia,
80138 Naples, Italy

Abstract

The term "acute abdomen" defines a clinical syndrome characterized by the sudden onset of severe abdominal pain, requiring early medical or surgical treatment. The acute abdominal pain may be due to trauma or non-trauma diseases and it is a frequent condition in patients presenting to the hospital emergency department. Computed Tomography is universally considered the key imaging modality for the evaluation of severe trauma patients and patients with non-traumatic acute abdominal disease. In case of acute abdomen unenhanced CT scan is not performed routinely. The contrast enhanced CT study is performed with a two-phase protocol, in arterial and portal venous phases; in trauma patients excretory phase is done only in cases of suspected urinary track lesions (renal pelvis, ureter and bladder). Multiplanar reconstruction (MPRs) are useful for interpretation of abdominal diseases as they allow the scanned volume to be viewed in any arbitrary plane interactively determined by the viewer. These reconstructions are especially useful when tubular structures, such as vessels, ureters, and bowel, are followed. Maximum intensity projections (MIPs) are useful for CT angiography and CT urography. The reconstruction of volume rendered (VR) images is particularly helpful for visualization of complex anatomy and pathology of visceral vasculature and best delineates a tortuous course of vessels and small branches.

M. Scaglione et al. (eds.), *Emergency Radiology of the Abdomen*,
Medical Radiology. Diagnostic Imaging,
DOI: 10.1007/174_2011_465, © Springer-Verlag Berlin Heidelberg 2012

1   Trauma

Trauma patients presenting to the hospital emergency department frequently suffer from acute abdominal pain. The "acute abdomen" represents a clinical syndrome characterized by the sudden onset of severe abdominal pain, requiring early medical or surgical treatment (Silen 1996).

Although computed tomography (CT) is universally considered the key imaging modality for the evaluation of severe trauma patients, the major role of sonography (ultrasound, US) for the early demonstration of hemopericardium, hemothorax, or hemoperitoneum in the initial assessment of hemodynamically unstable patients is also widely recognized. US has gained broad acceptance as an effective triage tool to evaluate trauma victims with suspected blunt abdominal injuries, because it is repeatable, non-invasive, non-irradiating and inexpensive (Poletti et al. 2007). In clinical practice, two main trends have recently emerged with regard to the utilization of US in the setting of blunt abdominal trauma in adults: the first consists of using US as a rapid diagnostic test mainly for the depiction of free fluid. This method has been termed FAST "focused assessment sonography for trauma" (Shackford 1993). The second trend consists of using US in association with a second-generation US contrast medium. Despite this and other important improvements in US technology, the presence of life-threatening visceral injuries not detected by contrast-enhanced US, as reported in the literature (Poletti et al. 2007), suggests that this approach cannot be recommended yet to replace CT in the triage of hemodynamically stable trauma patients.

The use of CT in blunt trauma was originally reported in the 1980s (Milia and Brasil 2011), but the long acquisition times and poor resolution limited its use. Since then, newer technologies have expanded the role of CT in the evaluation of injured patients. The first multidetector CT (MDCT) scanner, based on a 4-slice detector array, was developed in 1998. Since then, 16-, 32-, and 64- slice MDCTs, and recently, 128- and 256-slice MDCTs have become available (Rogalla et al. 2009). When combined with helical scanning, MDCT significantly reduces scan times. This reduction allows imaging with a thinner collimation (1–2 mm), yielding rapidly acquired higher-resolution images with a concomitant reduction of motion artifacts due to patient movement and cardiac activity. The use of MDCT has allowed for greater flexibility in image reformatting and in applications such as CT angiography.

In multitrauma patients, radiological investigation is necessary to detect or exclude injuries in all body regions. Given the recent advances in CT technology, a corresponding "whole-body" radiological survey can be obtained within a short time, thereby revealing critical occult injuries and decreasing the number of overlooked lesser injuries. Whole-body CT is the fastest possible radiological investigation permitting "complete" body coverage in the multitrauma patient. A single contiguous scanning pass from the vertex to the pubis symphysis not only results in all of the expected traditional transverse images of the head, neck, chest, abdomen, and pelvis but also provides data that enable the extraction of off-axial or focused images of the entire spine, aorta, facial bones, orbits, and hips without the need for rescanning. These images are readily obtained using a 64-detector row MDCT scanner with a minimum rotation time of 0.35 s, a maximum table speed of 175 mm/s, and maximum volume coverage of 200 cm. The isotropic design of the 40-mm detector delivers 0.35-mm isotropic resolution and thin-slice (64 × 0.625 and 32 × 1.25 mm) imaging in all scan modes and at all scan speeds. This allows fast whole-body scanning of a polytraumatized patient from tip-to-toe. All patients receive a single intravenous bolus of 120 mL of intravenous contrast medium injected through an 18- or 20-gauge cannula in an antecubital vein at a rate of 5 mL/s by using a dual-syringe power injector. The administration of saline solution (30 mL) as a bolus chaser, also injected at a rate of 5 mL/s, after the intravenous contrast material injection, is also recommended (Table 1).

Unenhanced CT scans. These are appropriate for the head and face. The neck, chest, abdomen, and pelvis are not routinely explored by this route to avoid unnecessary radioexposure.

Contrast-enhanced CT. Used in examinations of the neck, chest, abdomen, and pelvis. A multiphasic study is performed consisting of arterial, portal-venous and, if necessary, excretory phases. An arterial phase study of the whole body begins at the circle of Willis and extends to the pubis symphysis, using the bolus tracking technique with the region of interest (ROI)

Table 1 Whole body MDCT protocol in trauma patient

	CM concentration	CM volume	Injection rate	Delay	Rotation time	Pitch	Detector width
16-slice MDCT	350 mg I/ml	150 ml	4 ml/sec	Arterial phase: bolus track (ascending aorta)	0.7 s	1,375	1.25 mm
				Portal phase (abdomen): 40″ after a.p.			
	Saline	30 ml	4 ml/sec	Excretory phase (abdomen): 180″ after p.p.			
64-slice MDCT	370–400 mg I/ml	120 ml	5 ml/sec	Arterial phase: bolus track (ascending aorta)	0.5 s	0.938	0.625 mm
				Portal phase (abdomen): 35″ after a.p.			
	Saline	30 ml	5 ml/sec	Excretory phase (abdomen): 180″ after p.p.			

Unhenanced CT: Head, Face
CT + IV cm: Neck, Chest, Abdomen, Pelvis

positioned in the ascending aorta. This phase can detect serious vascular injuries, such as active bleeding of arterial origin, post-traumatic pseudoaneurysms, and acute arterial thrombosis (e.g., in the carotid). In the portal-venous phase, only the abdomen, from the dome of the diaphragm to the iliac bones, is routinely studied. This phase provides evidence of traumatic lesions involving the parenchymal organs as well as effusion into the peritoneal cavity. The excretory phase is done only in patients of injuries to the urinary tract (renal pelvis, ureter, and bladder) are suspected based on evidence of parenchymal renal damage or in case of hematuria. It is performed 180 s after the end of the portal venous phase and well demonstrates the leakage of urine from the urinary tract, with collection in the retroperitoneal space or, less commonly, in the intraperitoneal space.

Multiplanar reconstructions (MPRs) in coronal and sagittal planes are routinely obtained to evaluate the cervical, thoracic, and lumbar spine as well as thoracic and abdominal structures. Maximum-intensity projections (MIPs) and volume-rendering (VR) reconstructions are performed in cases of vascular lesions or fractures of the spine or pelvis.

The practice of whole-body CT in multitrauma patients is increasing rapidly, especially in the emergency setting. One consideration in assessments of the value of this technique is the risk of radiation exposure associated with a full-body CT examination. Radiation risk from diagnostic imaging is a subject of substantial controversy, and estimates of cancer induction and

death should be evaluated with caution (Ptak et al. 2003). The risk of cancer development and of the deterministic effects of radiation was recently pointed out in a series of publications and has resulted in attempts to reduce the radiation dose through modulation of the CT technique itself (Fanucci et al. 2007). Moreover, in emergency radiology, CT scanning is being increasingly used for the evaluation of trauma, which typically involves younger population in most instances. As children and young patients are at greater risk than older patients in developing cancer following radiation exposure, the radiation dose associated with CT scanning in these patients has become a cause of concern. Although it is prudent to maintain image quality to reach a satisfactory diagnosis, an immediate benefit with greater priority than the delayed risk of cancer associated with radiation exposure, radiologists, including those in emergency radiology departments, must also ensure that the ALARA (as low as reasonably achievable) radiation dose is used. Recent studies have documented that satisfactory image quality can be achieved with CT scanning performed at radiation dose lower than commonly used (Kalra et al. 2002, 2003). Indeed, low-dose CT scanning has been validated in different regions of the body, including the paranasal sinuses, face, chest, abdomen, and pelvis (Kalra et al. 2003; Frush 2002; Prasad et al. 2002). Amongst emergency CT indications, low-dose CT scanning has been recommended for imaging in children and for the evaluation of facial trauma, chest trauma, appendicitis, renal colic, and flank pain and diverticulosis (Hagtvedt et al. 2003). A weight- and cross-sectional dimensions-based adaptation of scanning parameters (tube current and tube potential) has also been recommended to reduce the radiation dose associated with CT scanning (Kalra et al. 2002, 2003; Frush 2002).

During CT scanning, a user can manually set the scanning parameters to reduce or adjust the radiation dose according to patient size, clinical indications and body region being scanned. These scanning parameters may include tube voltage, tube current, gantry rotation time, pitch, and beam collimation or detector configuration. The manual selection of a lower tube current (milliampere) is the most commonly used method to reduce the radiation dose associated with CT scanning (Kalra et al. 2005). Several studies have demonstrated that low-dose CT with reduced tube current is a useful alternative to standard tube current scanning and can provide satisfactory image quality (Kalra et al. 2002, 2003; Frush 2002; Prasad et al. 2002; Hagtvedt et al. 2003).

Few studies have investigated the role of magnetic resonance imaging (MRI) in the work-up of hemodynamically stable trauma patients for non-neurological indications (Poletti et al. 2007). Indeed, beside its limited availability in most emergency centers, MRI is difficult to use in uncooperative patients and in the presence of metallic components such as skin ECG electrodes and life-support equipment. Some authors reported that MRI can be used as a complement to non-enhanced CT in patients with major contraindications for the injection of iodinated contrast agent (Hedrick et al. 2005), or to evaluate the integrity of the pancreatic ducts (Fulcher and Turner 1999). Unfortunately, such reports remain anecdotal and the MRI is not yet integrated into the current diagnostic management of trauma patients, except for neurological indications (Poletti et al. 2007).

Although caution must be exerted regarding the radiation dose, the value of CT in deceleration traumatic injuries is well-established, not only in the diagnosis of these patients but also in decisions regarding their management. Contrast-enhanced MDCT allows a fast and accurate evaluation of all body regions in polytraumatized patients, thus safely directing the patient toward non-operative management (NOM), selective embolization, or surgery. Furthermore, one of the most important achievements of the latest MDCT scanners is the rapid diagnosis of vascular injuries, which are the primary cause of early death in polytraumatized patients.

2   Non-Traumatic Diseases

Acute abdominal pain unrelated to trauma is one of the most common conditions in patients presenting to the hospital emergency department. A wide variety of disorders, ranging from benign, self-limited diseases to conditions that require immediate surgery, can cause acute abdominal pain. Eight conditions account for over 90% of patients who are referred to the hospital and seen on surgical wards: acute appendicitis, acute cholecystitis, small-bowel obstruction, urinary colic, perforated peptic ulcer, acute pancreatitis, acute diverticular disease, and non-specific, non-surgical abdominal pain (dyspepsia, constipation) (Marincek 2002). A confident and accurate diagnosis can be made solely on the basis of medical history, physical examination, and laboratory test findings in only a small proportion of patients. The clinical manifestations of the various causes of acute abdominal pain usually are not straightforward. For proper treatment, a diagnostic work-up that enables the clinician to differentiate between the various causes of acute abdominal pain is important, and imaging plays an important role in this process (Stoker et al. 2009). Due to the impact of cross-sectional imaging, the need for plain abdominal radiographs has declined (Kellow et al. 2008). Although ultrasonography (US) has gained widespread acceptance for evaluating the gallbladder in affected patients and the pelvis in children and women of reproductive age, CT is considered to be one of the most valued tools for triaging patients with acute abdominal pain (Mindelzun and Jeffrey 1997; Novelline et al. 1999; Gore et al. 2000; Rosen et al. 2000; Urban and Fishman 2000). In recent years, most emergency centers have been equipped with newer helical CT scanners that permit imaging procedures to be performed in less time, with greater accuracy, and with less patient discomfort. The introduction of MDCT technology, with substantial improvements in scan speed and z-axis resolution, has further enhanced the utility of CT in abdominal imaging.

In patients with an acute abdomen, unenhanced CT scan is not performed routinely. Instead, the contrast-enhanced CT study, with a two-phase protocol

Table 2 MDCT protocol in acute abdomen

	CM concentration	CM volume	Injection rate	Delay	Rotation time	Pitch	Detector width
16-slice MDCT	350 mg I/ml	140 ml	4 ml/sec	Arterial phase: bolus track (abdominal aorta)	0.7 s	1,375	1.25 mm
	Saline	30 ml	4 ml/sec	Portal phase: 40″ after a.p.			
64-slice MDCT	370-400 mg I/ml	120 ml	5 ml/sec	Arterial phase: bolus track (abdominal aorta)	0.5 s	0.938	0.625 mm
	Saline	30 ml	5 ml/sec	Portal phase: 35″ after a.p.			

consisting of arterial and portal-venous phases, is the preferred approach (Table 2).

The interpretation of abdominal diseases is well accomplished with MPRs, as they allow the scanned volume to be viewed in any arbitrary plane interactively determined by the viewer. These reconstructions are especially useful when tubular structures, such as vessels, ureters, and bowel, are followed. MIPs are obtained by the projection onto an image plane of the highest-attenuation voxels encountered through a volume, which allows structures not lying in a single plane to be evaluated. Thus, MIP has found many applications in CT angiography and CT urography (Leschka et al. 2005). The reconstruction of VR images is particularly helpful for visualizing the complex anatomy and pathologies of the visceral vasculature and better delineates a tortuous course of vessels and small branches than MPR or axial images alone (Leschka et al. 2005).

According to the American College of Radiology (ACR) appropriateness criteria (2006), contrast-enhanced CT of the abdomen and pelvis is the most appropriate examination for patients with fever, non-localized abdominal pain, and no recent surgery. Non-enhanced CT, US, and conventional radiography are considered less appropriate initial imaging examinations for these patients. In the right upper quadrant, acute cholecystitis is by far the most common disease. In such cases, US is the preferred imaging method for evaluating patients with acute right upper abdominal pain. The ACR criteria also recommend the use of US in patients suspected of having acute calculous cholecystitis (Bree et al. 2000). The primary criterion is the detection of gallstones. Secondary signs include the sonographic Murphy sign, gallbladder-wall thickening ≥3 mm,

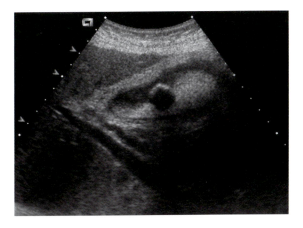

Fig. 1 Acute calculous cholecystitis. Sonography shows a gallstone and sludge in the gallbladder lumen. Gallbladder wall thickening is also evident

and peri-cholecystic fluid (Fig. 1). In acute calculous cholecystitis a calculus typically obstructs the cystic duct. Gallbladder perforation and complicating peri-cholecystic abscess usually occur adjacent to the gallbladder fundus because of the sparse blood supply. MDCT may be useful for confirmation of the sonographic diagnosis (Marincek 2002). Emphysematous cholecystitis is a rare complication of acute cholecystitis and is associated with diabetes mellitus. US or MDCT demonstrate gas in the wall and/or lumen of the gallbladder, which implies underlying gangrenous changes (Marincek 2002) (Fig. 2).

Acute abdomen with left upper quadrant pain is an infrequent complaint. Splenic infarction, splenic abscess, gastritis, and gastric ulcer are the most important causes. US is mostly reserved for screening, with CT enabling accurate further evaluation. The diagnosis of gastric pathology is established by endoscopy, with imaging playing a minor role.

Fig. 2 Acute emphysematous cholecystitis. CT scan (**a**) demonstrates gas in the lumen of the gallbladder, with air-fluid level, and in the gallbladder wall, more evident using a lung window (**b**)

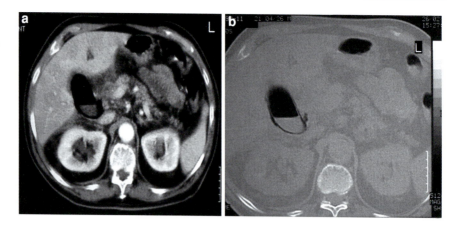

Acute pain in the right lower quadrant is also a common complaint in clinical practice. The differential diagnosis includes a broad spectrum of clinical entities, from benign self-limited disorders to those with high morbidity. Acute appendicitis is not only the most frequent cause of acute right lower quadrant pain, but also the most commonly encountered cause of an acute abdomen (Marincek 2002). Other diseases manifesting as acute right lower quadrant pain include acute terminal ileitis (Crohn's disease), acute typhilitis, and, in women, pelvic inflammatory disease, complications of ovarian cyst (hemorrhage, torsion, leak), endometriosis, and ectopic pregnancy. Recent advances in US and CT have greatly improved the preoperative diagnostic accuracy in these patients (Birnbaum and Jeffrey 1998). US has become an important imaging option in the evaluation of acute appendicitis, particularly in children. Demonstration of a swollen, non-compressible appendix >7 mm in diameter with a target configuration is the first sonographic criterion (Fig. 3). Generally, the normal appendix cannot be defined with US; thus, clear visualization of the appendix is suggestive of inflammation. Appendicitis may be diagnosed in indeterminate cases based on increased appendiceal perfusion on color Doppler examination. Gangrenous appendicitis is suggested when there is a loss of the echogenic submucosal layer and color Doppler flow to that segment of the appendix is absent (Birnbaum and Jeffrey 1998). The advantages of US include the lack of ionizing radiation, relatively low cost, and widespread availability. On the other hand, US requires considerable skill and is difficult to perform in obese patients, patients with severe pain, and

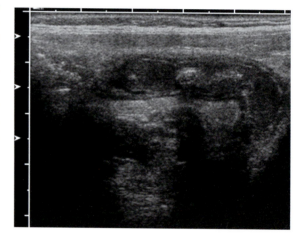

Fig. 3 Phlegmonous appendicitis. Sonography shows a completely visualized thickened appendix with an appendicolith; a peri-appendiceal fat infiltration is also observed

patients likely to have a complicating peri-appendiceal abscess. When the sonographic findings are unclear, MDCT can provide a rapid and definitive diagnosis (Fig. 4).

In the left lower quadrant, diverticular disease is the most common cause of acute abdominal pain. Diverticulitis occurs in up to 25% of patients with known diverticulosis and typically involves the sigmoid colon (Marincek 2002). MDCT is very sensitive and approaches 100% specificity and accuracy in the diagnosis or exclusion of diverticulitis; it has thus largely replaced barium enema examinations (Rao et al. 1998). The advent of CT has revolutionized the diagnosis and management of patients with diverticulitis. Fulfillment of the following four criteria is considered diagnostic: presence of diverticula,

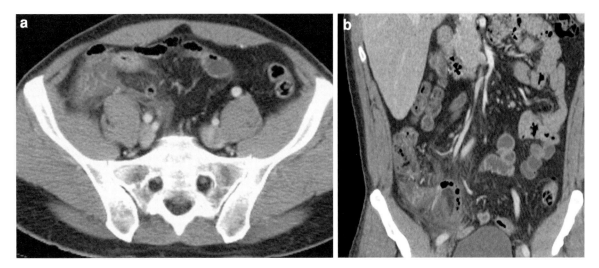

Fig. 4 Gangrenous appendicitis. Axial CT scan (**a**) and multiplanar coronal reconstruction (**b**) show a distended thickened appendix. Peri-appendiceal and peri-cecal fat infiltration is also evident. Note the involvement of the cecum in the inflammatory peri-appendiceal fat changes

Fig. 5 Acute diverticulitis. Axial CT scan (**a**) and multiplanar coronal reconstruction (**b**) show thickening of the sigmoid wall with inflammatory pericolic fat changes and the presence of a pericolic abscess (**a**)

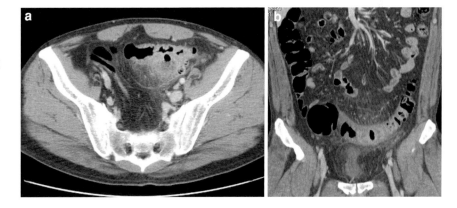

thickening of the bowel wall >4 mm, inflammatory pericolic fat, and pericolic abscess (Pradel et al. 1997). The CT findings in complicated diverticulitis may include the presence of an abscess (defined as a fluid-containing mass with or without air and an enhancing wall) and contained or free extraluminal air bubbles or pockets (Fig. 5). Other complications, such as bowel obstruction, hepatic abscess, fistula and inferior mesenteric vein thrombosis, can often be demonstrated with CT. Fistulas frequently communicate with an abscess or other hollow viscus, with colovesicular fistulas as the most common type (DeStigter and Keating 2009).

MDCT is also very useful in differentiating sigmoid diverticulitis from carcinoma, the most common condition in the differential diagnosis of colonic thickening.

Acute diffuse abdominal pain may be caused by any disorder that irritates a large portion of the GI tract and/or the peritoneum. The most frequently seen disorder is gastroenterocolitis but other important disorders are bowel obstruction, acute mesenteric ischemia, and GI tract perforation. Bowel obstruction is a frequent reason for abdominal pain and accounts for approximately 20% of surgical admissions for acute abdominal conditions (Marincek 2002). The small

Fig. 6 Small-bowel
obstruction. Axial CT scan
(**a**) and multiplanar coronal
reconstruction (**b**) show
dilated jejunal loops and
collapsed ileal loops.
The transition point
with the "beak sign"
is also evident (**a**)

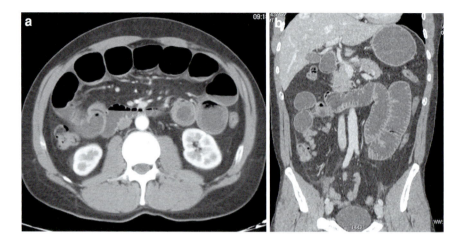

Fig. 7 Small-bowel
obstruction. Axial CT scan
(**a**) and multiplanar coronal
reconstruction (**b**) show
dilated jejunal loops at the
level of the mesogastrium and
collapsed ileal loops. The
small-bowel feces sign is
observed near the point
of obstruction

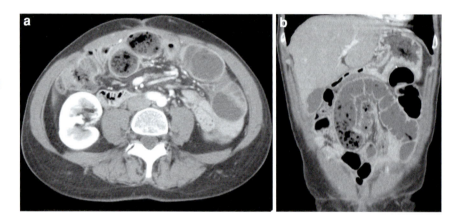

bowel is involved in 60–80% of cases. Small-bowel obstruction (SBO) are typically the result of adhesions, hernias, and neoplasms. In the large bowel, mechanical obstruction is very often due to carcinoma and diverticular disease; sigmoid volvulus, although relatively infrequent, ranks third among all causes of large-bowel obstruction (Marincek 2002). The diagnosis of bowel obstruction is established on clinical grounds and usually confirmed with plain abdominal radiographs. However, because of the diagnostic limitations of plain films, MDCT is increasingly used to identify the site, severity, and cause of obstruction and to determine the presence or absence of associated complications, particularly bowel ischemia (Ha et al. 1997; Caoili and Paulson 2000; Furukawa et al. 2001; Boudiaf et al. 2001). The essential CT finding of bowel obstruction is the delineation of a transition zone between the prestenotic, dilated bowel and the poststenotic, decompressed bowel (Fig. 6).

A helpful sign for identifying the point of obstruction is the small-bowel feces sign, i.e., feces-like material in the distended small bowel (Lazarus et al. 2004) (Fig. 7). The transition point should be scrutinized for the source of the obstruction. Additional reformatted images using sagittal, coronal, oblique, or curved planes help to trace the intestine and to determine the transition point (Caoili and Paulson 2000). MDCT facilitates this task substantially.

Patients with bowel ischemia often have a short clinical history of prominent abdominal pain, while other possible symptoms, such as nausea, vomiting, diarrhea, and distended abdomen, are substantially less prominent. Nonetheless, all of these symptoms are non-specific. A diagnosis of bowel ischemia is often made after the usual diagnoses, i.e., those with similar associated symptoms, are excluded. Bowel ischemia should be considered especially in elderly patients with known cardiovascular disease

Fig. 8 Small-bowel ischemia due to arterial occlusion. Axial CT scan (**a**) and multiplanar coronal reconstruction (**b**) demonstrate the presence of dilated small-bowel loops with thin walls. Embolic occlusion of the superior mesenteric artery is evident (*arrowheads*)

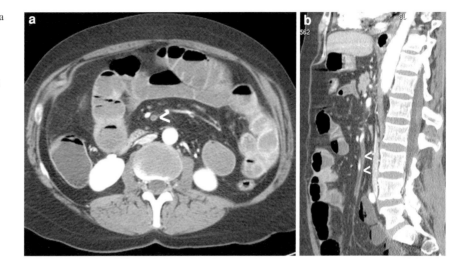

Fig. 9 Small-bowel ischemia due to venous thrombosis. Multiplanar coronal CT reconstructions (**a, b**) show the presence of dilated small-bowel loops in the left upper quadrant. In the pelvis, an ileal loop demonstrates an abnormal bowel-wall thickening associated with bowel-wall hypoattenuation. Free fluid is visible in the peritoneal cavity. Mesenteric venous thrombosis is observed (**b**)

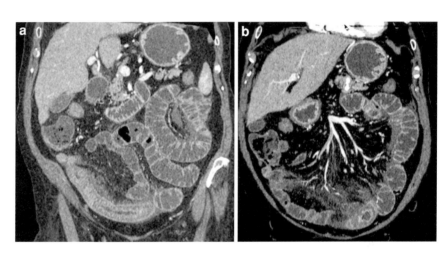

(e.g., atrial fibrillation) and in younger patients known to have diseases that may give rise to inadequate mesenteric blood flow, such as vasculitis, hereditary or familial coagulation disorders (e.g., antiphospholipid syndrome), and protein C or S deficiency. Causes of acute mesenteric ischemia are arterial occlusion (thromboembolism; external compression by adhesion, volvulus, hernia, intussusception; vasculitis), hypotension (congestive heart failure; hypovolemia; sepsis), vasoconstrictive medications, or impaired venous drainage; often, a combination of these conditions is observed. Colonic ischemia generally results from hypoperfusion or hypotension; a mesenteric thrombus is rare. The predominance of one condition determines the outcome and the findings on MDCT. Although several CT signs are associated with bowel ischemia, they are not very frequent nor are they specific. Visualized occluded mesenteric arteries or venous thrombus is a clear sign of mesenteric ischemia (Fig. 8). The bowel wall may be thickened (>3 mm) because of mural edema, hemorrhage, congestion, or superinfection. Thickening owing to edema, congestion, or hemorrhage is a frequent manifestation of venous obstruction (Fig. 9). Bowel-wall hypoattenuation (edema), hyperattenuation (hemorrhage), abnormal enhancement (target sign), and absence of enhancement are features of bowel ischemia. The absence of bowel-wall enhancement is highly specific but is often missed (Stoker et al. 2009). The wall may become paper thin, which may indicate impending perforation. Luminal dilatation and fluid levels (fluid exudation of the ischemic bowel segments) are common in irreversible bowel ischemia, whereas mesenteric stranding and ascites are

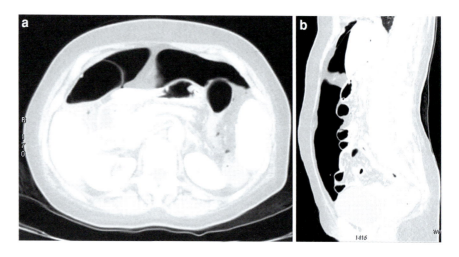

Fig. 10 Intestinal perforation. Axial CT scan (**a**) and multiplanar sagittal reconstruction (**b**) show the presence of pneumoperitoneum, which is more evident with a lung window

non-specific CT findings of this condition. Pneumatosis cystoides intestinalis can be present, manifesting as a single gas bubble or a broad rim of air dividing the bowel wall into two layers.

When pneumatosis cystoides intestinalis occurs in combination with portal-venous gas, especially in the liver periphery, it is definitely associated with bowel ischemia but is not a pathognomonic finding (Stoker et al. 2009). Portal-venous gas is an ominous sign that is generally seen in patients with a poor prognosis.

In patient with clinically suspected GI-tract perforation, pneumoperitoneum can be recognized by the presence of subdiaphragmatic air on an erect chest radiograph or an erect or left lateral decubitus radiograph of the abdomen (Grassi et al. 1996; Cho and Baker 1994; Levine et al. 1991). An abundant pneumoperitoneum is indicative of a perforation complicating a large-bowel obstruction. With perforation of the small bowel, only small quantities of gas escape because the small bowel usually does not contain gas (Grassi et al. 1998). The detection of subtle pneumoperitoneum is often difficult. MDCT is far more sensitive than conventional radiography in identifying a small pneumoperitoneum and has thus become the modality of choice in cases that are unclear on a conventional radiograph (Grassi et al. 2004; Pinto et al. 2000, 2004; Imuta et al. 2007). To enhance the sensitivity of CT for extraluminal gas, the scans are also viewed at "lung window" settings (Fig. 10).

Acute flank or epigastric pain is commonly a manifestation of retroperitoneal pathology, especially urinary colic, acute pancreatitis, or leaking abdominal

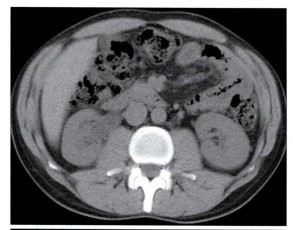

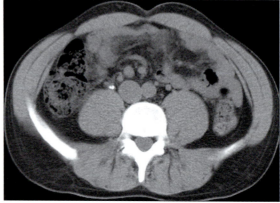

Fig. 11 Urolithiasis. Axial CT sections, without intravenous contrast material, at the levels of the kidneys and the ureteral abdominal tract. Multiplanar coronal reconstruction performed with low-dose technique show a right hydro-uretero-nephrosis with evidence of an obstructing calculus located at the level of the ureteral abdominal portion

Fig. 12 Necrotizing
pancreatitis. Axial CT
scan (**a**) and multiplanar
coronal reconstruction
(**b**) show a pancreatic
parenchymal distruction
with pancreatic exudate
extending at the level
of the perisplenic
space

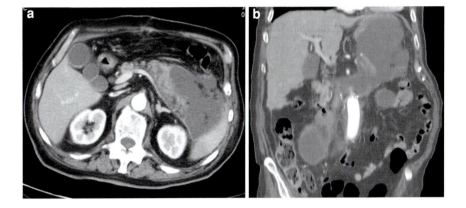

Fig. 12 Necrotizing
pancreatitis. Axial CT
scan (**a**) and multiplanar
coronal reconstruction
(**b**) show a pancreatic
parenchymal distruction
with pancreatic exudate
extending at the level
of the perisplenic
space

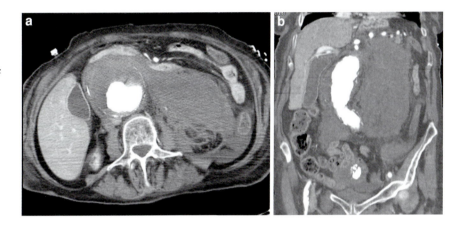

Fig. 13 Abdominal aortic
aneurysm. Axial CT scan
(**a**) and multiplanar coronal
reconstruction (**b**) show the
rupture of an abdominal aortic
aneurysm, with a large
hemoretroperitoneum

aortic aneurysm. For several decades, intravenous urography has been the primary imaging technique used in patients with flank pain caused by a suspected urolithiasis-induced urinary colic. Abdominal US is considered useful in patients with contraindications to irradiation or contrast media. However, because of the low sensitivity of US for urinary-tract calculi, the role of unenhanced CT has grown rapidly (Smith et al. 1995, 1996) (Fig. 11). MDCT examination at reduced exposure factors maintains the diagnostic accuracy. Unenhanced, low-dose MDCT provides a rapid and accurate diagnosis of ureteral stones, because almost all calculi are radio-opaque at CT (Leschka et al. 2005). Obstructing ureteral calculi are typically located at the ureteropelvic or ureterovesical junction. Subtle calculi may be detectable by the presence of focal peri-ureteral stranding. Secondary CT signs of urolithiasis include hydro-ureter, hydrone-phrosis, peri-nephric stranding, and renal enlarge-ment. The use of oblique–coronal reconstructions is more effective for precise stone localization and measurement than axial slices (Leschka et al. 2005). With MDCT, high-resolution, cine-viewing recon-structions can be obtained from thin-collimation acquisitions. The use of curved reformations provides unequivocal images focused on the ureteral stone.

An important disease causing epigastric pain is acute pancreatitis. US is helpful for the demonstration of gallstones as a cause of acute pancreatitis and for the follow-up of known fluid collections. The CT findings correlate well with the clinical severity of acute pan-creatitis, such that MDCT has become the imaging modality of choice to stage the extent of disease and to detect complications (Marincek 2002). Pancreatic enlargement due to interstitial parenchymal edema may progress to pancreatic exudate collecting in the anterior pararenal space, the transverse mesocolon, the mesenteric root, and the lesser sac. Necrosis or hem-orrhage may develop within the pancreas itself, in addition to extending to adjacent organs, which can be further compromises by thrombosis of the splenic and portal veins (Marincek 2002) (Fig. 12).

One of the most life-threatening alternative diagnoses in acute flank pain is a leaking aneurysm of the abdominal aorta. In a suspected rupture of an abdominal aortic aneurysm, US is the initial imaging technique. The examination can be performed rapidly with portable equipment in the emergency room. In hemodynamically stable patients, contrast-enhanced MDCT accurately delineates the para-aortic hemorrhage and can directly visualize the actual site of the leaking aortic aneurysm (Fig. 13).

Even though the ACR Appropriateness Criteria still rate MRI below CT and US for the evaluation of acute abdominal and pelvic conditions (Miller et al. 2008), MRI is an excellent alternative to CT in patients in whom the use of iodinated contrast agents or radiation is not desirable (Heverhagen and Klose 2009). In addition, when US findings are non-diagnostic or equivocal, MRI is an appropriate modality for the evaluation of acute lower abdominal and pelvic pain, especially in pregnant or younger patients. Depending on local availability, MRI may be considered as the modality of first choice in all patients with acute lower abdominal and pelvic pain. In general, high costs, long imaging times, and limited availability are considered to be its major drawbacks in this setting. However, its value has been assessed in many acute conditions of the lower abdomen and pelvis, for example, appendicitis, diverticulitis, bowel obstruction, chronic inflammatory disease (Crohn disease and ulcerative colitis), vascular disease, and gynecologic disorders (Patel et al. 2007). The body of scientific research on the use of MRI in patients with acute abdominal pain is relatively limited. Therefore, the availability of and expertise with this examination are limited, and the cost-effectiveness has not been studied. Further research should be directed toward better defining the role of MRI in the setting of acute abdominal pain, especially compared with US and CT. Attention to proper technique and the use of tailored protocols are essential for optimizing the effectiveness of the MRI examination and maximizing its diagnostic accuracy. The recently increased awareness and attending concern regarding radiation-related health risks warrant the adoption of a flexible approach to imaging in the emergency setting, particularly in pregnant and pediatric patients.

References

ACR appropriateness criteria (2006) American College of Radiology Web site. http://www.acr.org/SecondaryMain MenuCategories/quality_safety/app_criteria/pdf/Expert PanelonGastrointestinalImaging/AcuteAbdominalPainand FeverorSuspectedAbdominalAbscessDoc1.aspx. Accessed 15 Oct, 2008

Birnbaum BA, Jeffrey RB (1998) CT and sonographic evaluation of acute right lower quadrant abdominal pain. Am J Roentgenol 170:361–371

Boudiaf M, Soyer P, Terem C et al (2001) CT evaluation of small bowel obstruction. Radiographics 21:613–624

Bree RL, Ralls PW, Balfe DM et al (2000) Evaluation of patients with acute right upper quadrant pain: American College of Radiology—ACR appropriateness criteria. Radiology 215 (suppl):153–157

Caoili EM, Paulson EK (2000) CT of small-bowel obstruction: another perspective using multiplanar reformations. Am J Roentgenol 174:993–998

Cho KC, Baker SR (1994) Extraluminal air: diagnosis and significance. Radiol Clin North Am 32:829–844

DeStigter KK, Keating DP (2009) Imaging update: acute colonic diverticulitis. Clin Colon Rectal Surg 22:147–155

Fanucci E, Fiaschetti V, Rotili A et al (2007) Whole-body 16-row multislice CT in emergency room: effects of different protocols on scanning time, image quality and radiation exposure. Emerg Radiol 13:251–257

Frush DP (2002) Pediatric CT: practical approach to diminish the radiation dose. Pediatr Radiol 32:714–717

Fulcher AS, Turner MA (1999) Magnetic resonance pancreatography (MRP). Crit Rev Diagn Imaging 40:285–322

Furukawa A, Yamasaki M, Furuichi K et al (2001) Helical CT in the diagnosis of small bowel obstruction. Radiographics 21:341–355

Gore RM, Miller FH, Scott Pereles F et al (2000) Helical CT in the evaluation of the acute abdomen. Am J Roentgenol 174:901–913

Grassi R, Di Mizio R, Pinto Pinto A et al (1996) Comparative adequacy of conventional radiography, ultrasonography and computed tomography in sixty-one consecutive patients with gastrointestinal perforation. Radiol Med 91:747–755

Grassi R, Pinto A, Rossi G et al (1998) Conventional plain-film radiology, ultrasonography and CT in jejuno-ileal perforation. Acta Radiol 39:52–56

Grassi R, Romano S, Pinto A et al (2004) Gastro-duodenal perforations: conventional plain film, US and CT findings in 166 consecutive patients. Eur J Radiol 50:30–36

Ha HK, Kim JS, Lee MS et al (1997) Differentiation of simple and strangulated small-bowel obstructions: usefulness of known CT criteria. Radiology 204:507–512

Hagtvedt T, Aalokken TM, Notthellen J et al (2003) A new low-dose CT examination compared with standard-dose CT in the diagnosis of acute sinusitis. Eur Radiol 13:976–980

Hedrick TL, Sawyer RG, Young JS (2005) MRI for the diagnosis of blunt abdominal trauma: a case report. Emerg Radiol 11:309–311

Heverhagen JT, Klose KJ (2009) MR imaging for acute lower abdominal and pelvic pain. RadioGraphics 29:1781–1796

Imuta M, Awai K, Nakayama Y et al (2007) Multidetector CT findings suggesting a perforation site in the gastrointestinal tract: analysis in surgically confirmed 155 patients. Radiat Med 25:113–118

Kalra MK, Prasad S, Saini S et al (2002) Clinical comparison of standard-dose and 50% reduced-dose abdominal CT: effect on image quality. AJR Am J Roentgenol 179:1101–1106

Kalra MK, Maher MM, Prasad SR et al (2003) Correlation of patient weight and cross-sectional dimensions with subjective image quality at standard dose abdominal CT. Korean J Radiol 4:234–238

Kalra MK, Rizzo SMR, Novelline RA (2005) Reducing radiation dose in emergency computed tomography with automatic exposure control techniques. Emerg Radiol 11:267–274

Kellow ZS, MacInnes M, Kurzencwyg D et al (2008) The role of abdominal radiography in the evaluation of the nontrauma emergency patient. Radiology 248:887–893

Lazarus DE, Slywotsky C, Bennett GL et al (2004) Frequency and relevance of the "small-bowel feces" sign on CT in patients with small-bowel obstruction. Am J Roentgenol 183:1361–1366

Leschka S, Alkadhi H, Wildermuth S et al (2005) Multidetector computed tomography of acute abdomen. Eur Radiol 15:2435–2447

Levine MS, Scheiner JD, Rubesin SE et al (1991) Diagnosis of pneumoperitoneum on supine abdominal radiographs. Am J Roentgenol 156:731–735

Marincek B (2002) Nontraumatic abdominal emergencies: acute abdominal pain: diagnostic strategies. Eur Radiol 12:2136–2150

Milia DJ, Brasil K (2011) Current use of CT in the evaluation and management of injured patients. Surg Clin N Am 91:233–248

Miller F, Bree R, Rosen M, et al. ACR Appropriateness Criteria® October (2008) American College of Radiology Web site. http://www.acr.org/. Accessed 10 Apr 2009

Mindelzun RE, Jeffrey RB (1997) Unenhanced helical CT for evaluating acute abdominal pain: a little more cost, a lot more information. Radiology 205:43–45

Novelline RA, Rhea JT, Rao PM et al (1999) Helical CT in emergency radiology. Radiology 213:321–339

Patel SJ, Reede DL, Katz DS et al (2007) Imaging the pregnant patient for nonobstetric conditions: algorithms and radiation dose considerations. RadioGraphics 27:1705–172

Pinto A, Scaglione M, Pinto F et al (2000) Helical computed tomography diagnosis of gastrointestinal perforation in the elderly patient. Emerg Radiol 7:259–262

Pinto A, Scaglione M, Giovine S et al (2004) Comparison between the site of multislice CT signs of gastrointestinal perforation and the site of perforation detected at surgery in forty perforated patients. Radiol Med 108:208–217

Poletti P-A, Platon A, Becker CD (2007) Role of imaging in the management of trauma victims. In: Marincek B, Dondelinger RF (eds) Emergency radiology. Imaging and Intervention, Chap. 1.1. Springer, Berlin, pp 3–23

Pradel JA, Adell JF, Taourel P et al (1997) Acute colonic diverticulitis: prospective comparative evaluation with US and CT. Radiology 205:503–512

Prasad SR, Wittram C, Shepard JA et al (2002) Standard-dose and 50%-reduced-dose chest CT: comparing the effect on image quality. Am J Roentgenol 179:461–465

Ptak T, Rhea JT, Novelline RA (2003) Radiation dose is reduced with a single-pass whole-body multi-detector row CT trauma protocol compared with a conventional segmented method: initial experience. Radiology 229:902–905

Rao PM, Rhea JT, Novelline RA et al (1998) Helical CT with only colonic contrast material for diagnosing diverticulitis: prospective evaluation of 150 patients. Am J Roentgenol 170:1445–1449

Rogalla P, Kloeters C, Hein P (2009) CT technology overview: 64-slice and beyond. Radiol Clin North Am 47:1–11

Rosen MP, Sands DZ, Esterbrook Longmaid H et al (2000) Impact of abdominal CT on the management of patients presenting to the emergency department with acute abdominal pain. Am J Roentgenol 174:1391–1396

Shackford SR (1993) Focused ultrasound examinations by surgeons: the time is now. J Trauma 35:181–182

Silen W (1996) Cope's early diagnosis of the acute abdomen, 19th edn. Oxford University Press, New York

Smith RC, Rosenfield AT, Choe KA et al (1995) Acute flank pain: comparison of non-contrast-enhanced CT and intravenous urography. Radiology 194:789–794

Smith RC, Verga M, McCarthy S et al (1996) Diagnosis of acute flank pain: value of unenhanced helical CT. Am J Roentgenol 166:97–101

Stoker J, van Randen A, Lameris W et al (2009) Imaging patients with acute abdominal pain. Radiology 253:31–46

Urban BA, Fishman EK (2000) Tailored helical CT evaluation of acute abdomen. Radiographics 20:725–749

Liver and Bile Ducts

Gerd Schueller

Contents

Abstract

Hepatic and biliary emergencies have an important impact on the workload of an emergency unit. However, the symptoms are likely to be unspecific in the non-traumatic acute abdomen. Most patients present with right upper quadrant pain and tenderness, fever, and jaundice. Rapidly establishing the diagnosis is mandatory and, in experienced hands, the chosen imaging techniques are powerful tools by which to narrow the diagnosis.

1 Introduction

Hepatic and biliary emergencies have an important impact on the workload of an emergency unit. However, the symptoms are likely to be unspecific in the non-traumatic acute abdomen. Most patients present with right upper quadrant pain and tenderness, fever, and jaundice. Rapidly establishing the diagnosis is mandatory and, in experienced hands, the chosen imaging techniques are powerful tools by which to narrow the diagnosis.

In the trauma setting, the management of hepatic injuries in adults has changed considerably within the last few decades, rendering conservative strategies successful in most cases. This development parallels the advent of multidetector computed tomography (MDCT) scanners, which in dedicated trauma centers are physically linked to the emergency ward. Radiologic diagnosis is carefully established at the earliest possible time. The introduction of CT-based organ injury scales is of further help for individual treatment planning. In biliary trauma, magnetic resonance

G. Schueller (✉)
Department of Radiology, Medical University of Vienna,
General Hospital of Vienna, Währinger Gürtel 18-20,
1090 Vienna, Austria
e-mail: gerd.schueller@meduniwien.ac.at

M. Scaglione et al. (eds.), *Emergency Radiology of the Abdomen*,
Medical Radiology. Diagnostic Imaging,
DOI: 10.1007/174_2011_466, © Springer-Verlag Berlin Heidelberg 2012

imaging (MRI)-based diagnosis has proved its potential to replace invasive techniques, which are widely reserved as a therapeutic tool.

In this chapter, diseases and trauma to the liver and the biliary tree are discussed, each including the major differential diagnoses. For cholelithiasis and cholecystitis, also see "Gallbladder", and for detailed technical considerations, "Acute Abdomen: Rational Use of US, MDCT, and MRI".

2 The Liver

2.1 Polycystic Liver Disease

2.1.1 Terminology and Clinical Issues
Dysontogenic hepatic cysts occur commonly in patients with autosomal dominant polycystic kidney disease, types 1 and 2. This entity is seldom seen in patients without renal involvement. Its incidence cannot be determined definitively, since there are various degrees of expression. Associated pathologies are hepatic fibrosis and biliary hamartomas (Qian et al. 2003).

The cysts have a variable appearance, many are clustered, and some lack smooth margins. They lead to a substantial distortion and enlargement of the liver. Most of the patients are asymptomatic; however, in some cases, abdominal distension and pain are apparent, primarily in the right upper quadrant. The extrinsic compression of the bile ducts and of venous outflow lead to cholestasis, venous intrahepatic thrombosis, and the generation of portal hypertension and ascites. Rarely, failure of liver function and Budd-Chiari syndrome are reported. Other causes of an acute abdomen are hemorrhage, spontaneous cyst rupture, and infection. Treatment options range from simple interventional cyst aspiration to surgical fenestration and resection, as well as orthotopic liver transplantation.

2.1.2 Imaging
In the acute abdomen setting, ultrasound (US) and CT suitably delineate the extent of the disease, as well as demonstrate hepatic thrombosis, portal hypertension, ascites, and hemorrhage. In CT, the unruptured cysts have an attenuation of 0–20 HU and do not enhance after IV contrast administration. In some cases, wall calcifications are seen as remnants of old hemorrhage. Complicated cysts show wall enhancement and

septatitis. MRI is unequivocally excellent (Fig. 1). The age of cystic hemorrhage can be quantified according to the morphology of blood products in T1w- and T2w images (Mortele and Ros 2001). Magnetic resonance cholangiopancreatography (MRCP) shows no communication of cysts or connections with the biled ducts (Morgan et al. 2006).

2.1.3 Differentials
Multiple abscesses. Commonly, patients have a history of infection or surgery. Multiple hypodense lesions are seen with CT (Fig. 2), which present with wall thickness, the presence of septa, and characteristic enhancement patterns.

Caroli discase. This disease originates from a congenital cavernous dilatation of the biliary tree. The evidence of a communication between the lesions and the bile ducts is pathognomonic (Fig. 3). In many cases, multiple intrasaccular calculi are observed.

Biliary hamartoma. Von Meyenburg complexes show variable imaging patterns according to the amount of cystic and solid components (Fig. 4).

Cystic metastases. Depending on the presence of metastasis from adenocarcinoma, some lesions show no or very little enhancement (Fig. 5); additional peritoneal implants are frequently seen.

2.2 Infection

2.2.1 Hepatitis

2.2.1.1 Terminology and Clinical Issues
Hepatitis has multiple causes, primarily viral infection and alcohol. It is defined as a nonspecific inflammation of the liver parenchyma. In the acute setting, imaging is often requested since hepatitis appears with symptoms that may mimic an acute abdomen. In chronic disease, imaging is requested to detect associated cirrhosis and hepatocellular carcinoma (Murakami et al. 1996).

Typically, young and middle-aged patients appear with a history of fever, unspecific pain in the upper right quadrant, jaundice, and anorexia.

2.2.1.2 Imaging
Imaging findings may be as equivocal as the clinical symptoms (Murakami et al. 1996). The most

Fig. 1 Polycystic liver disease. Ubiquitous cysts enlarge and distort the liver (**a**, **b**). Note the associated polycystic kidney disease in (**b**). Multiple hemorrhagic cysts led to right upper quadrant pain. Blood is isointense on T1w and hypointense on T2w, which is characteristic of acute bleeding. US sagittal view (**a**), coronal T2w (**b**), axial T1w in-phase (**c**), and axial T2w (**d**) MRI

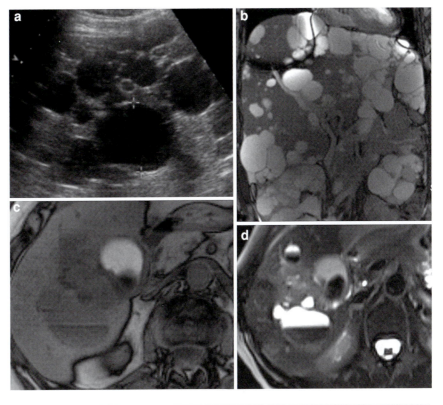

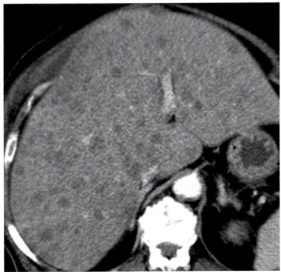

Fig. 2 Multiple hepatic abscesses are hyperdense compared to cysts, lesions are smaller, and show at least moderate peripheral enhancement. Axial pv CECT

Fig. 3 Multiple saccular cystic dilatations in the central right liver lobe in Caroli disease. Axial fat-saturated T2w MRI

frequently encountered US findings are a so-called starry-sky appearance (based on the painting by Vincent Van Gogh), which describes an increased echogenicity of the portal-venous walls, as well as a periportal tracking , suggesting periportal edema. In acute viral and alcoholic hepatitis, in particular, an enlarged and diffusely hypoechoic liver is suggestive. In some cases, the gallbladder wall is thickened.

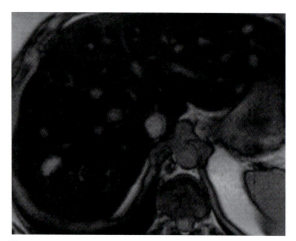

Fig. 4 Multiple hamartomas in both liver lobes are less hyperintense than cysts. Axial T2w MRI

CT findings correlate well with US pathologies (Fig. 6a); in addition, in contrast-enhanced CT (CECT), heterogeneous enhancement patterns may be present. In chronic disease, lymphadenopathy is common along the hepatoduodenal ligament. T1w in- and out-of-phase MRI adequately depicts the fatty infiltrated parenchyma (Bahl et al. 2008; Reeder and Sirlin 2010).

2.2.1.3 Differentials

Steatosis hepatis. The patterns of fatty infiltration in steatosis hepatis are difficult to differentiate from hepatitis (Fig. 7). However, with US, the starry-sky appearance will not be present.

Lymphoma. In rare cases, lymphoma may mimic the clinical signs of an acute abdomen. The imaging findings will also resemble those of fatty liver disease, as well as hepatitis, except for lobulated areas that represent focal solid infiltration (Fig. 8).

2.2.2 Hepatic Abscess

2.2.2.1 Terminology and Clinical Issues

Abscesses of the liver most commonly are pyogenic or amoebic in origin. They are defined as a collection of pus and the concomitant destruction of liver tissue. A pyogenic abscess is the result of biliary (cholangitis), portal-venous (most often, diverticulitis), or arterial (i.e., septic) infection (Mortele et al. 2004). With portal-venous infection, most commonly, the right liver lobe is affected; with a biliary genesis, both lobes are involved equally. Abscesses are also observed subsequent to surgery and after blunt or

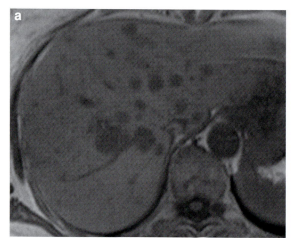

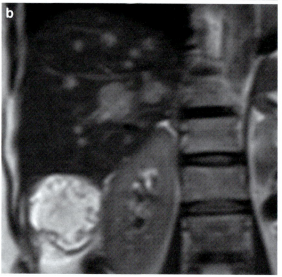

Fig. 5 Multiple cystically transformed metastases after systemic therapy show MRI features characteristic of dysontogenic cysts (**a**, **b**). Note: large subcapsular adenoma in (**b**). Axial T1w (**a**) and coronal T2w (**b**) MRI

penetrating trauma, most commonly during conservative treatment of marked liver injury.

Patients usually present with fever and pain in the right upper abdominal quadrant. Parasympathetic symptoms, such as nausea and vomiting, also render the diagnosis of an acute abdomen feasible. Amoebic abscesses are often accompanied by diarrhea. Rarely, vascular complications occur (Sodhi et al. 2008).

2.2.2.2 Imaging

Typically, small hypodense lesions progress to form a large, partially septated, sharply defined liquefied mass (Benedetti et al. 2008). When abscesses are

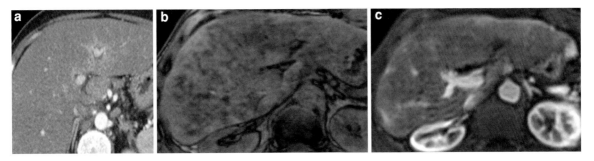

Fig. 6 Marked steatotic infiltration of the liver parenchyma and periportal hypervascularization in acute hepatitis (**a**). Scattered fat distribution correlates with inhomogenous attenuation (**b**, **c**). Axial art CECT (**a**); axial T1w out-of-phase (**b**), and T1w fat saturated, contrast-enhanced (**c**) MRI

Fig. 7 Sharply demarcated steatosis hepatis with hypointensity on axial T1w in-phase (**a**) and hyperintense signal on axial T2w (**b**) MRI

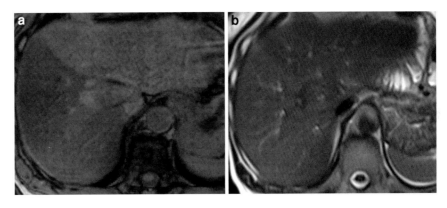

Fig. 8 Lobulated confluent solid lesions in hepatic lymphoma. Axial T1 (**a**) and T1w contrast enhanced, fat saturated (**b**) MRI

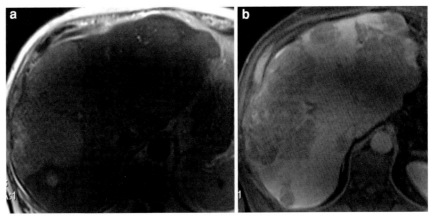

multiple, they have a clustered appearance (cluster sign). On US, most abscesses are anechoic; however, about 30% have marked hyperechogenicity, dependent on the amount of debris. The rim and septations always show a marked contrast enhancement on CT and MRI (Balci and Sirvanci 2002) (Fig. 9). Very small abscesses will sometimes show a homogeneous enhancement (which renders the differentiation from a small hemangioma difficult). Particularly with *Klebsiella* infection, intralesional gas formation is observed (Alsaif et al. 2011) (Fig. 9c). Amoebic abscesses most often involve the right liver lobe and abut the liver capsule.

2.2.2.3 Differentials

Hepatic infarction. Lobar infarction is rarely seen; however, segmental hypoperfusion is commonly observed with arterial emboli. The infarcted parenchyma usually is peripherally located and wedge-shaped (Fig. 10). Along its border, no significant

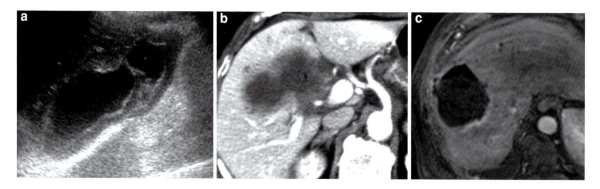

Fig. 9 Abscesses of the right liver lobe. Moderate internal hyperechogenicity due to debris, and a thickened and irregular wall (**a**) with marked enhancement (**b**). Intralesional gas formation in another patient with *Klebsiella* infection (**c**). Sagittal view US (**a**), axial pv CECT (**b**), axial T1w contrast-enhanced, fat saturated MRI (**c**)

contrast enhancement is detectable, except for the so-called subcapsular luxury perfusion in persisting disease.

Hepatic candidiasis. A systemic fungal infection that affects the liver and leads to disseminated small abscesses of both liver lobes. Commonly, immuno-compromised patients are vulnerable. On US, multiple small "bull's eye" lesions with hyperechoic centers and hypoechoic rims are seen. On CT, multiple hypo-dense nonenhancing lesions are distributed throughout the parenchyma (Fig. 11). However, in some cases, there is a central structure within the lesions, repre-senting the fungal hyphae. Contrast-enhanced MRI improves the detection of small lesions.

Hydatid cyst . The larvae of the dog tapeworm *Echinococcus granulosus* are seen in the liver in up to 75% of cases of infection. Patients present with allergic reactions, particularly when the cysts rupture. Extrinsic compression of the bile ducts next to the cysts leads to the dilation of peripheral segments of the biliary tree. In rare cases, the hepatic portal vein is partially compressed, with concomitant portal hyper-tension in long-standing disease. The hepatic lesions are well demarcated and have a three-layer appearance: the outer pericyst; the middle membrane; and the inner germinal layer. Cysts have water density, but due to hydatid sand some are hyperdense (up to 50 HU) on non-enhanced CT (NECT). Smaller peripheral daugh-ter cysts have a lower density than the mother cyst (Fig. 12). Rim calcifications are frequent; however, in therapy monitoring, only dense calcification suggests avitality of the cyst. The "water lily" sign describes a cyst with a floating detached inner layer. It is readily seen with every imaging modality, but was first described as an US feature. With MRI, the floating membrane has a low to intermediate signal on both T1w and T2w images. Hepatic lesions from *Echinococcus multilocularis*, however, have an infiltrative appear-ance, and the walls are correspondingly not well-demarcated. CECT shows partially enhancing solid and cystic masses as well as marked calcifications. Hepatic hydatid cysts also appear in the lung parenchyma with similar imaging patterns.

Biliary hamartomas. These represent benign biliary malformations. No communication with the biliary tree is visible. Multiple, small cyst-like lesions have a diffuse distribution in both liver lobes. Most commonly, the lesion walls do not enhance on CT or MRI (Fig. 13).

Hepatic metastasis. These account for the most common liver tumor. Dependent on the characteristics of the primary lesions, metastases are hypo- or hypervascularized. The former typically shows a low attenuation and a low peripheral enhancement on CT (Fig. 14). Cystic metastases or cystically transformed lesions, especially subsequent to systemic therapy, can have an attenuation of <20 HU. In rare cases, the discrimination between these and benign cysts or abscesses can be difficult.

Hepaticneoplasms. With the multifocal imaging appearance of hepatic neoplasms, primary liver tumors may be indistinguishable from multiple abscess formation. Particularly if the central tumor parts are necrotic and the periphery is at least moderately hypervascularized, the findings may be equivocal (Fig. 15).

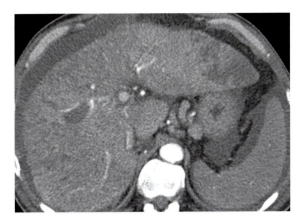

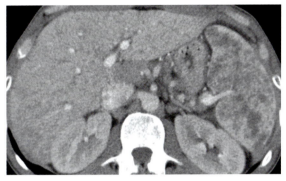

Fig. 11 Disseminated non-enhancing abscesses in hepatic candidiasis. Note the extensive splenic involvement. Axial pv CECT

Fig. 10 Hypoperfusion in the subcapsular left liver lobe. No rim enhancement on axial art CECT

2.3 Vascular

2.3.1 Portal-Vein Obstruction

2.3.1.1 Terminology and Clinical Issues

Most often, portal-vein occlusion is associated with hepatic cirrhosis. In addition, extrinsic tumor compression or tumor invasion, caused by thrombosis, results in portal-vein occlusion, which leads to acute symptoms ranging from abdominal pain, liver dysfunction, and bowel congestion to ileus, venous infarction, and massive ascites. Due to the pathologic occlusion of the portal vein, portosystemic collaterals develop; bleeding from esophageal varices, and elsewhere, is a major reason for morbidity in these patients (Pieters et al. 1997).

2.3.1.2 Imaging

The direction of portal venous flow is appropriately determined with US. The extent of thrombosis and intravascular tumor tissue is also readily detectable. However, detailed information about the extent of portosystemic collaterals and the amount of ascites is best visualized with CT (Hidajat et al. 2005) (Fig. 16). With arterial (art) CECT, the hypervascularized appearance of the involved segments is dependent on the extent of the arterioportal shunt volume. Usually, portal-venous (pv) CECT provides a detailed image of a low-density thrombus within a portal vein, the extent of involvement of the intrahepatic branches or the superior mesenteric and the splenic veins, and the cavernous transformation ,

i.e., portal thrombosis and periportal collaterals along the hepatoduodenal ligament (Fig. 16c). In addition, mesenteric congestion is readily interpretable by means of indirect signs, e.g., mesenteric edema, bowel wall thickening, and congestion of non-obstructed veins (Acosta et al. 2009).

2.3.1.3 Differentials

Budd-Chiari syndrome. This disease is associated with thrombosis of the hepatic veins and/or the inferior vena cava (IVC) (Fig. 17). On CECT, diminished peripheral contrast enhancement and a hypertrophy of the caudad lobe are visible. The latter is due to its separate venous drainage into the IVC.

Streaming artifact. During the early pv phase, contrast-enhanced blood from the splenic vein partially fills the portal vein while the mesenteric vein is comparably less opacified. The result is an incomplete mixture and, hence, the risk of a false-positive diagnosis of a filling defect. In patients with hepatic cirrhosis, in particular, proper timing is crucially important in the detection of portal venous thrombosis: it is present at a homogeneous attenuation of the liver parenchyma (equilibrium phase).

Lymphoma of the porta hepatis. The biologic patterns of lymphoma are ubiquitous and so are the imaging characteristics. When lymphoma arises along the hepatoduodenal ligament, it usually does not compress the portal vessels or the bile duct in the early stages (Fig. 18). However, thrombosis of the portal vein may occur as a consequence of tumor invasion.

Fig. 12 Septated hydatid cysts of the right liver lobe; partially marked hyperdensity in (**a**) due to hydatid sand; density of daughter cysts in (**b**) is lower than that of the mother cyst. Axial pv CECT

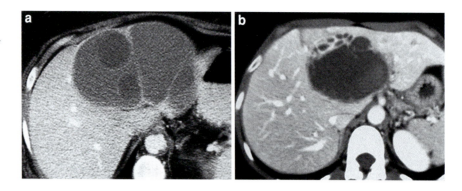

2.3.2 Budd-Chiari Syndrome

2.3.2.1 Terminology and Clinical Issues

Hepatic venous outflow obstruction increases post-sinusiodal pressure and leads to the dilatation of the central veins, a delay in portal vein inflow and, as a result, blood flow reversal. The Budd-Chiari syndrome is rare, but it is a major cause of hepatic venous obstruction. It is predominantly due to hypercoagulable states, tumor obstruction, and trauma. About one-third of the patients present with acute symptoms ranging from sudden abdominal pain to ascites and liver failure (Cura et al. 2009).

2.3.2.2 Imaging

Depending on the level of obstruction, with pv CECT, thrombi are seen in the hepatic part of the IVC (type I) and/or the major hepatic veins (type II), or the small centrilobar veins (type III, i.e., veno-occlusive disease); eventually, these vessels are narrowed and finally non-opacified during the sequelae of the disease (Fig. 19). The caudad lobe is commonly unaffected because of its private drainage into the IVC; thus, it is enlarged compared to the pathologically altered and eventually shrinking lobes. As a result of the increased arterial inflow, with art CECT, patchy areas of parenchymal hyperattenuation are seen in the occluded segments and liver lobes (transient hepatic attenuation difference). On US, the narrowed major hepatic veins have a diminished or absent flow. The dilated drainage of the caudad lobe is readily detectable, as is the reversed flow in later stages (Chaubal et al. 2006). In acute disease, further findings include diffuse fatty infiltration, hepatomegaly, and ascites. In subsequent stages, nodular hypervascularized regenerative nodules are typically seen throughout the affected liver lobes, best visualized with CECT and MRI (Brancatelli et al. 2002; Buckley et al. 2007).

2.3.2.3 Differentials

Decompensated liver cirrhosis. Ascites, a reversed portal venous flow, and diffuse hypervascularized parenchymal nodules are present. The nodules are smaller than those in Budd-Chiari syndrome and usually have a low signal on T2 GRE sequences because of iron depositions (Fig. 20). In contrast to the Budd-Chiari syndrome, in addition to the caudad lobe, the left liver lobe is hypertrophic. The hepatic veins are patent.

Vascular tumor invasion. In later stages of disease, vascular invasion may arise and thrombi are observed in major hepatic draining veins (Fig. 21).

2.3.3 Hepatic Infarction

2.3.3.1 Terminology and Clinical Issues

Hepatic infarction is uncommon because of the dual blood supply from the hepatic artery and the portal vein. Damage to the hepatic artery occurs after trauma and, less commonly, has an iatrogenic etiology, e.g., laparoscopic cholecystectomy, embolization. In addition, hepatic artery occlusion is a major complication after orthotopic liver transplantation. Rarely, it is observed in association with hypovolemic states and sepsis, as well as with the HELLP syndrome (hemolytic anemia, elevated liver enzymes, low platelets). With massive infarction, however, patients have severe symptoms, including right upper quadrant pain and ascites, as well as systemic disorders related to liver failure (Stewart et al. 2008).

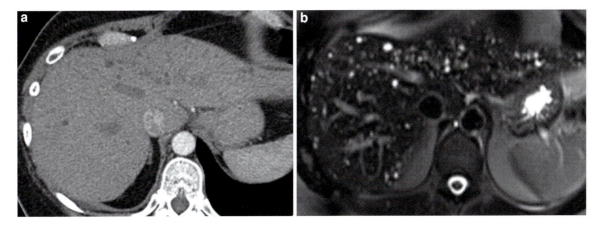

Fig. 13 Multiple hamartomas in both liver lobes mimic small abscesses; however, they lack confluency and peripheral enhancement. Axial art CECT (**a**), axial T2w fat saturated MRI

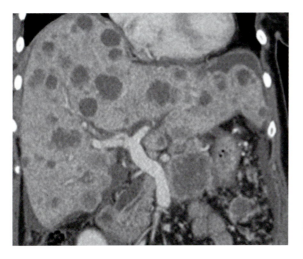

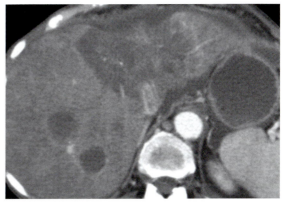

Fig. 15 Large HCC involving the liver segments II, III, and IV; multifocal disease with large secondary lesions in the posterior segments of the right liver lobe. Note the compression of the inferior vena cava. Axial pv CECT

Fig. 14 Disseminated hepatic metastases show confluency and peripheral enhancement. In particular, large lesions are centrally necrotic. Coronal pv CECT

2.3.3.2 Imaging

New, peripheral wedge-shaped hypovascularized areas are suggestive of arterial infarction. With US, hypoechogenic lesions with indistinct margins are observed. On duplex US, the absence of a hepatic-artery signal is pathognomonic. NECT shows low-density wedge-shaped or round lesions. In some cases, however, these lesions can resemble the bile ducts. In the acute setting, they are poorly demarcated. CECT better delineates the extent of hypo-vascularization, particularly in the portal-venous phase (Fig. 22); lesions that are hypodense to the liver parenchyma in each phase of CECT are suggestive of

necrosis; art CECT (i.e., CT angiography of the visceral aortic branches) shows a contrast abruption or a dissection of the hepatic artery (Smith et al. 1998; Torabi et al. 2008) (Fig. 22b).

2.3.3.3 Differentials

Focal steatosis hepatis. Various etiologies, including focal hypoxia and metabolic causes, lead to focally varying fatty infiltration of the liver parenchyma. Fatty infiltration most commonly assumes geographic or rounded patterns, affecting regions with an atypical portal venous supply. In particular, tissue surrounding the falciform ligament, the hilus, and the gallbladder,

Fig. 16 Thrombosis of the portal vein confluence, extending into the distal splenic vein (**a**); intrahepatic thrombosis of the right portal vein branch in a patient with liver cirrhosis (**b**); concomitant cavernous transformation (**c**) and extensive esophageal varices (**d**). Axial pv CECT

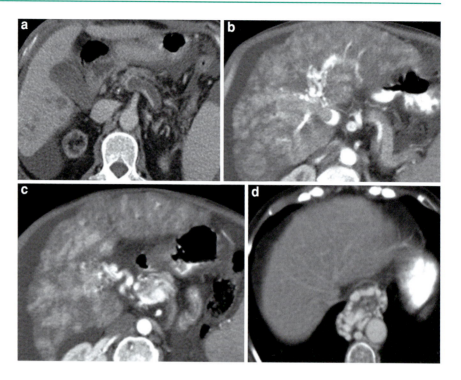

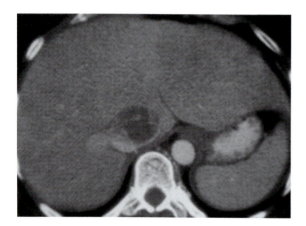

Fig. 17 Thrombosis of the intrahepatic IVC in a patient with Budd-Chiari syndrome. Axial pv CECT

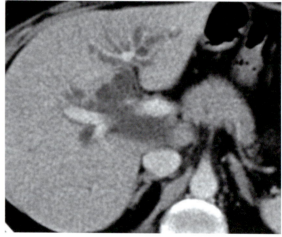

Fig. 18 Lymphoma of the porta hepatis causes marked intrahepatic cholangiectasis; no compression or thrombosis of the portal vein. Axial pv CECT

is involved. T1 out-of-phase MRI show a pathognomically diminished signal intensity compared to T1 in-phase images (Fig. 23).

Hepatic abscess. The rim of an abscess virtually always shows a marked enhancement. An abscess is well-demarcated and has a round shape (Fig. 24). Large abscesses have a substantial volume and compress the surrounding parenchyma, which is not seen with hepatic infarction.

2.4 Hepatic Neoplasms

2.4.1 Terminology and Clinical Issues

Although primary malignant hepatic tumors are ranked fourth in malignancy occurrence worldwide (Liu et al. 2010), it is the benign disorders that play the larger role as a cause for the acute abdomen.

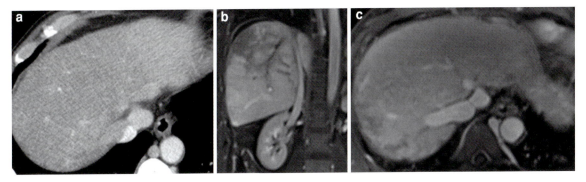

Fig. 19 Absent perfusion of the central hepatic veins in Budd-Chiari syndrome (**a**); inhomogeneous parenchymal attenuation in the affected right liver lobe (**b**); and onset of large regenerative nodules (**c**). Axial pv CECT (a), coronal (b), and axial (c) T1w contrast-enhanced, fat-saturated MRI

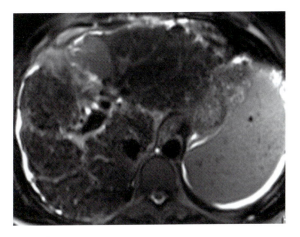

Fig. 20 Hypertrophy of the left liver lobe and small parenchymal nodules in liver cirrhosis. Axial T2w fat-saturated MRI

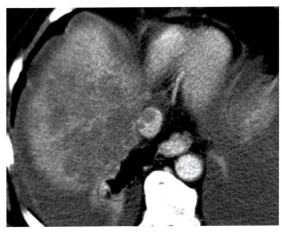

Fig. 21 Intrahepatic cholangiocarcinoma of the right liver lobe causes tumor invasion of the IVC, as well as ascites characteristic of liver insufficiency. Axial pv CECT

The most common symptom is pain. Fever appears with the hemorrhage or infection of large masses. An acute onset of pain in the right upper quadrant is commonly caused by hemorrhage from cysts (Vachha et al. 2011), adenoma, or giant cavernous hemangioma (Danet et al. 2003), the latter being the most common liver tumor after metastasis. In rare cases, hemoperitoneum is observed from epithelioid hemangioendothelioma, as well as from hepatic vein invasion in Budd-Chiari syndrome. In hepatic cholangiocellular carcinoma, symptoms are rare at the early stage of disease (Chung et al. 2009; Han et al. 1997). Later, a palpable mass and jaundice are the most common clinical symptoms; the latter is due to the obstruction of the central biliary tree.

2.4.2 Imaging

Mass lesions are readily seen with US, and the extent of bile duct dilatation and hepatic venous congestion are depicted elegantly. In addition, portal venous flow is best visualized with US. Hemoperitoneum is also easily detected; however, this finding is equivocal in terms of a clinical treatment decision.

CT and MRI are best suited for a one-step evaluation in these patients. Most importantly, the discrimination between benign and malignant tumors can be made in the majority of cases (Zondervan PE 2002) (Fig. 25). MRI shows the varied signal intensity of hemorrhage, dependent on the extent of mixed blood products. Although art and pv CECT are recommended, NECT visualizes hemorrhage as well, and the level of HU is suggestive of the age of hemorrhage.

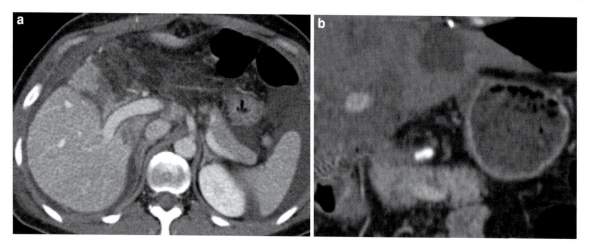

Fig. 22 Extensive infarction of the left liver lobe after traumatic dissection of the left hepatic artery branch (**a**). Abrupt termination of the common hepatic artery attenuation due to thrombosis. Axial pv CECT (**a**), coronal art CECT (**b**)

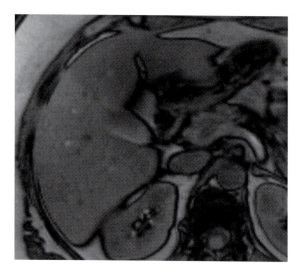

Fig. 23 Geographic patterns of steatosis hepatis. Axial T1w out-of-phase MRI

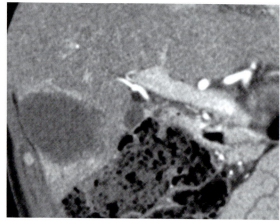

Fig. 24 Round-shaped abscess of the right liver lobe. Coronal pv CECT

2.4.3 Differentials

Liver cirrhosis. The liver has a nodular contour, the right lobe is atrophic, and the caudad and the left lobes are enlarged. Splenomegaly, portosystemic collaterals, and ascites are present at late stages. CECT sometimes reveals a persistent enhancement due to confluent fibrosis. Associated intrahepatic biliary obstruction may be present, based on the extent of the fibrotic, wedge-shaped lesions radiating from the porta hepatis to the liver capsule. MRI depicts siderotic regenerative nodules through the

paramagnetic effect of intranodular iron deposition. The discrimination between a regenerative dysplastic nodule and an incipient hepatocellular carcinoma (HCC) is made by T1w and T2w images: the first is hyperintense on T1w images and hypointense on T2w images, compared to liver parenchyma (Fig. 26). HCC is hyperintense on T2w images and iso- or hypointense on T1w images.

Hepatic abscess. Usually, small hypodense lesions progress to form a large, partially septated, sharply defined mass (Fig. 27). The rim and septations always show a marked contrast enhancement on CT and MRI. Abscesses may present with fluid-debris levels.

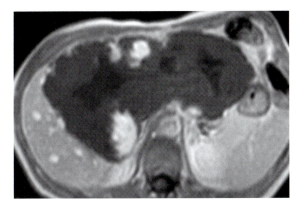

Fig. 25 Giant cavernous hemangioma of both liver lobes with recent intralesional hemorrhage. Axial T1w contrast-enhanced MRI

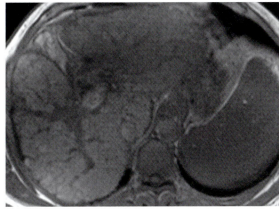

Fig. 26 Disseminated nodules in liver cirrhosis are hyperintense on T1w images, with no evidence of malignancy. Axial T1w in-phase MRI

2.5 Hepatic Trauma

2.5.1 Terminology and Clinical Issues

The liver is the second most-injured abdominal organ after the spleen. Injuries occur in 25% of patients following blunt trauma, and in up to 70% of patients following penetrating trauma from stab and gunshot injuries (Moore et al. 1995). Rarely, iatrogenic side effects develop after a liver biopsy or malpositioning of a chest tube. The most common injury mechanism in blunt trauma is rapid acceleration, followed by rapid deceleration, most likely sustained during a motor vehicle accident. The most common clinical signs are right upper quadrant pain and tenderness. However, because liver trauma is frequently sustained as a part of multiple severe trauma, often these symptoms are not evaluable as the patient is unconscious. In all cases, hypotension and tachycardia due to hemorrhagic hypovolemia are important diagnostic clues.

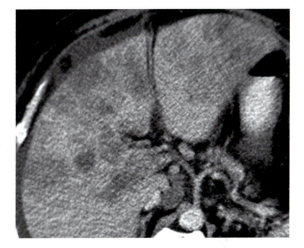

Fig. 27 Multiple abscesses in both liver lobes, indistinguishable from multifocal malignancy unless clinical presentation is considered. Axial pv CECT

2.5.2 Imaging

Characteristic US findings of intraparenchymal hematoma include round, echogenic lesions and irregular, mostly hypoechoic abnormalities that are indicative of lacerations (Korner et al. 2008). However, in dedicated trauma centers, US is predominantly performed as FAST, i.e., Focused Assessment with Sonography for Trauma . This type of US is considered an adjunct during the first 5 min after the arrival in the emergency room of the multiply and severely injured patient (Poletti et al. 2003). Its goal is the detection of gross free abdominal fluid. However, compared to CT imaging,

US has a markedly lower sensitivity of 42–69% for the detection of intraperitoneal blood. To be detected by US, about 500 ml of free fluid must be present in the peritoneal cavity. In contrast, with CT imaging, as little as 10 ml of fluid are readily seen (Yoon et al. 2005). In addition, up to half of all liver injuries occur without the presence of a hemoperitoneum. Instead, CT scanning is performed at a very early time point after the trauma, i.e., at the time of the primary patient survey, according to the Advanced Trauma Life Support (ATLS) report.

Dedicated injury severity scales (OIS) have been developed to facilitate clinical research (Becker et al. 1998). A detailed scaling system has been proposed by the American Association of the Surgery of Trauma (AAST) that includes an injury description for each individual abdominal organ. The system is based on the findings of clinical, CT-based radiologic and pathologic findings. Indeed, the trauma team is aware that, in each patient, the vital-sign stability is of the greatest relevance for the treatment plan. However, the OIS help the trauma team to predict whether the patient will need surgery or could be managed with a wait-and-see strategy.

Direct CT findings include lacerations, subcapsular and parenchymal hematomas, as well as active hemorrhage. While the extent of lacerations and hematomas is readily seen with pv CECT, the detection of active arterial bleeding or pseudoaneurysm often requires art CECT (Fig. 28). Lacerations are hypodense lesions that commonly parallel the venous branches. Early after trauma, in NECT, parenchymal hematomas are hyperdense to the surrounding unaffected liver tissue. The injuries are graded according to the extent of capsular tear, parenchymal laceration, hematoma, and parenchymal devascularization. The OIS for the liver comprises six grades, depending on the extent of hematoma and lacerations, as well as the presence of vascular hepatic avulsion (Table 1, Figs. 29, 30, 31, 32, and 33).

CT findings suggestive of hepatic trauma are hemoperitoneum and periportal tracking. The latter comprises linear hypodense lines along the central periportal zones and is commonly caused by blood or bile from multiple parenchymal microtraumas. Based on the typically benign course of liver hematomas, most blunt traumas are managed conservatively. If CT imaging reveals active bleeding, or if a hepatic lobe is completely damaged, surgical repair is indicated. MRI is not indicated at an early time point in the adult patient. In equivocal findings in children, however, it may be considered a valuable alternative.

2.5.3 Differentials

HELLP syndrome. HELLP is the abbreviation for hemolysis, elevated liver enzymes and low platelets, and occurs within the first trimester of pregnancy. It is considered a variant of eclampsia. Parenchymal and/or subcapsular fluid in the HELLP syndrome patient can mimic trauma-related liver lesions. Right upper quadrant pain is caused by the hepatic distension due to hepatocyte destruction and liver enlargement. Active hemorrhage from the liver parenchyma occurs as well, rendering the condition impossible to differentiate from

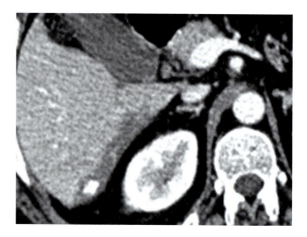

Fig. 28 Active arterial hemorrhage from a subcasular vessel of the liver segment VI. Axial art CECT

trauma in some cases. However, infarction frequently accompanies HELLP disorders, which is not typical for trauma; conversely, lacerations are not observed in the HELLP syndrome. Major US findings are irregular or wedge-shaped infarcted areas or hematomas, as well as periportal tracking due to dissecting blood or bile along the bile ducts. A low platelet count helps to narrow the differentials, together with elevated bilirubin and lactate dehydrogenase. CT and MRI reveal typical patterns of parenchymal and/or subcapsular hemorrhage. However, in most cases, a marked fatty infiltration of the parenchyma is obvious.

Hepatic hemangioma. These lesions are the most common benign tumors of the liver. Since they are located in the posterior area of the right lobe subcapsularly, in conjunction with right-sided rib fractures they can be mistaken for a parenchymal hematoma. This is even more likely when only pv CECT is performed. However, most hemangiomas with a size between 2 and 15 cm pathognomically show an early peripheral nodal enhancement pattern on art CECT, as well as a centripetal progression of enhancement on pv CECT. Hemangiomas are isodense to blood vessels in art and pv CECT, which distinguishes them from hematomas. MRI visualizes a central scar in large hemangiomas, which is hypointense on T1w and hyperintense on T2w images. After IV contrast administration, the enhancement pattern is comparable to CT imaging; however, the central scar remains unenhanced. US shows a hyperechoic lesion with posterior acoustic enhancement. The pattern is more lobulated the larger the hemangioma is (Fig. 34).

Table 1 Classification of liver injuries according to the organ injury scale (OIS)

Grade	Morphology	Description
I	Hematoma	Subcapsular, <10% of surface area
	Laceration	<1 cm in depth
II	Hematoma	Subcapsular, 10–50% of surface area OR intraparenchymal <10 cm in width
	Laceration	1–3 cm in depth OR <10 cm in length
III	Hematoma	Subcapsular, >50% of surface OR intraparenchymal > 10 cm in width
	Laceration	>3 cm in depth
IV	Laceration	Disruption of 25–75% of one lobe OR 1–3 segments of one lobe
V	Laceration	Disruption of > 75% of one lobe OR >3 segments of one lobe
	Vascular	Juxtahepatic venous injury involving the IVC and/or central hepatic veins
VI	Vascular	Hepatic avulsion

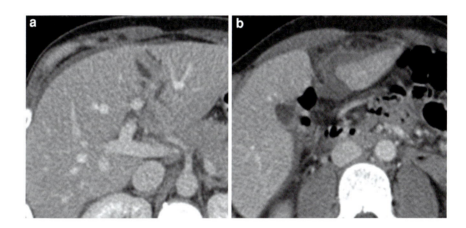

Fig. 29 Small lacerations within the liver segments IVb and III (**a**); subcapsular hematoma < 10% of the surface area (**b**): OIS grade I. Axial pv CECT

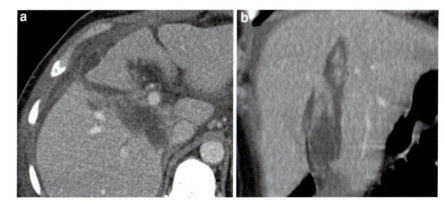

Fig. 30 Intraparenchymal hematoma of <10 cm (**a**); parenchymal laceration <10 cm in length (**b**): OIS grade II. Axial (**a**) and coronal (**b**) pv CECT

3 The Biliary System

3.1 Caroli Disease

3.1.1 Terminology and Clinical Issues

Caroli disease is a rare disorder and represents one variant of fibropolycystic liver disease. The others include congenital fibrosis, polycystic liver disease, and cystic dilatation of the choledochal duct (Brancatelli et al. 2005; Levy et al. 2002). Characteristically, multifocal cystic dilatations of the intrahepatic bile ducts are found, varying in size from a few millimeters to several centimeters. Clinically, most commonly, adolescents and young adults present with recurrent episodes of right upper quadrant

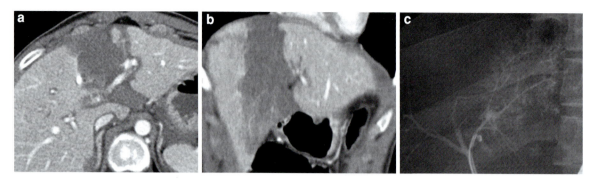

Fig. 31 Multiple deep lacerations (>3 cm in width) and a large hematoma of the central right liver lobe (**a**, **b**): OIS grade III. Severe damage to the intrahepatic bile ducts, with multisegmental extraductal contrast material (**c**). Axial (**a**) and coronal (**b**) pv CECT, ERCP (**c**)

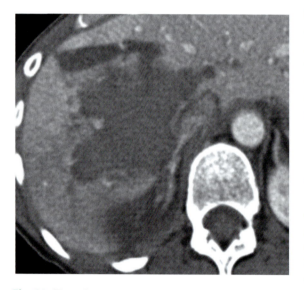

Fig. 32 Extensive parenchymal disruption involving < 25% of the right liver lobe: OIS grade IV. Axial pv CECT

pain, fever, and jaundice. Acute symptoms are aggravated by hepatic abscesses and sepsis.

3.1.2 Imaging

In most cases, portal branches are surrounded by markedly dilated cysts, which is referred to as the "central dot" sign. The cysts show communication with the bile ducts or with one another (Vachha et al. 2011). US is the primary imaging modality (Fig. 35a). Homogeneous septa and central portal branches are suggestive. In some patients, intraductal calculi may be seen. Complications, such as abscesses, are better discriminated by CECT. MRI

has an important role in chronic disease, since most patients are young and would sustain a marked radiation dose from repetitive CT. MRCP shows multiple, oval-shaped, sometimes beaded cysts that follow the course of the portal structures (Mortele and Ros 2001; Guy et al. 2002) (Fig. 35b). Intraluminal sludge or calculi are recognized as a loss of signal in all sequences.

3.1.3 Differentials

Cholangitis. Bile duct obstruction caused by stones, strictures, parasitic infestation, or by malignant disease can cause ascending cholangitis. Intrahepatic abscesses differ from the cystically dilated bile ducts of Caroli disease in that the ducts are ill-defined and have thick walls with a characteristic enhancement pattern in CECT and MRI (Fig. 36).

Biliary hamartomas. Von Meyenburg complexes represent benign biliary malformations. They internalize a variable degree of cystic and fibrous tissue. A pathognomonically relevant feature is the lack of communication with the biliary tree. Most commonly, multiple small cyst-like lesions are present in both liver lobes and show a diffuse distribution (Fig. 37). Depending on the amount of fibrous stroma along the lesion walls, there is little or no enhancement on CECT and MRI.

Polycystic liver disease. Non-communicating multiple dysontogenic cysts are found in both lobes. These cysts have characteristic water density and intensity on CT and MRI, respectively (Fig. 38). However, some cysts may appear with inhomogeneous margins and wall calcification may be seen.

Fig. 33 Massive parenchymal disruption involving >75% of the right liver lobe: OIS grade V. Note the lacerations extending along the major hepatic veins and the IVC, consistent with a juxtahepatic injury. Axial art CECT

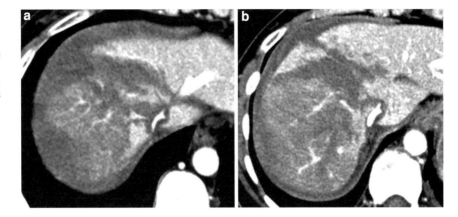

3.2 Cholangitis

3.2.1 Terminology and Clinical Issues

Biliary tree obstruction, an increased intraluminal pressure, and infection of the bile are considered the main pathogenetic factors in acute bacterial cholangitis. Biliary obstruction is believed to increase small-bowel bacterial colonization by the retrograde ascent of bacteria from the duodenum or from portal venous blood. An increased biliary pressure pushes the infection into the biliary canaliculi, the hepatic veins, and the perihepatic lymphatics, potentially leading to suppurative infection and bacteremia (Catalano et al. 2009).

Recurrent pyogenic cholangitis, also termed Oriental cholangiohepatitis, is endemic in southeast Asia. It is characterized by the formation of multiple intra- and extrahepatic bile stones, hepatic abscesses, and dilatation and stricturing of the intrahepatic and extrahepatic bile ducts (Wani et al. 2011). This variant is most commonly due to the parasitic infection from *Ascaris lumbrocoides.*

Patients with acute cholangitis present with right upper quadrant pain, fever, and jaundice (i.e., Charcot triad), and, at a later stage, with sepsis.

3.2.2 Imaging

The irregular shape and the dilatation of bile ducts are readily visualized with US. Stenosis, thickened duct walls, and associated duct stones are better seen with CT and MRI (Arai et al. 2003) (Fig. 39). High-attenuation intraductal debris also suggests the presence of purulent bile. Abscesses are considered a complication, and CECT as well as MRI are the modalities of choice for their detection (Fig. 39c, d). MRCP detects stones as low-signal filling defects, as well as irregular bile-duct calipers with stenotic and dilatated segments (Yeh et al. 2009). If stones are seen in the intra- and extrahepatic bile ducts, involving the left lobe more than the right lobe but without evidence of stones within the gallbladder, recurrent pyogenic cholangitis is the most likely diagnosis (Kim et al. 1999). ERCP is highly suggestive when intrahepatic bile duct segments are not filled with contrast material.

3.2.3 Differentials

Primary sclerosing cholangitis. The disease is considered to have an autoimmune etiology. It is characterized by a progressive inflammatory and fibrotic cholangiopathy of the intra- and extrahepatic bile ducts. The common bile duct is virtually always involved. Portal hypertension and liver cirrhosis are frequent sequelae, rendering orthotopic liver transplantation the only promising therapy. CT and MRI show diffusely thickened duct walls and a typical beaded pattern of the concomitant strictures and dilatations (Vitellas et al. 2000) (Fig. 40). Periportal fibrosis is also seen as hypodense and hypointense areas along the major ducts. Calculi are most often found in the periphery of strictures. At later stages, the typical patterns of cirrhosis, ascites, portosystemic collaterals, and splenomegaly are readily visible.

Cholangiocarcinoma. Extrahepatic bile duct carcinoma is far more common than intrahepatic cancer, which is also referred to as cholangiocarcinoma. A solid hypovascularized mass, intrahepatic

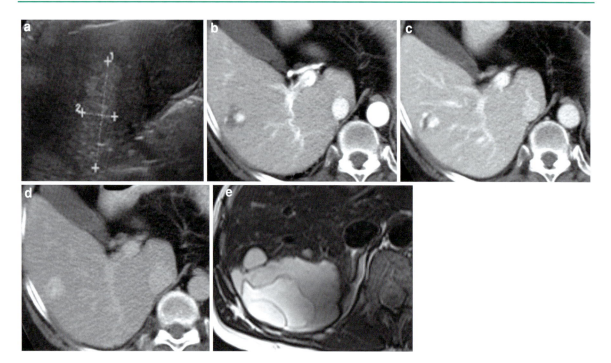

Fig. 34 Hemangiomas of the posterior right liver lobe. US shows a homogeneous hyperechoic lesion (**a**); characteristic early peripheral nodal enhancement pattern and centripetal progression on CECT (**b, c, d**); hyperintense central scar on T2w MRI (**e**)

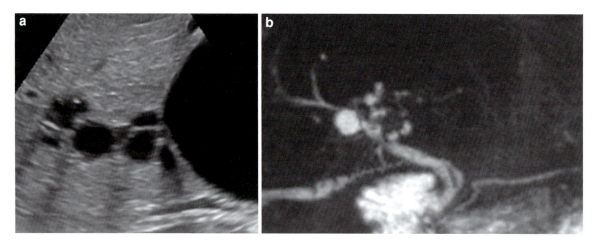

Fig. 35 Caroli disease: cystic dilatation of the choledochal duct (**a**) and multiple beaded cysts along the intrahepatic bile duct (**a, b**). Sagittal view US (**a**), MRCP (**b**)

secondary tumors, as well as the extent of concomitant cholangiectasis are readily seen with either US, CT, or MRI (Fig. 41).

3.3   Cholelithiasis and Cholecystitis

See Sects. 2– 4 in "Gallbladder"

3.4   Biliary System Neoplasms

3.4.1   Terminology and Clinical Issues

Intra- and extrahepatic biliary tumors are rare causes of an acute abdomen in patients who present with right upper quadrant pain. Bile duct carcinoma is referred to as extrahepatic carcinoma. It is more common than intrahepatic cholangiocarcinoma

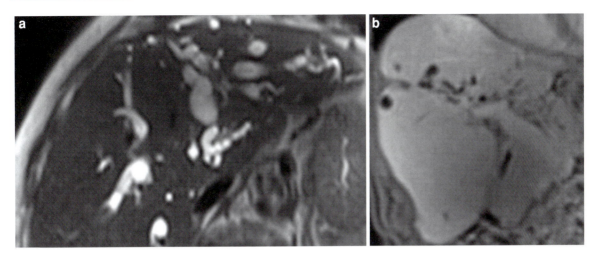

Fig. 36 Ascending cholangitis is associated with bile duct dilatation (**a**) and multiple small abscesses in both liver lobes (**a**, **b**). Axial T2w (**a**) and coronal T1w contrast-enhanced, fat-saturated (**b**) MRI

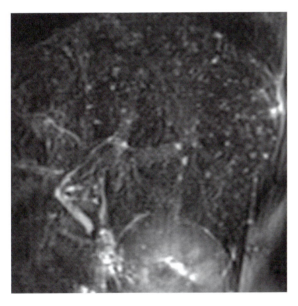

Fig. 37 Diffuse distribution of biliary hamartomas in both liver lobes without communication between von Meyenburg complexes and bile ducts. MRCP

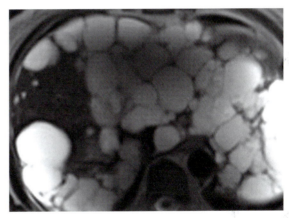

Fig. 38 Disseminated dysontogenic cysts in both liver lobes in polycystic disease. Axial T2w MRI

(Chung et al. 2009; Gore and Shelhamer 2007). Most patients with these entities present with painless jaundice. In up to 25% of patients, the confluence of the main hepatic bile ducts is involved (Klatskin's tumor), and in half the cases, the tumor is found in the common bile duct (Vogl et al. 2006). However, the most common malignant tumor of the biliary tree is gallbladder carcinoma. Its appearance is associated with long-standing chronic cholecystitis and porcelain gallbladder. The prevalence of gallstones, however, is overinterpreted: <1% of patients with cholecystolithiasis develop gallbladder carcinoma.

3.4.2 Imaging

In many patients, CT has false-negative results for extrahepatic tumors; it is therefore not the modality of choice. This is particularly true for the detection of polypoid intraductal tumor spread. A bile duct tumor that is visible on CT, however, has an extraductal component and is, in general, associated with a poor prognosis. ERCP is the method that allows the diagnosis, while US commonly only depicts dilatation of

Fig. 39 Cholangitis: irregularly shaped, dilated intra- and extrahepatic bile ducts (**a**) and duct stones in the left main branch (**b**); dilation of the intrahepatic bile ducts and associated abscesses of the right liver lobe (**c**, **d**). MRCP (**a**, **b**), axial T2w MR (**c**), axial pv CECT (**d**)

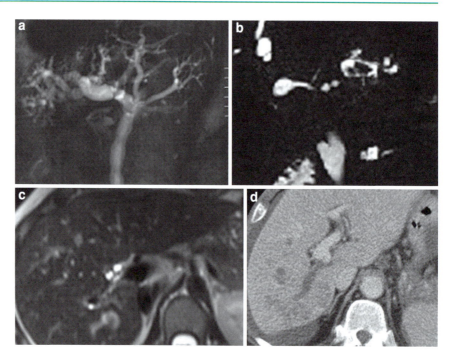

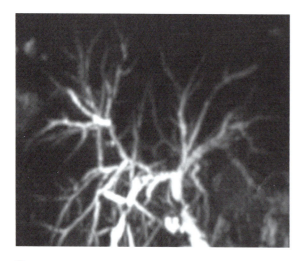

Fig. 40 Beaded pattern of bile duct strictures and dilatations in primary sclerosing cholangitis. MRCP

the prestenotic bile ducts, at least in extrahepatic disease (Fig. 42). Gallbladder carcinoma is best diagnosed with CECT and MRI. The extent of the invasion of the right liver lobe and the porta hepatis is readily visualized.

3.4.3 Differentials

Xanthogranulomatous cholecystitis. An irregular gallbladder wall thickening may resemble a lobulated mass (Fig. 43). Rarely, intralesional calcifications are observed (Enomoto et al. 2003). The chronically affected pericholecystic tissue and adenomyomatosis of the gallbladder may simulate carcinoma.

Complicated cholecystitis. The gallbladder wall is sometimes asymmetrically thickened, and pericholecystic abscesses are seen (Fig. 44).

Pancreatic carcinoma and chronic pancreatitis. Hypovascularized adenocarcinomas are the most frequent pancreatic malignancies. Tumors arising from the pancreatic head may cause obstructions of the common bile duct and the pancreatic duct ("double duct" sign). Tumor spread along the bile duct leads to irregular wall alterations, best visible with MRI (Fig. 45). Chronic pancreatitis may not be distinguishable from carcinoma in cases in which the tumor does not infiltrate adjacent vessels or the duodenum. However, in this entity, dilatation of the pancreatic duct is often due to calculi, which are best seen with CT and MRI.

3.5 Biliary Trauma

3.5.1 Terminology and Clinical Issues

Most injuries of the biliary system have their cause in blunt or penetrating trauma. In rare cases, iatrogenic injuries occur with cholecystectomy, percutaneous

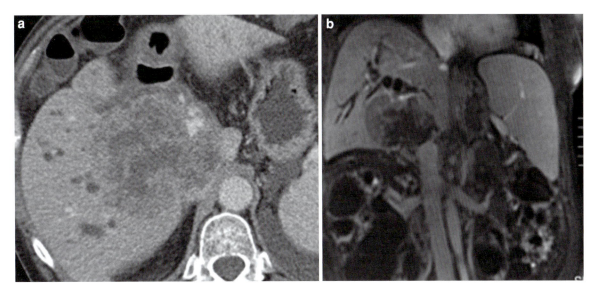

Fig. 41 Cholangiocarcinoma: large centrally nectrotic mass of the right liver lobe and marked bile duct dilatation (**a**, **b**). Note: polycystic kidney disease in (**b**). Axial pv CECT (**a**), coronal T1w contrast-enhanced, fat-saturated MRI (**b**)

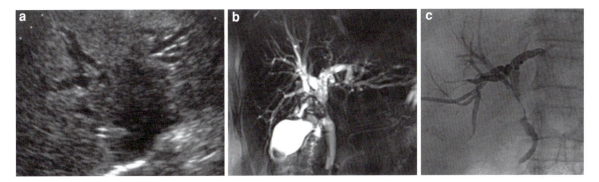

Fig. 42 Klatskin's tumor: inhomogenous echotexture along the porta hepatis (**a**), stenosis of the proximal hepatic duct, and incipient dilatation of the intrahepatic bile ducts (**b**, **c**). Axial view on US (**a**), MRCP (**b**), ERCP (**c**)

Fig. 43 Asymmetrical thickening of the gallbladder wall in xanthogranulomatous cholecystitis. Axial (**a**) and coronal (**b**) pv CECT

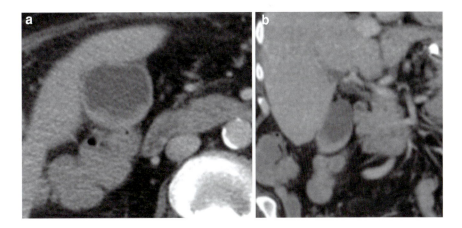

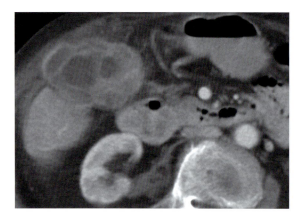

Fig. 44 Pericholecystic abscess along the gallbladder bed. Axial pv CECT

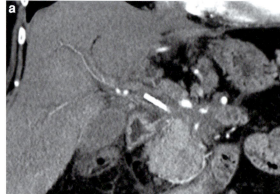

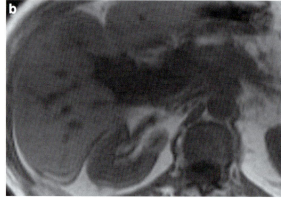

Fig. 45 Pancreatic carcinoma extending along the hepatoduodenal ligament; implanted stent of the common choledochal duct due to symptomatic cholangiectasis. Coronal art CECT (**a**), axial T1w MR (**b**)

bile-duct drainage, or following percutaneous liver biopsy. Acute symptoms are caused by the damage to the liver parenchyma and the associated hemoperitoneum rather than by bile-duct damage alone. However, subacute and chronic symptoms are due to biliary peritonitis as a consequence of bile leakage and to bile-duct strictures. Hemobilia is a severe clinical problem; in most cases, these patients present with the triad of blood loss, jaundice, and colic. It is usually recognized within the first week after trauma.

3.5.2 Imaging

With either US, CT, or MRI, visualization of direct signs of injury is limited to the complete transection or occlusion of the main bile ducts and to the disruption of the gallbladder wall (Gupta et al. 2004). US reveals blood as echogenic clots within the biliary tree (Fig. 46). The dilatation of bile ducts proximal to the trauma is seen. Complications, such as bilioma, are easily seen. CT is recommended as pv and delayed CECT. MRCP is suitable for the detection of strictures and the delineation of disorders of the major bile ducts (Tkacz et al. 2009). CECT detects blood in the biliary tree and the gallbladder as high-attenuation clots (> 60 HU), and can help to suggest a biliary-enteric fistula, when contrast media is found in the biliary tree as well as in the bowel. However, ERCP is

often necessary when leaks and fistulas from small ducts are suspected (Fig. 46d). These lesions are commonly suspected in the subacute phase of trauma, at the earliest. Therefore, nuclear medicine, in the form of with ^{99}Tc scans, can contribute to the detection of fistulas.

3.5.3 Differentials

Hepatic arterial thrombosis. This is a rare condition. Embolic material occluding the main branches of the intrahepatic artery is the main cause of ischemia of the bile ducts. However, the absence of either trauma or iatrogenic manipulation of the liver is suggestive.

Fig. 46 Iatrogenic gallbladder trauma during percutaneous bile drainage. Hyperechogenic blood within the bladder (**a**); hemobilia of the central right intrahepatic bile duct, with the blood clot hyperintense on T1w and hypointense on T2w images (**b**, **c**); rupture of the central left bile duct subsequent to trauma, marked extravasation of contrast material, and dilatation of the distal left duct (**d**). Axial view US (**a**); axial T1w (**b**); and T2w (**c**) MRI; ERCP (**d**)

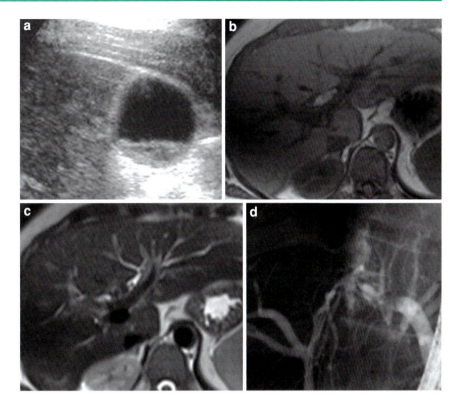

References

Acosta S, Alhadad A, Ekberg O (2009) Findings in multi-detector row CT with portal phase enhancement in patients with mesenteric venous thrombosis. Emerg Radiol 16(6):477–482

Alsaif HS, Venkatesh SK, Chan DS, Archuleta S (2011) CT Appearance of pyogenic liver abscesses caused by Klebsiella pneumoniae. Radiology 260:129–138

Arai K, Kawai K, Kohda W, Tatsu H, Matsui O, Nakahama T (2003) Dynamic CT of acute cholangitis: early inhomogeneous enhancement of the liver. AJR Am J Roentgenol 181(1):115–118

Bahl M, Qayyum A, Westphalen AC et al (2008) Liver steatosis: investigation of opposed-phase T1-weighted liver MR signal intensity loss and visceral fat measurement as biomarkers. Radiology 249(1):160–166

Balci NC, Sirvanci M (2002) MR imaging of infective liver lesions. Magn Reson Imaging Clin N Am 10(1):121–135 vii

Becker CD, Mentha G, Terrier F (1998) Blunt abdominal trauma in adults: role of CT in the diagnosis and management of visceral injuries. Part 1 liver and spleen Eur Radiol 8(4):553-62

Benedetti NJ, Desser TS, Jeffrey RB (2008) Imaging of hepatic infections. Ultrasound Q 24(4):267–278

Brancatelli G, Federle MP, Grazioli L, Golfieri R, Lencioni R (2002) Benign regenerative nodules in Budd-Chiari syndrome and other vascular disorders of the liver: radiologic-pathologic and clinical correlation. Radiographics 22(4):847–862

Brancatelli G, Federle MP, Vilgrain V, Vullierme MP, Marin D, Lagalla R (2005) Fibropolycystic liver disease: CT and MR imaging findings. Radiographics 25(3):659–670

Buckley O, OB J, Snow A et al (2007) Imaging of Budd-Chiari syndrome. Eur Radiol 17(8):2071–2078

Catalano OA, Sahani DV, Forcione DG et al (2009) Biliary infections: spectrum of imaging findings and management. Radiographics 29(7):2059–2080

Chaubal N, Dighe M, Hanchate V, Thakkar H, Deshmukh H, Rathod K (2006) Sonography in Budd-Chiari syndrome. J Ultrasound Med 25(3):373–379

Chung YE, Kim MJ, Park YN et al (2009) Varying appearances of cholangiocarcinoma: radiologic-pathologic correlation. Radiographics 29(3):683–700

Cura M, Haskal Z, Lopera J (2009) Diagnostic and interventional radiology for Budd-Chiari syndrome. Radiographics 29(3):669–681

Danet IM, Semelka RC, Braga L, Armao D, Woosley JT (2003) Giant hemangioma of the liver: MR imaging characteristics in 24 patients. Magn Reson Imaging 21(2):95–101

Enomoto T, Todoroki T, Koike N, Kawamoto T, Matsumoto H (2003) Xanthogranulomatous cholecystitis mimicking stage IV gallbladder cancer. Hepatogastroenterology 50(53):1255–1258

Gore RM, Shelhamer RP (2007) Biliary tract neoplasms: diagnosis and staging. Cancer Imaging 7 Spec No A:S15–23

Gupta A, Stuhlfaut JW, Fleming KW, Lucey BC, Soto JA (2004) Blunt trauma of the pancreas and biliary tract: a multimodality imaging approach to diagnosis. Radiographics 24(5):1381–1395

Guy F, Cognet F, Dranssart M, Cercueil JP, Conciatori L, Krause D (2002) Caroli's disease: magnetic resonance imaging features. Eur Radiol 12(11):2730–2736

Han JK, Choi BI, Kim TK, Kim SW, Han MC, Yeon KM (1997) Hilar cholangiocarcinoma: thin-section spiral CT findings with cholangiographic correlation. Radiographics 17(6):1475–1485

Hidajat N, Stobbe H, Griesshaber V, Felix R, Schroder RJ (2005) Imaging and radiological interventions of portal vein thrombosis. Acta Radiol 46(4):336–343

Hussain SM, JN IJ, Zondervan PE, Schalm SW, de Man RA, Krestin GP (2002) Benign versus malignant hepatic nodules: MR imaging findings with pathologic correlation. Radiographics 22(5):1023–1036 (discussion 37-9)

Kim MJ, Cha SW, Mitchell DG, Chung JJ, Park S, Chung JB (1999) MR imaging findings in recurrent pyogenic cholangitis. AJR Am J Roentgenol 173(6):1545–1549

Korner M, Krotz MM, Degenhart C, Pfeifer KJ, Reiser MF, Linsenmaier U (2008) Current role of emergency US in patients with major trauma. Radiographics 28(1):225–242

Levy AD, Rohrmann CA Jr, Murakata LA, Lonergan GJ (2002) Caroli's disease: radiologic spectrum with pathologic correlation. AJR Am J Roentgenol 179(4):1053–1057

Liu QY, Huang SQ, Chen JY et al (2010) Small hepatocellular carcinoma with bile duct tumor thrombi: CT and MRI findings. Abdom Imaging 35(5):537–542

Moore EE, Cogbill TH, Jurkovich GJ, Shackford SR, Malangoni MA, Champion HR (1995) Organ injury scaling: spleen and liver (1994 revision). J Trauma 38(3):323–324

Morgan DE, Lockhart ME, Canon CL, Holcombe MP, Bynon JS (2006) Polycystic liver disease: multimodality imaging for complications and transplant evaluation. Radiographics 26(6):1655–1668 (quiz)

Mortele KJ, Ros PR (2001) Cystic focal liver lesions in the adult: differential CT and MR imaging features. Radiographics 21(4):895–910

Mortele KJ, Segatto E, Ros PR (2004) The infected liver: radiologic-pathologic correlation. Radiographics 24(4):937–955

Murakami T, Baron RL, Peterson MS (1996) Liver necrosis and regeneration after fulminant hepatitis: pathologic correlation with CT and MR findings. Radiology 198(1):239–242

Pieters PC, Miller WJ, DeMeo JH (1997) Evaluation of the portal venous system: complementary roles of invasive and non-invasive imaging strategies. Radiographics 17(4):879–895

Poletti PA, Kinkel K, Vermeulen B, Irmay F, Unger PF, Terrier F (2003) Blunt abdominal trauma: Should US be used to detect both free fluid and organ injuries? Radiology 227(1):95–103

Qian Q, Li A, King BF et al (2003) Clinical profile of autosomal dominant polycystic liver disease. Hepatology 37(1):164–171

Reeder SB, Sirlin CB (2010) Quantification of liver fat with magnetic resonance imaging. Magn Reson Imaging Clin N Am 18(3):337–357 (9)

Smith GS, Birnbaum BA, Jacobs JE (1998) Hepatic infarction secondary to arterial insufficiency in native livers: CT findings in 10 patients. Radiology 208(1):223–229

Sodhi KS, Ojili V, Sakhuja V, Khandelwal N (2008) Hepatic and inferior vena caval thrombosis: vascular complication of amebic liver abscess. J Emerg Med 34(2):155–157

Stewart BG, Gervais DA, O'Neill MJ, Boland GW, Hahn PF, Mueller PR (2008) Imaging and percutaneous treatment of secondarily infected hepatic infarctions. AJR Am J Roentgenol 190(3):601–607

Tkacz JN, Anderson SA, Soto J (2009) MR imaging in gastrointestinal emergencies. Radiographics 29(6):1767–1780

Torabi M, Hosseinzadeh K, Federle MP (2008) CT of nonneoplastic hepatic vascular and perfusion disorders. Radiographics 28(7):1967–1982

Vachha B, Sun MR, Siewert B, Eisenberg RL (2011) Cystic lesions of the liver. AJR Am J Roentgenol 196(4):W355–W366

Vitellas KM, Keogan MT, Freed KS et al (2000) Radiologic manifestations of sclerosing cholangitis with emphasis on MR cholangiopancreatography. Radiographics 20(4):959–975 (quiz 1108-9, 12)

Vogl TJ, Schwarz WO, Heller M et al (2006) Staging of Klatskin tumours (hilar cholangiocarcinomas): comparison of MR cholangiography, MR imaging, and endoscopic retrograde cholangiography. Eur Radiol 16(10):2317–2325

Wani NA, Robbani I, Kosar T (2011) MRI of oriental cholangiohepatitis. Clin Radiol 66(2):158–163

Yeh BM, Liu PS, Soto JA, Corvera CA, Hussain HK (2009) MR imaging and CT of the biliary tract. Radiographics 29(6):1669–1688

Yoon W, Jeong YY, Kim JK et al (2005) CT in blunt liver trauma. Radiographics 25(1):87–104

Gallbladder

Jorge A. Soto

Contents

J. A. Soto (✉)
Department of Radiology, Boston Medical Center,
Boston University School of Medicine,
FGH Building, 3rd Floor 820 Harrison Avenue,
Boston, MA 02118, USA
e-mail: Jorge.Soto@bmc.org

Abstract

Acute biliary tract pathology remains as one of the most common worldwide causes of emergency room visits. Emergency room physicians, surgeons and radiologists devote considerable time and effort to rapidly and accurately diagnose these conditions in order to avoid mistakes that may lead to considerable morbidity and mortality. Fortunately, rapid advances in technology and refinements in invasive and non-invasive methods have improved our ability to provide precise and timely diagnoses. Ultrasonography (US) remains as the premier modality for initial (and often definitive) evaluation, but in order to maximize the accuracy of this technique, a meticulous and thorough evaluation by the operator is necessary. As the utilization of computed tomography (CT) in the emergency setting has grown exponentially in recent years, it is not surprising that many patients ultimately diagnosed with acute biliary diseases are evaluated initially with CT. Magnetic resonance (MR) and nuclear scintigraphy are usually second tier examinations, reserved for specific clinical situations or as complementary tests following an initial US or CT. However, the use of MR cholangiopancreatography (MRCP) in the emergency setting has also increased substantially in recent years. Endoscopic retrograde and percutaneous cholangiography are reserved mainly for therapeutic interventions after a precise diagnosis has been reached through a judicious use of imaging tests. This chapter reviews the appearance of common acute biliary conditions on the various imaging modalities. Emphasis is placed

M. Scaglione et al. (eds.), *Emergency Radiology of the Abdomen*,
Medical Radiology. Diagnostic Imaging,
DOI: 10.1007/174_2011_467, © Springer-Verlag Berlin Heidelberg 2012

on discussing the most appropriate test for each disease. Potential sources of error and imaging pitfalls are also discussed in detail.

1   Introduction and Imaging Techniques

As the volume of emergency department visits continues to increase, so has the number of patients in whom the biliary tract is suspected as being the cause of acute abdominal symptoms. Acute biliary tract pathology is common, and clinicians, surgeons, and radiologists expend considerable effort to rapidly and accurately diagnose these conditions in order to avoid mistakes that are result in considerable morbidity and mortality. Fortunately, rapid advances in technology and refinements in invasive and non-invasive methods have improved the ability of imaging techniques to provide a more complete visualization of the biliary tract and gallbladder, and consequently allow a more precise diagnosis.

Due to its widespread availability and relative ease of performance, as well as its excellent diagnostic capabilities for the biliary tract, ultrasonography (US) is still the modality most often relied upon for initial and, in many instances, definitive evaluation. An adequate US examination requires a careful evaluation of the gallbladder, biliary tree, and pancreas in multiple positions. Evaluation with color Doppler is also helpful for the assessment of vascular flow to the gallbladder wall and liver.

The utilization of computed tomography (CT) in the emergency setting has grown exponentially in recent years, and many reasons have been offered to explain its increased use in the emergency room. CT is widely available and, in fact, at many institutions CT scanners have been installed either inside or in very close proximity to the emergency room itself. In addition, CT is a very powerful diagnostic tool, with a very high accuracy for detecting acute diseases affecting the abdominal solid organs and hollow viscera. The biliary tract is no exception. Patients with acute signs and symptoms or with abnormal laboratory exams suggestive of abnormalities of the gallbladder or bile ducts are usually evaluated initially with US; however, the reality is that the clinical presentation is often non-specific. In these circumstances, CT is usually the next logical step in the diagnostic workup. Although concerns about radiation exposure have brought unprecedented scrutiny to the use of CT in the emergency setting, in the vast majority of cases the expected benefits outweigh the largely theoretical risks of exposure from a single CT examination. Nonetheless, proper technique is essential in order to ensure that diagnostic images are acquired following the ALARA (as low as reasonably achievable) principle for controlling radiation exposure. At our institution, all emergent CT examinations are currently performed with a 64-row multi-detector CT scanner, obtaining 1.25 mm thick images and using a 1.25 mm reconstruction interval. Orthogonal (coronal and sagittal) reformations are generated for all patients, with a 2.5 mm slice thickness and a 2.5 mm reconstruction interval. Additional post-processing tools are helpful for delineating the anatomy of the bile ducts. Specifically, minimum intensity pixel projection reformations can be generated with minimal operator effort to produce excellent quality images of the biliary tract, with an accuracy for depicting the bile ducts that rivals that of magnetic resonance cholangiopancreatography (MRCP) (Denecke et al. 2006). Unless there is a specific contraindication, intravenous contrast (100–120 ml) is administered to all patients and a 70 s delay is used in the acquisition of the portal venous phase. Non-contrast, arterial phase (25–30 s after the initiation of the contrast bolus injection) or delayed phase (5–7 min) images are obtained selectively on an individual basis, depending upon the specific indication for the examination. The use of oral contrast material in the emergency setting in patients with non-traumatic acute abdominal pain has been the subject of much debate in recent years (Laituri et al. 2011; Wang et al. 2011; Lee et al. 2006; Mun et al. 2006; Keyzer et al. 2009; Anderson et al. 2009). In general, oral contrast material is not considered necessary for patients with clinical suspicion of hepatic, biliary tract, or pancreatic pathology. At our institution, we are increasingly moving towards omitting oral contrast administration from abdominal-pain CT protocols and currently reserve its use for patients with suspected bowel or pelvic diseases who have a calculated body mass index (BMI) <25. This approach was instituted following evidence that patients with higher BMIs (>25) usually have enough intra-abdominal fat to serve as intrinsic contrast to adequately assess the bowel wall and detect disease (Anderson et al. 2010; Wolfe et al. 2006).

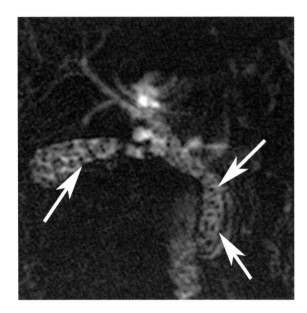

Fig. 1 MRCP (single-shot thick-slab sequence) image demonstrating multiple hypointense stones (*arrows*) in the distal common bile duct (CBD) and gallbladder

However, patients who are unable to receive intravenous contrast should always undergo a complete preparation with oral contrast material (typically 900 ml of barium sulfate or diluted water-soluble contrast agent), administered over a 2 h period, to ensure adequate filling of the complete small bowel and, at least, the proximal colon and appendiceal region.

Magnetic resonance (MR) and especially MRCP have become integral components of the diagnostic armamentarium for patients with suspected acute biliary tract disease. MRCP is an extremely accurate test (Fig. 1). Additionally, its non-invasive nature and the fact that no ionizing radiation is used make MRCP a very appealing test. In fact, in the vast majority of settings, MRCP has virtually replaced endoscopic retrograde cholangiopancreatography (ERCP) in the diagnosis of biliary disease. Although access to this modality is more limited compared to US or CT, a growing number of MR scanners are being installed worldwide. The indications for using MR to evaluate acute abdominal conditions, including those affecting the gallbladder and biliary tract, are growing continuously (Pedrosa and Rofsky 2003; Varghese et al. 1999; Tkacz et al. 2009).

Other diagnostic tests that are used for evaluating the gallbladder and biliary tract in the emergency setting include nuclear biliary scintigraphy, ERCP, and percutaneous transhepatic cholangiography (both used almost exclusively for therapeutic purposes given their invasive nature), endoscopic US and, in some countries, CT cholangiography.

In the remaining sections, a detailed description of the diseases affecting the biliary tract that are often seen in clinical emergency practice is provided. Emphasis is placed on the relative merits and weaknesses of each imaging technique for the diagnosis of the various diseases.

2 Acute Cholecystitis

2.1 Acute Calculous Cholecystitis

2.1.1 Terminology and Clinical Issues

Acute cholecystitis is defined as an acute inflammation of the gallbladder wall, regardless of the cause. In the majority of cases, the underlying etiology is obstruction of the cystic duct by an impacted stone in either the neck of the gallbladder or the cystic duct (acute calculous cholecystitis). Acute cholecystitis can also occur without associated cholelithiasis (acute acalculous cholecystitis). Although the pathophysiologies leading to acute cholecystitis differ based on the presence or absence of gallstones, the complications that may develop when the condition is not diagnosed in a timely fashion are the same.

Calculous cholecystitis occurs more commonly in women than in men, reflecting the higher prevalence of gallstones in females. The process usually begins with a stone located strategically in the gallbladder neck or cystic duct, causing impaired drainage of bile into the extrahepatic ducts and duodenum. Progressive gallbladder dilatation and increased intraluminal pressure ensue. If cystic duct patency is reestablished, acute cholecystitis may resolve spontaneously within 5–7 days after the onset of symptoms. However, this is not usually the case. Instead, if the cholecystitis is not detected and treated, inflammatory cell infiltration occurs in the gallbladder wall, followed by mural and mucosal hemorrhagic necrosis. Gangrenous cholecystitis and superimposed infection may then develop and are found in as many as 20% of patients undergoing emergency cholecystectomy. Microorganisms are identified in 80% of acute cholecystitis cases, although infection is considered a secondary event rather than a primary one. Gangrenous cholecystitis is discussed in detail later in this section.

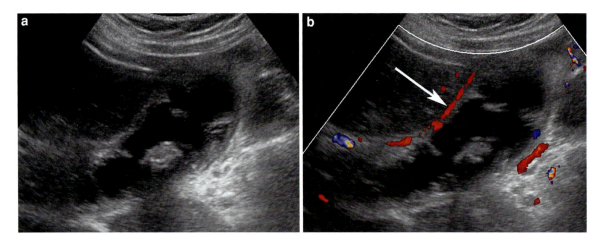

Fig. 2 Longitudinal images (**a**, *gray* scale; **b**, *color* Doppler) of an ultrasonographic examination of the gallbladder demonstrate the characteristic findings of acute cholecystitis. There are multiple stones in the gallbladder, with associated diffuse wall thickening and wall hyperemia (**b**, *arrow*). The patient also complained of exquisite pain in the region of the gallbladder (positive US Murphy sign)

In most patients with acute cholecystitis, a history of multiple prior episodes of colicky pain of a biliary type can be elicited. Frequently, the pain begins in the epigastric region and then localizes focally in the right upper quadrant. Although the pain is initially described as colicky in many instances, it becomes constant in virtually all cases. Fever, chills, leukocytosis, and other laboratory evidence of acute infection are commonly present once acute cholecystitis has established. Approximately 20% of these patients have mild jaundice. In the elderly and in diabetic patients, however, the clinical presentation can be very non-specific or atypical, with only minimal, vague, or even absent pain. Fever may also be absent, with localized tenderness as the only presenting sign. Cholecystitis is differentiated from biliary colic by the persistence nature of the pain. Constant pain lasting for more than 6 h should immediately raise the suspicion of acute cholecystitis. Deep palpation of the right subcostal area often reveals exquisite tenderness which often worsens when the patient takes a deep inspiration, leading to a sudden inspiratory arrest; this is the Murphy sign. In approximately one third of patients, a distended, tender gallbladder may be palpable. The Murphy sign may be elicited with an US probe as well (Trowbridge et al. 2003; Nino-Murcia and Jeffrey 2001).

2.1.2 Imaging

Ultrasound is the preferred imaging examination for the diagnosis of acute cholecystitis and is the first method used when the clinical presentation is suggestive of biliary pathology. The main findings of acute calculous cholecystitis on US include, in addition to the presence of stones: distention of the gallbladder lumen, gallbladder wall thickening, a positive US Murphy sign , pericholecystic fluid (Trowbridge et al. 2003; Nino-Murcia and Jeffrey 2001), and a hyperemic wall upon evaluation with color Doppler (Schiller et al. 1996; Paulson et al. 1994) (Fig. 2). All of these findings are suggestive but none of them is diagnostic of acute cholecystitis. The US Murphy sign is absent in as many as 70% of patients with acute cholecystitis. Patients with less specific clinical presentations (diffuse or non-localized abdominal pain, unexplained liver function test abnormalities, or unexplained fever or leukocytosis) may undergo CT as the initial imaging test. CT can also clearly depict the gallbladder changes characteristic of acute inflammation (Shakespear et al. 2010; Paulson 2000) (Fig. 3). Inflammatory changes in the gallbladder fossa and pericholecystic fat are often better depicted with CT than with US (Fig. 4). CT is also useful in making the specific diagnosis when obesity or gaseous distention limits the use of US. MR with MRCP may be requested to rule out coexisting bile duct stones in patients with known or suspected acute cholecysititis. MR demonstrates the same morphologic alterations as CT, i.e., inflammatory changes in the gallbladder wall and pericholecystic fat (Park et al. 1998; Altun et al. 2007; Watanabe et al. 2007) (Fig. 5). Biliary scintigraphy is a highly sensitive diagnostic modality for diagnosing

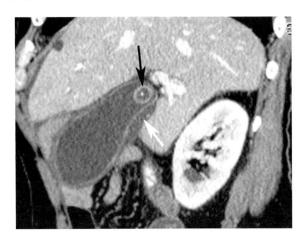

Fig. 3 CECT shows a distended gallbladder with wall thickening and pericholecystic fluid (*white arrow*). Note also the stone impacted in the gallbladder neck (*black arrow*)

acute cholecystitis (Flancbaum and Choban 1995; Ziessman 2003) (Fig. 6), although the findings are non-specific. It is important to remember that all imaging tests can be associated with false-negative and false-positive diagnoses of acute cholecystitis (Brook et al. 2011); therefore, close correlation with the clinical presentation is critical in order to avoid these pitfalls.

2.1.3 Differentials

Mirizzi syndrome. The CBD is obstructed by an impacted gall stone in the cystic duct or in the infundibulum of the gallbladder. Chronic inflammation is present around the site of impaction. MRCP and ERCP show a filling defect of the common bile duct, which is sometimes associated with dilatation of the intrahepatic bile ducts (Fig. 7).

Pancreatic and ampullary neoplasms. Most commonly, on CT and MR a moderately vascularized mass is present around the distal CBD, the ampulla, or in the pancreatic head (Fig. 8). Dilatation of the CBD and the pancreatic duct may be present, referred to as the "double duct" sign.

2.2 Acalculous Cholecystitis

2.2.1 Terminology and Clinical Issues

Acute acalculous cholecystitis is a severe condition that most commonly occurs in hospitalized, debilitated patients with multiple comorbidities, such as coronary artery or peripheral vascular disease, sepsis, severe burns, and multiple trauma, and in patients on mechanical ventilation in the intensive care unit and in those with poorly controlled diabetes. The main cause of acalculous cholecystitis is thought to be chronic bile stasis that leads to overdistention of the gallbladder (Barie and Eachempati 2010; Shapiro et al. 1994). Critically ill patients are more prone to developing acute acalculous cholecystitis because of prolonged fasting, resulting in a decrease or absence of cholecystokinin-induced gallbladder contraction. In fact, acalculous cholecystitis is particularly common in patients on prolonged total parenteral nutrition. Over time, multiple factors lead to the development of gallbladder wall ischemia and secondary infection. Dehydration and a slow flow state (such as heart failure) also play a role.

Acalculous cholecystitis accounts for approximately 5–10% of all cases of acute cholecystitis and the mortality rate (10–50%) is considerably higher than that associated with calculous cholecystitis (1–2%). In addition, compared to cholecystitis caused by stone disease, acalculous cholecystitis is associated with a higher incidence of complications, such as gangrene, emphysema, and perforation.

In patients with acute acalculous cholecystitis, routine laboratory tests usually demonstrate an elevated white blood cell count and altered liver function tests. However, the results are not specific in these very sick patients. Blood cultures may be positive but do not localize the focus of the infection. Therefore, the diagnostic evaluation usually leads to the request for imaging tests.

2.2.2 Imaging

The examinations most commonly performed in these severely ill, hospitalized patients with unexplained sepsis or leukocytosis are US and CT. The usual finding is a distended gallbladder with thickened walls (>3–4 mm), with or without pericholecystic fluid, often with intraluminal sludge but without stones (Summers et al. 2010) (Fig. 9). Unfortunately, these findings are not specific and can be mimicked by myriad diseases and conditions, such as hepatitis, cirrhosis, heart failure, and hypoalbuminemia (Puc et al. 2002). Nuclear scintigraphy can be used to assess the patency of the cystic duct (Fig. 9) but this test also has numerous potential pitfalls, leading to false-negative and, especially, false-positive results. In this setting, the failure of the gallbladder to fill with

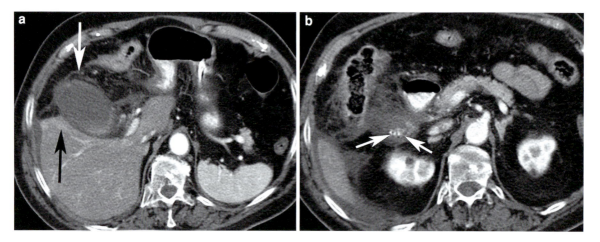

Fig. 4 CECT images demonstrate inflammatory changes in the gallbladder wall and pericholecystic fat (**a**, *white arrow*). Note also a focal area of hyperenhancement in the liver parenchyma adjacent to the gallbladder (**a**, *black arrow*). This transient hyperemia occurs secondary to the acute gallbladder inflammation. There are small calcified stones in the gallbladder neck (**b**, *arrows*)

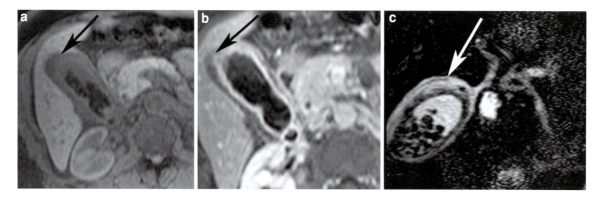

Fig. 5 T1-weighted (T1w) fat-suppressed MR images obtained before (**a**), and after (**b**), the administration of intravenous contrast and coronal heavily T2w MR image (**c**), together demonstrate the characteristic changes of acute calculous cholecystitis. The gallbladder is distended, with wall thickening and hyperenhancement on **b**. There is also intramural and pericholecystic fluid (**a, b,** and **c**, *arrows*) seen as a halo of low signal on the T1w images and as high signal on the T2w image

nuclear scintigraphy is suggestive, but not diagnostic, of acute cholecystitis (Ananian et al. 2006). Definitive therapy is achieved with cholecystectomy (open or laparoscopic). Non-surgical candidates often undergo percutaneous cholecystostomy under US guidance (Morse et al. 2010). This procedure also serves to confirm the diagnosis in complex or questionable cases. Because of concurrent antibiotic therapy, bile culture results are positive in only approximately 50% of patients with acalculous cholecystitis.

3　Complicated Acute Cholecystitis

3.1　Terminology and Clinical Issues

Complications of untreated acute cholecystitis include gallbladder empyema, mural hemorrhage, gangrenous cholecystitis, emphysematous cholecystitis, gallbladder perforation, pericholecystic abscess, and bilio-enteric fistula. All of them are more common in

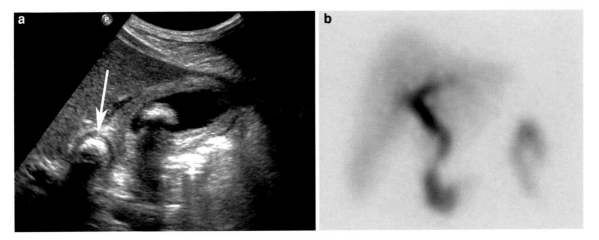

Fig. 6 **a** US image demonstrates the findings of acute cholecystitis: an impacted stone in the gallbladder neck (*arrow*), gallbladder wall thickening, and a large stone in the gallbladder lumen. **b** The HIDA (hepatobiliary iminodiacetic acid) scan demonstrates findings of acute cholecystitis. The image was acquired 60 min after radiotracer injection. There is adequate filling of the extrahepatic bile ducts and passage of the tracer to the duodenum, but no filling of the gallbladder. In the proper clinical setting, these findings are highly consistent with acute cholecystitis

Fig. 7 Mirizzi syndrome. Impacted stone in the cystic duct obliterates the common choledochal duct, accompanied by marked dilatation of the intrahepatic bile ducts: Axial T1w fat-saturated, out-of-phase MR (**a**), ERCP (**b**)

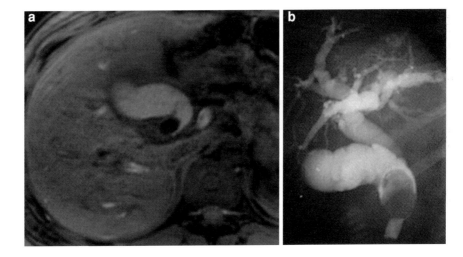

the elderly and in patients with significant comorbidities. As mentioned previously, as inflammation of the gallbladder wall progresses the bile becomes infected. In 85% of patients, relief of the cystic duct obstruction occurs and inflammation in the gallbladder settles. However, if the cystic duct remains obstructed, the process may progress to gallbladder empyema and eventually to wall gangrene or perforation.

3.2 Imaging

On US, gallbladder gangrene is typically seen as a thickened wall with a multi-layered, striated appearance (Simeone et al. 1989; Jeffrey et al. 1983) (Fig. 10). Doppler US may demonstrate absent perfusion either focally or diffusely (Schiller et al. 1996; Ziessman 2003). On contrast-enhanced CT or MR, the

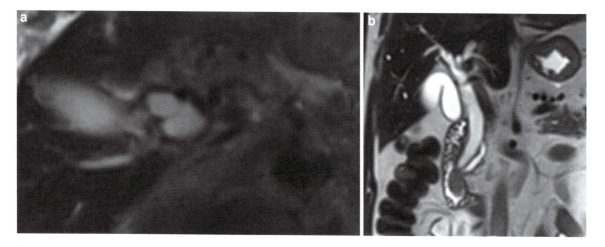

Fig. 8 a Hypovascularized mass of the pancreatic head, with marked distension of the common choledochal duct, which is filled with mucinous material. **b** Mass at the ampulla Vateri with moderate dilatation of the extrahapatic bile duct. Axial (**a**) and coronal (**b**) T2w MR

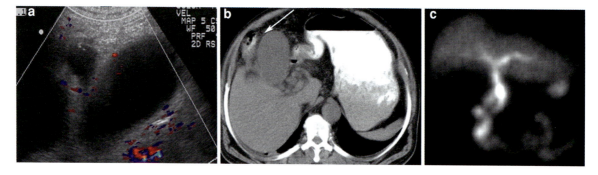

Fig. 9 A 75-year-old male patient in the coronary intensive care unit exhibited new-onset *low-grade* fever and an elevated white blood cell count, both appearing one week after he suffered a myocardial infarction. **a** *Color* Doppler US image shows a distended gallbladder with thickened walls. These findings are not specific. **b** Non-contrast-enhanced CT image demonstrates the distended gallbladder with thickened walls and inflammatory changes in the pericholecystic fat (*arrow*). **c** An HIDA scan static image obtained 60 min after radiotracer injection shows patent bile ducts, but no filling of the gallbladder, confirming the clinical diagnosis of acute cholecystitis

wall is indistinct, with an absence of enhancement in the gangrenous areas (Pedrosa et al. 2003) (Fig. 11). This focally or diffusely decreased (or absent) enhancement of the gallbladder has been shown to be highly predictive of wall gangrene (Pedrosa et al. 2003; Singh and Sagar 2005). Gallbladder wall ischemia can also cause hemorrhage. Demonstration of blood contents in the wall and/or the lumen of the gallbladder is also a highly specific sign of complicating gangrenous cholecystitis (Singh and Sagar 2005) (Fig. 12).

In gallbladder perforation, the wall of the gallbladder is not well delineated on imaging tests and a localized defect in the wall may be noted at the site of perforation. Perforation may be either localized, producing an intramural or pericholecystic abscess (Fig. 13), or free, resulting in peritonitis. A pericholecystic abscess can be demonstrated on cross-sectional imaging as a localized fluid collection, with surrounding hyperemia or hyperenhancement, usually at the site of a focal gallbladder wall defect (Takada et al. 1989). An inflamed gallbladder may also perforate through the wall of the colon or duodenum because of the close proximity of the gallbladder to these structures. This allows passage of infected bile and gallstones into the lumen of these hollow viscera, which may subsequently lead to gallstone ileus (impaction of a gallstone in the ileocecal valve with

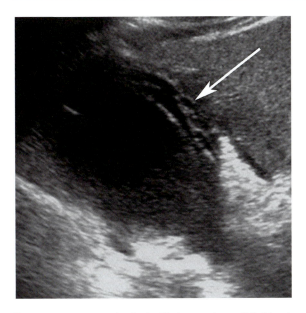

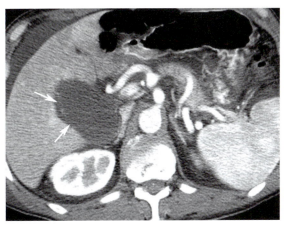

Fig. 11 CT image obtained with intravenous contrast shows areas of absent enhancement in the gallbladder wall (*arrows*). These findings are typical of gangrenous cholecystitis

Fig. 10 On this longitudinal US image the gallbladder is distended by echogenic debris/sludge and shows a focal area with a striated appearance (*arrow*), consistent with gangrenous cholecystitis

bowel obstruction) or, rarely, to Bouberet's syndrome (impaction of a stone in the duodenum).

Emphysematous cholecystitis can complicate acute calculous or acalculous cholecystitis and is especially common in poorly controlled diabetic patients. Ischemia of the gallbladder wall is followed by infection with gas-forming organisms that produce gas in the gallbladder lumen (Fig. 14), wall, or both. In 30–50% of patients, diabetes mellitus is a predisposing condition. The mortality rate of emphysematous cholecystitis is 15%. Clinical symptoms can be deceptively mild in these patients. The imaging hallmark of emphysematous cholecystitis is the presence of intramural or intraluminal gas in the gallbladder (Garcia-Sancho Tellez et al. 1999).

4 Choledocholithiasis

4.1 Terminology and Clinical Issues

Choledocholithiasis complicates cholelithiasis in 10–15% of these patients, either at the time of cholecystectomy or following gallbladder removal. The frequency may be even higher in patients older than 60 years. The presence of choledocholithiasis contributes to increased morbidity and mortality associated with gallstone disease. The clinical suspicion of choledocholithiasis complicates the workup and management of simple cholelithiasis, leading to additional diagnostic and therapeutic procedures. The vast majority of cases of choledocholithiasis occur as a result of the passage of stones from the gallbladder through the cystic duct into the CBD (secondary choledocholithiasis). The primary formation of stones within the CBD is much less common.

Patients with choledocholithiasis may be completely asymptomatic; in approximately 7% of cases, the stones are found incidentally during cholecystectomy. Approximately 25–50% of CBD stones eventually cause symptoms and require treatment. Patients become symptomatic after biliary obstruction ensues, and the clinical presentation will depend on both the degree of obstruction and the presence or absence of biliary infection (ascending cholangitis, discussed later in this chapter). Laboratory tests, such as elevated bilirubin, alkaline phosphatase and γ-glutamyl transpeptidase levels, can suggest biliary obstruction but the results are not specific. The white blood cell count is elevated in patients with associated ascending cholangitis.

4.2 Imaging

Although US is highly accurate for detecting biliary ductal dilatation, the direct depiction of bile duct stones as intraductal echogenic foci with acoustic

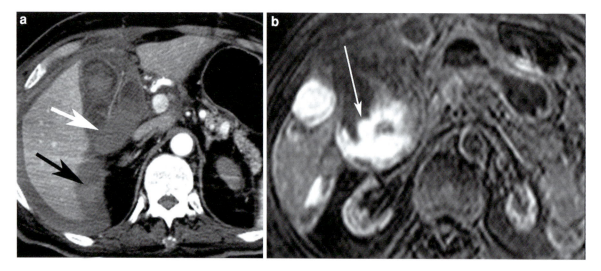

Fig. 12 a CECT image in a patient with chronic renal failure shows hyperattenuating material in the lumen (*white arrow*) of the gallbladder and in the peritoneal cavity (*black arrow*). **b** The T1w fat-suppressed image shows intraluminal content of high signal intensity (*arrow*). These findings are indicative of gallbladder hemorrhage, associated with advanced acute cholecystitis

Fig. 13 CECT image demonstrates multiple intramural and pericholecystic fluid collections, consistent with abscesses. The gallbladder itself is poorly defined. Advanced cholecystitis with perforation and walled-off abscesses were found at laparotomy

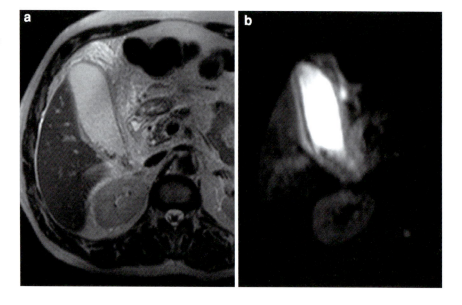

shadowing (Fig. 15) is often suboptimal. The reported sensitivity of US for the detection of CBD stones is variable (15–70%) (Baron et al. 1982; Mitchell and Clark 1984; Wermke and Schulz 1987). Duodenal gas frequently limits the ability to visualize the distal CBD (Fig. 16).

CT is equally useful for detecting ductal dilatation and is more precise than US for identifying the site and the cause of the obstructing lesion. The sensitivity of CT for the detection of choledocholithiasis varies between 60 and approximately 90% (Soto et al. 2000a; Neitlich et al. 1997; Anderson et al. 2006; Baron et al. 1988; Anderson et al. 2008). Multidetector CT technology with thin slices and high spatial resolution improves the ability to detect small stones. The appearance of biliary stones on CT depends upon stone composition: predominantly cholesterol, predominantly pigment, or mixed cholesterol and pigment. Pigment is associated with a higher calcium content and a hyperattenuating appearance on CT (Fig. 17), while cholesterol stones are low in attenuation (Fig. 16). Most stones contain

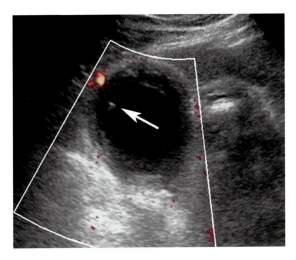

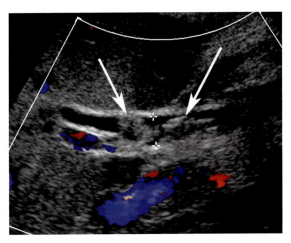

Fig. 14 Transverse US image demonstrates a highly echogenic focus in the lumen of the distended gallbladder (*arrow*). The finding was considered consistent with acute emphysematous cholecystitis. The diagnosis was confirmed at laparotomy

Fig. 15 Color Doppler US image, obtained along the long axis of the CBD, demonstrates multiple intraluminal echogenic stones (*arrows*)

both pigment and cholesterol and therefore have a variable appearance on CT (Neitlich et al. 1997; Anderson et al. 2006; Baron et al. 1988; Anderson et al. 2008; Chan et al. 2006). Exposure parameters, especially the kVp used, also affect the appearance of biliary stones on CT (Chan et al. 2006). Although oral and intravenous contrast may obscure small intraductal stones, the clinical indication of CT usually mandates the administration of one or both contrast materials. MRCP is the ultimate non-invasive test for detecting bile duct stones. It has a very high sensitivity and specificity (approximately 95–98%, comparable to ERCP) (Griffin et al. 2003; Soto et al. 2000b; Kim et al. 2002; Chan et al. 1996; Becker et al. 1997; Regan et al. 1996; Reinhold et al. 1998). On heavily T2w images, all stones, regardless of their composition, are depicted as intraductal foci of low signal intensity, either completely or partially surrounded by high signal intensity bile (Fig. 18). State of the art MR scanners and pulse sequences allow the acquisition of fast sequences for MRCP during short breath-hold periods. Radiologists must be aware of the albeit rare potential pitfalls and causes of false-negative and false-positive MRCP images and interpretations.

Currently, ERCP is usually reserved for patients with confirmed bile duct stones demonstrated on other imaging tests. In this scenario, ERCP serves to confirm the diagnosis and, especially, as the preferred therapeutic approach to retained bile duct stones.

More recently, other tests such as endoscopic ultrasonography and choledochoscopy have been introduced into clinical practice. Their potential role in the pre-interventional diagnosis of choledocholithiasis has not been firmly established.

5 Cholangitis

See Sect. 3.2 in "Liver and Bile Ducts"

6 Mirizzi's Syndrome

6.1 Terminology and Clinical Issues

Mirizzi's syndrome occurs when a gallstone becomes impacted in the cystic duct or Hartmann's pouch. This situation develops as a result of chronic and/or acute cholecystitis, leading to contraction of the gallbladder. The inflammatory process extends beyond the gallbladder to involve the hepatoduodenal ligament, which then causes secondary stenosis of the common hepatic duct. In patients with cholelithiasis, anatomic variants, such as a long cystic duct coursing parallel with the common hepatic duct or a low insertion of the cystic duct into the CBD, increase the risk of developing Mirizzi's syndrome. A fistulous communication between the two involved ducts may be seen as well.

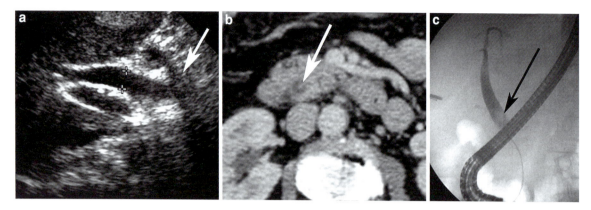

Fig. 16 The shadow arising from the duodenum (**a**, *arrow*) precludes visualization of the distal CBD on this US image obtained along the long axis of the duct. **b** Contrast-enhanced CT obtained the same day as the image in (**a**) demonstrates a small soft-tissue focus of attenuation (*arrow*) in the distal bile duct. The findings are consistent with a stone (composed predominantly of cholesterol) in the bile duct. **c** ERCP confirms the presence of a 6 mm intraductal filling defect (*arrow*) which represents a CBD stone

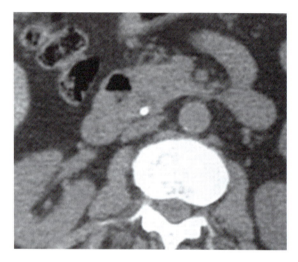

Fig. 17 Axial CT image acquired at the level of the head of the pancreas demonstrates a densely calcified stone (*arrow*) in the distal CBD. Dense calcification is explained by the stone's predominantly pigment composition

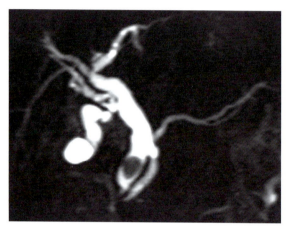

Fig. 18 MRCP (*single-shot thick-slab* sequence) image demonstrates a large hypointense stone in the distal CBD. There is associated biliary ductal dilatation

Accurate presurgical diagnosis of Mirizzi's syndrome determines the patient's prognosis. Chronic inflammation with extensive fibrosis and scarring can lead to serious surgical complications if not detected before the intervention. Adhesions may make visualization of the biliary anatomy in the hepatoduodenal ligament extremely difficult, especially during laparoscopic cholecystectomy. The CBD may be mistaken for the cystic duct, not uncommonly leading to ligation or permanent injury.

6.2   Imaging

Imaging studies are critical for a precise preoperative diagnosis of Mirizzi's syndrome (Abou-Saif and Al-Kawas 2002; Becker et al. 1984). US may demonstrate the impacted stone with dilated intrahepatic ducts and dilatation of the common hepatic duct and a distal CBD of normal caliber. Similar findings may be seen on CT, although direct visualization of the impacted stone is less predictable. MRCP is the most accurate non-invasive test for diagnosing Mirizzi's syndrome. Findings include direct demonstration of

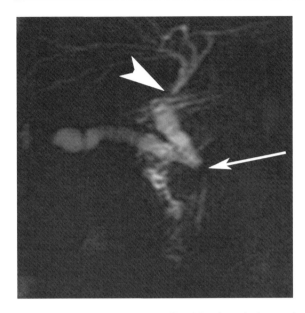

Fig. 19 MRCP demonstrates the dilated intrahepatic ducts and common hepatic duct, with a normal-caliber CBD. There is a focus of *low* signal intensity (stone, *arrow*) at the junction of the cystic duct and common hepatic duct, caused by an impacted stone. The combination of findings is characteristic of Mirizzi's syndrome. Note also a stricture affecting the left hepatic duct (*arrowhead*)

the impacted stone in the gallbladder neck or junction of the cystic duct with the common hepatic duct and a dilated biliary ductal system proximal to the site of impaction (Fig. 19). The gallbladder may be distended as well. On direct cholangiography (ERCP or percutaneous transhepatic cholangiography, PTC), a rounded or oval filling defect representing the calculus in the expected location of the cystic duct and/or a smooth extrinsic compression of the common hepatic duct are seen.

References

Abou-Saif A, Al-Kawas F (2002) Complications of gallstone disease: Mirizzi syndrome, cholecystocholedochal fistula, and gallstone ileus. Am J Gastroenterol 97:249–254

Altun E, Semelka RC, Elias J Jr, Braga L, Voultsinos V, Patel J, Balci NC, Woosley JT (2007) Acute cholecystitis: MR findings and differentiation from chronic cholecystitis. Radiology 244:174–183

Ananian C, Dunn A, Mansourian V, Caride VJ (2006) Scintigraphic gallbladder visualization with gangrenous acalculous cholecystitis. Clin Nucl Med 31:701–703

Anderson SW, Lucey BC, Varghese JC, Soto JA (2006) Accuracy of MDCT in the diagnosis of choledocholithiasis. AJR Am J Roentgenol 187:174–180

Anderson SW, Rho E, Soto JA (2008) Detection of biliary duct narrowing and choledocholithiasis: accuracy of portal venous phase multidetector CT. Radiology 247:418–427

Anderson SW, Soto JA, Lucey BC, Ozonoff A, Jordan JD, Ratevosian J, Ulrich AS, Rathlev NK, Mitchell PM, Rebholz C, Feldman JA, Rhea JT (2009) Abdominal 64-MDCT for suspected appendicitis: the use of oral and IV contrast material versus IV contrast material only. AJR Am J Roentgenol 193:1282–1288

Anderson SW, Rhea JT, Milch HN, Ozonoff A, Lucey BC, Soto JA (2010) Influence of body habitus and use of oral contrast on reader confidence in patients with suspected acute appendicitis using 64 MDCT. Emerg Radiol 17:445–453

Barie PS, Eachempati SR (2010) Acute acalculous cholecystitis. Gastroenterol Clin North Am 39:343–357

Baron RL, Stanley RJ, Lee JK et al (1982) A prospective comparison of the evaluation of biliary obstruction using computed tomography and ultrasonography. Radiology 145:91–98

Baron RL, Rohrmann CA Jr, Lee SP, Shuman WP, Teefey SA (1988) CT evaluation of gallstones in vitro: correlation with chemical analysis. AJR Am J Roentgenol 151:1123–1128

Becker CD, Hassler H, Terrier F (1984) Preoperative diagnosis of the Mirizzi syndrome: limitations of sonography and computed tomography. AJR 143:591–596

Becker CD, Grossholz M, Becker M et al (1997) Choledocholithiasis and bile duct stenosis: diagnostic accuracy of MR cholangiopancreatography. Radiology 205:523–530

Brook OR, Kane RA, Tyagi G, Siewert B, Kruskal JB (2011) Lessons learned from quality assurance: errors in the diagnosis of acute cholecystitis on ultrasound and CT. AJR Am J Roentgenol 196:597–604

Chan YL, Chan ACW, Lam WWM et al (1996) Choledocholithiasis: comparison of MR cholangiography and endoscopic retrograde cholangiography. Radiology 200:85–89

Chan WC, Joe BN, Coakley FV et al (2006) Gallstone detection at CT in vitro: effect of peak voltage setting. Radiology 241:546–553

Denecke T, Degutyte E, Stelter L, Lehmkuhl L, Valencia R, Lopez-Hänninen E, Felix R, Stroszczynski C (2006) Minimum intensity projections of the biliary system using 16-channel multidetector computed tomography in patients with biliary obstruction: comparison with MRCP. Eur Radiol 16:1719–1726

Flancbaum L, Choban PS (1995) Use of morphine cholescintigraphy in the diagnosis of acute cholecystitis in critically ill patients. Intensive Care Med 21:120–124

Garcia-Sancho Tellez L, Rodrigues-Montes JA, Fernandes LS et al (1999) Acute emphysematous cholecystitis: report of twenty cases. Hepatogastroenterology 46:2144–2148

Griffin N, Wastle ML, Dunn WK, Ryder SD, Beckingham IJ (2003) Magnetic resonance cholangiopancreatography versus endoscopic retrograde cholasngiopancreatography in the diagnosis of choledocholithiasis. Eur J Gastroenterol Hepatol 15:809–813

Jeffrey RB, Laing FC, Wong W, Callen PW (1983) Gangrenous cholecystitis: diagnosis by ultrasound. Radiology 148:219–221

Keyzer C, Cullus P, Tack D, De Maertelaer V, Bohy P, Gevenois PA (2009) MDCT for suspected acute appendicitis in adults:

impact of oral and IV contrast media at standard-dose and simulated low-dose techniques. AJR Am J Roentgenol 193: 1272–1281

Kim JH, Kim MJ, Park SII et al (2002) MR cholangiography in symptomatic gallstones: diagnostic accuracy according to clinical risk group. Radiology 224:410–416

Laituri CA, Fraser JD, Aguayo P, Fike FB, Garey CL, Sharp SW, Ostlie DJ, St Peter SD (2011) The lack of efficacy for oral contrast in the diagnosis of appendicitis by computed tomography. J Surg Res Mar 12. [Epub ahead of print]

Lee SY, Coughlin B, Wolfe JM, Polino J, Blank FS, Smithline HA (2006) Prospective comparison of helical CT of the abdomen and pelvis without and with oral contrast in assessing acute abdominal pain in adult emergency department patients. Emerg Radiol 12:150–157

Mitchell SE, Clark RA (1984) A comparison of computed tomography and sonography in choledocholithiasis. AJR Am J Roentgenol 142:729–733

Morse BC, Smith JB, Lawdalıl RB, Roettger RH (2010) Management of acute cholecystitis in critically ill patients: contemporary role for cholecystostomy and subsequent cholecystectomy. Am Surg 76:708–712

Mun S, Ernst RD, Chen K, Oto A, Shah S, Mileski WJ (2006) Rapid CT diagnosis of acute appendicitis with IV contrast material. Emerg Radiol 12:99–102

Neitlich JD, Topazian M, Smith RC, Gupta A, Burrell MI, Rosenfield AT (1997) Detection of choledocholithiasis: comparison of unenhanced helical CT and endoscopic retrograde cholangiopancreatography. Radiology 203:753–757

Nino-Murcia M, Jeffrey RB Jr (2001) Imaging the patient with right upper quadrant pain. Semin Roentgenol 36:81–91

Park MS, Yu JS, Kim YH, Kim MJ, Kim JH, Lee S, Cho N, Kim DG, Kim KW (1998) Acute cholecystitis: comparison of MR cholangiography and US. Radiology 209:781–785

Paulson EK (2000) Acute cholecystitis: CT findings. Semin Ultrasound CT MR 21:56–63

Paulson EK, Kliewer MA, Hertzberg BS, Paine SS, Carroll BA (1994) Diagnosis of acute cholecystitis with color Doppler sonography: significance of arterial flow in thickened gallbladder wall. AJR Am J Roentgenol 162:1105–1108

Pedrosa I, Rofsky NM (2003) MR imaging in abdominal emergencies. Radiol Clin North Am 41:1243–1273

Pedrosa I, Guarise A, Goldsmith J, Procacci C, Rofsky NM (2003) The interrupted rim sign in acute cholecystits: a method to identify the gangrenous form with MRI. J Magn Reson Imaging 18:360–363

Puc MM, Tran HS, Wry PW, Ross SE (2002) Ultrasound is not a useful screening tool for acute acalculous cholecystitis in critically ill trauma patients. Am Surg 68:65–69

Regan F, Fradin J, Khazan R, Bohlman M, Magnuson T (1996) Choledocholithiasis: evaluation with MR cholangiography. AJR Am J Roentgenol 167:1441–1445

Reinhold C, Taourel P, Bret PM (1998) Choledocholithiasis: evaluation of MR cholangiography for diagnosis. Radiology 209:435–442

Schiller VL, Turner RR, Sarti DA (1996) Color doppler imaging of the gallbladder wall in acute cholecystitis: sonographic-pathologic correlation. Abdom Imaging 21:233–237

Shakespear JS, Shaaban AM, Rezvani M (2010) CT findings of acute cholecystitis and its complications. AJR Am J Roentgenol 194:1523–1529

Shapiro MJ, Luchtefeld WB, Kurzweil S, Kaminski DL, Durham RM, Mazuski JE (1994) Acute acalculous cholecystitis in the critically ill. Am Surg 60:335–339

Simeone JF, Brink JA, Mueller PR, Compton C, Hahn PF, Saini S, Silverman SG, Tung G, Ferrucci JT (1989) The sonographic diagnosis of acute gangrenous cholecystitis: importance of the Murphy sign. AJR Am J Roentgenol 152:289–290

Singh AK, Sagar P (2005) Gangrenous cholecystitis: prediction with CT imaging. Abdom Imaging 30:218–221

Soto JA, Alvarez O, Munera F, Velez SM, Valencia J, Ramirez N (2000a) Diagnosing bile duct stones: comparison of unenhanced helical CT, oral contrast-enhanced CT cholangiography and MR cholangiography. AJR Am J Roentgenol 175:1127–1134

Soto JA, Barish MA, Alvarez O, Medina S (2000b) Detection of choledocholithiasis with MR cholangiography: comparison of three-dimensional fast spin-echo and single- and multisection half-Fourier rapid acquisition with relaxation enhancement sequences. Radiology 21:737–745

Summers SM, Scruggs W, Menchine MD et al (2010) A prospective evaluation of emergency department bedside ultrasonography for the detection of acute cholecystitis. Ann Emerg Med 56:114–122

Takada T, Yasuda H, Uchiyama K et al (1989) Pericholecystic abscess: classification of US findings to determine the proper therapy. Radiology 172:693–697

Tkacz JN, Anderson SA, Soto J (2009) MR imaging in gastrointestinal emergencies. Radiographics 29:1767–1780

Trowbridge RL, Rutkowski NK, Shojania KG (2003) Does this patient have acute cholecystitis. JAMA 289:80–86

Varghese JC, Farrell MA, Courtney G, Osborne H, Murray FE, Lee MJ (1999) A prospective comparison of magnetic resonance cholangiopancreatography with endoscopic retrograde cholangiopancreatography in evaluation of patients with suspected biliary tract disease. Clin Radiol 54:513–520

Wang ZJ, Chen KS, Gould R, Coakley FV, Fu Y, Yeh BM (2011) Positive enteric contrast material for abdominal and pelvic CT with automatic exposure control: What is the effect on patient radiation exposure? Eur J Radiol Apr 12. [Epub ahead of print]

Watanabe Y, Nagayama M, Okumura A, Amoh Y, Katsube T, Suga T, Koyama S, Nakatani K, Dodo Y (2007) MR imaging of acute biliary disorders. Radiographics 27: 477–495

Wermke W, Schulz HJ (1987) Sonographic diagnosis of bile duct calculi: results of a prospective study of 222 cases of choledocholithiasis. Ultraschall Med 8:116–120

Wolfe JM, Smithline H, Lee S, Coughlin B, Polino J, Blank F (2006) The impact of body mass index on concordance in the interpretation of matched noncontrast and contrast abdominal pelvic computed tomographic scans in ED patients with nontraumatic abdominal pain. Am J Emerg Med 24:144–148

Ziessman HA (2003) Acute cholecystitis, biliary obstruction, and biliary leakage. Semin Nucl Med 33:279–296

Spleen

Digna R. Kool, Ferco H. Berger, and Patrick M. Vos

Contents

Abstract

In this chapter non-traumatic and traumatic pathology of the spleen will be discussed. A variety of non-traumatic emergencies of the spleen are regularly encountered during emergency imaging of the abdomen. Sometimes diagnostic imaging is performed because the splenic pathology (infarcts, spontaneous rupture, abscess or splenomegaly) causes symptoms, more often these splenic abnormalities are encountered during diagnostic imaging for other indications. We will discuss the most common splenic findings that can be encountered during emergency imaging of the abdomen. The spleen is the most affected organ in patients with abdominal organ injury after blunt trauma. Imaging finding of traumatic injury to the spleen on Ultrasound and CT will be described and shown. The influence of imaging in selecting patients for non-operative management of splenic injuries and the value of the most frequently used grading systems in clinical decision making will be discussed.

D. R. Kool (✉)
Radiology, Jeroen Bosch Hospital, Henri Dunantstraat 1,
S Hertogenbosch, 5223 GZ, The Netherlands
e-mail: mscaglione@tiscali.it

F. H. Berger
Radiology, VU University Medical Center Amsterdam,
Boelelaan 1117, Amsterdam, 1081 HV, The Netherlands

P. M. Vos
Radiology, St. Pauls Hospital Vancouver BC,
1081 Burrard Street, Vancouver, BC V6z 1y6, Canada

1 Introduction

In this chapter, non-traumatic and traumatic pathologies of the spleen are discussed. For general considerations of multi-detector computed tomography (MDCT) scan protocols, the reader is referred to "Acute Abdomen: Rational use of US, MDCT, and MRI".

In contrast-enhanced CT (CECT), it must be kept in mind that if performed during the first 60 s after intravenous contrast administration, an inhomogeneous attenuation of the spleen, either diffuse

M. Scaglione et al. (eds.), *Emergency Radiology of the Abdomen*,
Medical Radiology. Diagnostic Imaging,
DOI: 10.1007/174_2011_468, © Springer-Verlag Berlin Heidelberg 2012

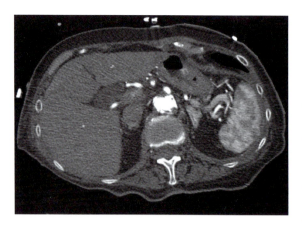

Fig. 1 Normal enhancement patterns. Arterial-phase CT, axial view, demonstrates a normal arterial "arciform" enhancement pattern

heterogeneity or a zebra-striped or leopard-spotted pattern, will be seen. Importantly, these inhomogeneous enhancement patterns may mimic or obscure underlying pathological conditions (Figs. 1, 2, 3) (Donnelly et al. 1999).

2 Non-Traumatic Emergencies

A variety of abnormalities including splenomegaly, infarcts, focal solid masses, and cystic lesions are regularly encountered during emergency imaging of the abdomen. Sometimes diagnostic imaging is performed because the splenic pathology (infarcts, spontaneous rupture, abscess or splenomegaly) causes symptoms. More often, these splenic abnormalities are encountered during diagnostic imaging for other indications. In the next section we discuss the most common splenic findings that may be encountered during emergency imaging of the abdomen.

2.1 Vascular

2.1.1 Splenic Infarct

2.1.1.1 Terminology and Clinical Issues
There are many recognized etiologies of splenic infarction, with the most prominent being hematological disorders, thromboembolic disorders, splenomegaly, and trauma (Robertson et al. 2001; Nores et al. 1998).

Moreover, splenic infarction can be caused by either arterial or venous compromise. It is usually segmental but can be multifocal or global.

The typical symptoms include the sudden onset of pain in the left upper abdominal quadrant, pleuritic chest pain, and referred pain to the left shoulder. Patients may develop fever and leukocytosis. However, 30–50% of patients are asymptomatic and splenic infarcts are seen during imaging of the upper abdomen for other indications (Nores et al. 1998; Goerg and Schwerk 1990). Complications of splenic infarction are more frequent in thromboembolic etiologies and include abscess formation, liquefaction, and hemorrhage, rarely causing splenic rupture (Nores et al. 1998).

2.1.1.2 Imaging
The radiologic appearance of a splenic infarction depends on the stage and size as well as on the degree of splenic involvement. The classic imaging appearance is that of a well-defined wedge-shaped defect with the base at the splenic capsule and the tip pointing towards the hilum. The size of the wedge depends on how peripheral the occlusion occurs.

On US, the wedge-shaped area is usually hypoechoic compared to the surrounding normal spleen (Fig. 4). On color Doppler examination, there may be decreased or absent flow in the affected area. However, in the acute phase, splenic infarcts are often isoechoic and the diagnostic accuracy of US is less than that of CT (Antopolsky et al. 2009). Non-enhanced CT usually shows the infarct as iso- or slightly hypodense compared to the normal parenchyma and typically hard to detect. Instead, infarcts are best visualized after intravenous contrast in the portal-venous phase. The classic appearance on CECT is a wedge-shaped, well-defined hypodense area (Fig. 5).

In the chronic phase, the infarct may resolve completely or the infarcted tissue may progress to a fibrotic scar, perhaps with volume loss and capsular retraction. On US, the fibrosis may be hyperechoic compared to the normal tissue, while on CECT the infarct will present as a well-defined hypoattenuated area.

The accurate characterization of an infarct can be difficult when it lacks the typical wedge-shaped appearance or is complicated by hemorrhage, infection, or rupture. If necrotic liquefaction occurs, the

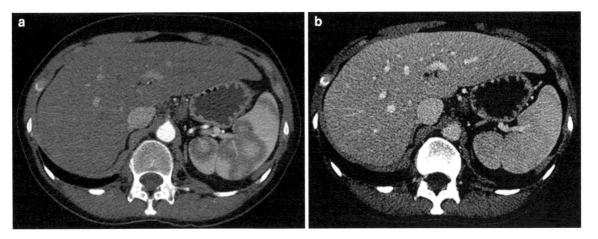

Fig. 2 CECT, axial views, shows atypical enhancement in arterial phase (**a**) and normal enhancement in the portal-venous phase (**b**) in the same patient. No splenic abnormalities were seen on subsequent US and MRI scan

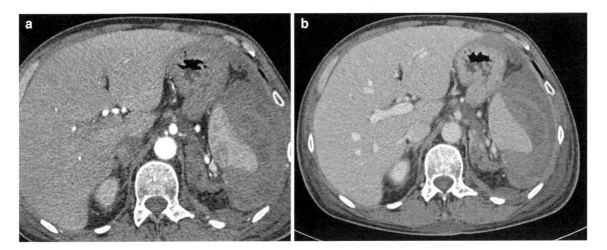

Fig. 3 CECT, axial views, shows normal enhancement patterns on arterial phase (**a**) and portal-venous phase (**b**). **a** Subcapsular hematoma and inhomogeneous enhancement of the splenic parenchyma mimicking a parenchymal injury is instead an artifact of the scan phase. **b** Homogenous enhancement of the splenic parenchyma. This patient also has a traumatic left adrenal hemorrhage

area of infarction will be seen as an anechoic area on US and a non-enhancing area with fluid attenuation on CT. Complications such as abscess formation and splenic rupture are discussed in later sections of this chapter.

Two atypical variants of splenic infarction that can be more difficult to appreciate on imaging, especially US, are global splenic infarction and infarction of an accessory spleen (splenunculus). Global splenic infarction typically appears as a diffuse, hypodense, non-enhancing spleen with possible persistent capsular enhancement (Fig. 6). On CECT, infarction of a splenunculus typically presents as a perisplenic hypoattenuating nodule with capsular enhancement surrounded by fat stranding.

2.1.1.3 Differentials

Focal splenic masses including lymphoma When infarcts lack the typical wedge-shaped appearance, are multifocal, or ill-defined, accurate differentiation from a splenic mass can be challenging.

Lymphoma Lymphomatous involvement of the spleen is often associated with splenomegaly and lymphadenopathy.

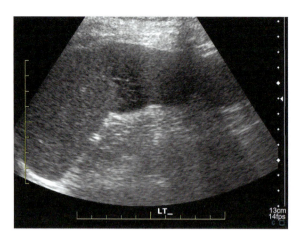

Fig. 4 Splenic infarction as seen on US. Longitudinal sonographic view of the spleen demonstrating splenomegaly and a segmental, hypoechoic, well-defined area in the mid-portion of the spleen, consistent with an infarct

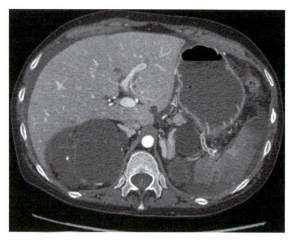

Fig. 6 Splenic infarction as seen on CECT, portal-venous phase, axial view. Acute, extensive splenic infarction in a patient with end-stage renal failure and severe atherosclerotic disease. There is also a thrombus in the distal splenic artery

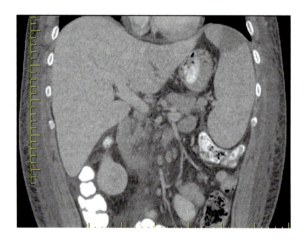

Fig. 5 Splenic infarction as seen on CECT, portal-venous phase, coronal view. Splenomegaly and a segmental, hypodense, well-defined, wedge-shaped area in the superior portion of the spleen, consistent with an infarct. Extensive lymphadenopathy is seen in this patient with advanced HIV

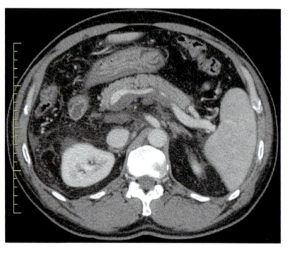

Fig. 7 Splenic vein thrombosis as seen on CECT, portal-venous phase, axial view. This 49-year-old male presented with pancreatitis and acute partial splenic vein thrombosis

Abscess Infarcts in which there is liquefaction or an infectious complication (e.g., endocarditis) may mimic or develop into a splenic abscess.

2.1.2 Splenic Torsion

2.1.2.1 Terminology and Clinical Issues

A potential albeit rare cause for splenic infarction is splenic torsion, typically encountered when the spleen is more mobile than usual, a condition commonly referred to as a "wandering spleen" (Soleimani et al. 2007; Ben Ely et al. 2006). This condition is caused by the absence or laxity of the supportive ligamentous structures and can be congenital or acquired. The wandering spleen may undergo torsion of its vascular supply, which can lead to infarction. This torsion may be acute, intermittent, or chronic. Treatment consists of splenectomy or splenopexy, depending on the

Fig. 8 Splenic artery aneurysm as seen on **a** CECT, arterial phase, coronal view, and **b** DSA. The aneurysm was found incidentally in this 47-year-old female and was subsequently embolized

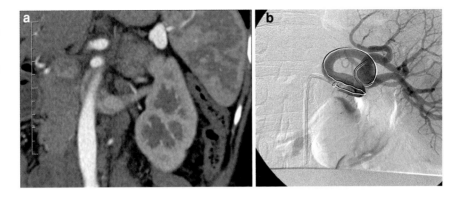

presentation and perioperative findings (Soleimani et al. 2007; Ben Ely et al. 2006).

2.1.2.2 Imaging

The typical imaging findings include the absence of the spleen at its normal location and/or a "whirl sign" of the vascular splenic pedicle, with or without associated findings of infarction.

2.1.2.3 Differentials

None.

2.1.3 Splenic Vein Thrombosis

2.1.3.1 Terminology and Clinical Issues

Splenic vein thrombosis is most often seen in patients with portal vein thrombosis. Isolated splenic vein thrombosis is rare; instead, it is typically associated with pancreatitis and pancreatic malignancies. Other causes include splenectomy, kidney disease, and infections.

2.1.3.2 Imaging

CECT in the portal venous phase demonstrates a non-enhancing splenic vein with or without collaterals (acute or subacute) or an absent splenic vein with collateral formation (chronic) (Fig. 7).

2.1.3.3 Differentials

Artifact In the arterial phase after intravenous contrast, the splenic vein is not yet enhanced.

2.1.4 Splenic Artery Aneurysm

2.1.4.1 Terminology and Clinical Issues

Aneurysms involving the splenic artery are the third most common abdominal aneurysm, after abdominal aortic and iliac artery aneurysms (Agrawal et al. 2007; Al-Habbal et al. 2010). Splenic artery aneurysms are more common in women, are usually located in the middle and distal segment of the artery, and can be fusiform or saccular. They are usually asymptomatic and an incidental finding during routine imaging; in other cases, patients may present with acute rupture and life-threatening hemorrhage. However, the rupture rate of these aneurysms is low, about 2%. Over half of those that rupture do so during pregnancy or in women who have had children. In the former, rupture is associated with very high maternal and fetal mortality rates (Ha et al. 2009). Treatment should be considered in patients with splenic artery aneurysms that are symptomatic, enlarging, >2 cm in diameter, or detected in pregnancy or following liver transplantation.

Pseudo-aneurysms are rare and usually occur as complications of pancreatitis or trauma, or they may be iatrogenic, after surgery. These false aneurysms are more often symptomatic, such that patients may present with pain or hemorrhage (Agrawal et al. 2007). The choice of endovascular or surgical therapy depends on the location of the (pseudo)-aneurysm, local practice, and patient characteristics (Abbas et al. 2002).

2.1.4.2 Imaging

On CECT and angiography, true splenic artery aneurysms appear as a focal arterial dilation, typically round to oval in shape (Fig. 8). Mural thrombus and calcification may be present. False aneurysms are more often ill-defined and may be surrounded by hemorrhage (Fig. 9). In addition, there may be associated findings of pancreatitis, pseudocysts, or post-traumatic changes.

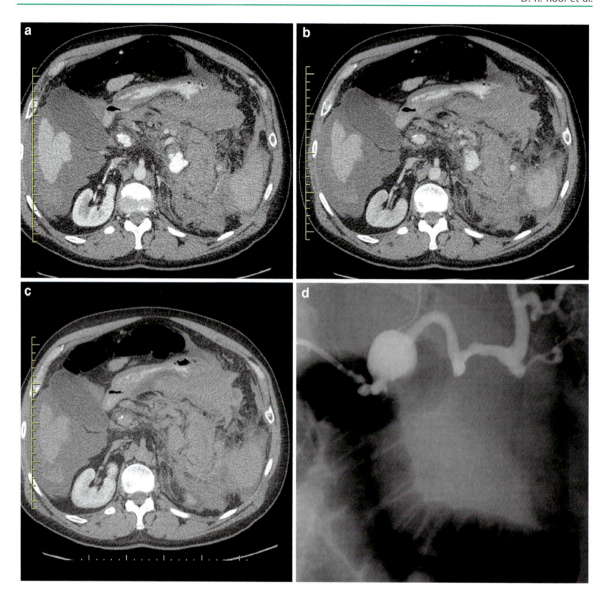

Fig. 9 Ruptured splenic pseudo-aneurysm. **a–c** CECT, axial views, in: arterial phase (**a**), portal-venous phase (**b**), and delayed phase (**c**). **d** DSA pre-embolization. This 49-year-old old male patient with acute pancreatitis had a ruptured splenic artery pseudo-aneurysm with a large surrounding hematoma and hemoperitoneum. The pseudo-aneurysm is best seen in the arterial phase and is not visible in the delayed phase

2.1.4.3 Differentials

Tortuous arteries can be difficult to differentiate from an aneurysm; multiplanar and maximum intensity reconstructions are often helpful problem-solving tools. Rarely, splenic artery aneurysms can mimic pancreatic tumors (Casadei et al. 2007).

2.2 Spontaneous Splenic Rupture

2.2.1 Terminology and Clinical Issues

Spontaneous splenic rupture, also referred to in the literature as spontaneous, non-traumatic, atraumatic, pathologic, occult, or idiopathic splenic rupture, is

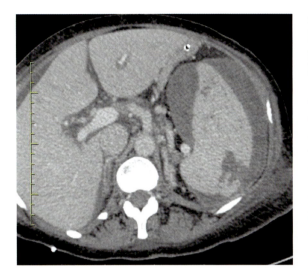

Fig. 10 Spontaneous splenic rupture as seen on CECT, portal-venous phase, axial view, in a 59-year-old female who presented with an acute abdomen. CECT demonstrated a splenic laceration and a large perisplenic hematoma. She was later diagnosed with acute myeloid leukemia

rare, with a mean of 30 cases published annually over the last three decades (Renzulli et al. 2009). The most common etiologies are infections and neoplastic and hematological disorders, causing congestion, spleno-megaly and pathological consistancy of the spleen. Worldwide, malaria is the leading cause of sponta-neous splenic rupture (Imbert et al. 2009). A true idiopathic rupture of a normal spleen is extremely rare (Renzulli et al. 2009).

Minimal events, such as sneezing, coughing, vomiting, or even stretching, may precede the rupture but often no significant traumatic event is reported (Renzulli et al. 2009; Safapor et al. 2007; Giagounidis et al. 1996). Clinical symptoms of atraumatic splenic rupture are related to intra-abdominal hemorrhage and their appearance is similar to that seen in traumatic splenic injuries. Hypotension, tachycardia, abdominal pain, pleuritic chest pain, and shoulder pain have all been described.

Spontaneous splenic rupture may lead to life-threatening hemorrhage. Morbidity and mortality are also related to the underlying splenic pathology and to advanced age of the patient (Renzulli et al. 2009).

Optimal management of spontaneous splenic

rupture depends on hemodynamic stability, under-lying splenic pathology, and local practice. Splenic preservation should be considered if the patient is hemodynamically stable and has a known self-limiting splenic disorder, such as infectious mononucleosis. On the other hand, splenectomy provides immediate definitive treatment and allows a surgical pathological diagnosis. Whether the same grading system applied to traumatic splenic rupture can be used is under debate (Testerman et al. 2011).

2.2.2 Imaging

Radiologic findings are similar to those seen in traumatic splenic injuries (see Sect. 3) (Fig. 10). The importance of imaging is the detection of underlying splenic pathology, such as splenomegaly or a mass.

2.2.3 Differentials

None Imaging findings and clinical history should lead to the diagnosis. Underlying splenic pathology should be suspected in the appropriate clinical setting, even if this is not apparent on initial diagnostic imaging.

2.3 Splenic Infection and Abscess

2.3.1 Terminology and Clinical Issues

The spleen, as part of the immune system, often enlarges during generalized infections (e.g., mononu-cleosis, tuberculosis, malaria). Imaging is used only to detect and quantify the splenomegaly, since the find-ings are not otherwise specific. Some infections may present with focal lesions or granulomas (tuberculosis, histoplasmosis, *Pneumocystis jirovecii*) (Fig. 11). In such cases, diagnostic imaging may reveal multiple focal nodular lesions ranging from a few millimeters to a few centimeters in diameter and frequently involving both the liver and spleen. These nodules may calcify after resolution of the acute infection.

Hydatid (echinococcus) disease is the most com-mon cause of splenic cysts in endemic areas. Knowledge of its prevalence and serology is para-mount (Adas et al. 2009). Isolated hydatid splenic involvement without liver and peritoneal disease is very rare (see below, "Cystic Lesions"). Splenic abscesses most commonly occur in a setting of met-

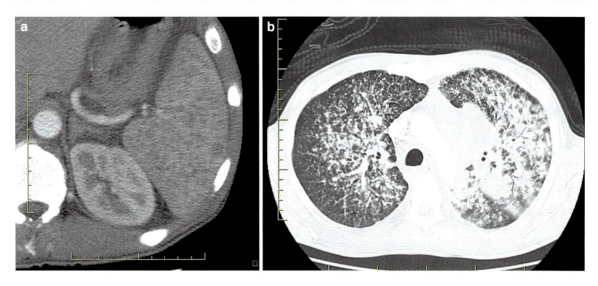

Fig. 11 Tuberculosis as seen on **a** CECT, portal-venous phase, axial view and **b** high-resolution CT. Numerous small nodular lesions throughout the spleen are seen in this 40-year-old male with disseminated miliary tuberculosis

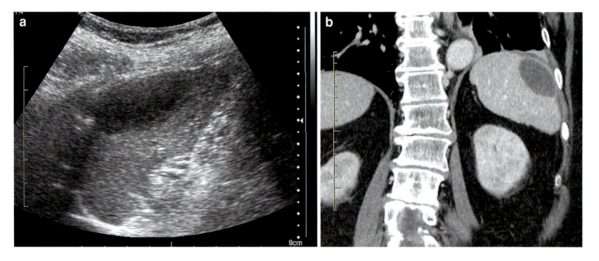

Fig. 12 Splenic abscess as seen on US (**a**) and CECT, portal-venous phase, coronal view (**b**) in a 71-year-old female with sepsis. Both modalities demonstrate a subcapsular splenic collection. Blood cultures and percutaneous aspiration revealed *Streptococcus intermedius* infection

astatic infection (septic emboli), contiguous infections (pancreatitis), or after splenic infarction (Fotiadis et al. 2008). Their typical clinical presentation is fever, occurring in 85%, and left upper quadrant abdominal pain, seen in 43%. Chills, nausea, vomiting, and/or anorexia may also be present (Fotiadis et al. 2008). On physical examination, splenomegaly is present in 50% and left upper quadrant tenderness in 45% of patients (Chang et al. 2006). If untreated, the condition can be life-threatening, especially in immunocompromised individuals. Multiple different organisms are found on cultures, depending on local endemic patterns and the patient's immune status (*Staphylococcus*, *Streptococci*, *E. coli*, *Salmonella, and Fungi*) (Ng et al. 2008; Joazlina et al. 2006; Krüger et al. 2011).

Splenic micro-abscesses caused by fungi are typically seen in patients with hematological malignancies or in immunocompromised patients. Imaging shows multiple small nodular lesions ranging from a few millimeters up to a few centimeters in size and often involving both liver and spleen.

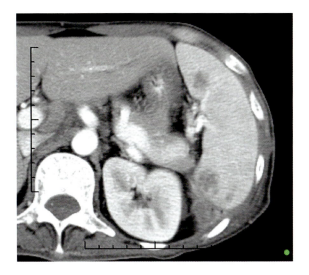

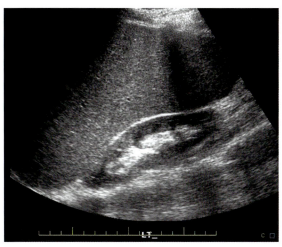

Fig. 13 Splenic abscess in a 40-year-old male with multifocal abscesses as seen on CECT, portal-venous phase, axial view. Multiple, ill-defined, hypodense areas in the spleen and a perisplenic collection with a few small gas bubbles. Diagnostic aspiration revealed a polymicrobial infection

Fig. 14 Splenomegaly. US image with extended field of view in a young female with marked splenomegaly due to portal hypertension

Complications of splenic abscess include free rupture into the peritoneal cavity and hemorrhage (Braat et al. 2009).

2.3.2 Imaging

Both US and CECT have a high sensitivity in the detection of splenic abscesses (Chang et al. 2006). In either modality, they are usually round or oval and can be unilocular or multilocular and multifocal. The imaging appearance of an abscess depends on the age and the degree of necrosis, varying from a simple cyst to a complex solid cystic structure (Fig. 12). The typical US appearance as a hypoechoic cystic structure with internal reflections and sediment in the dependent portion was only seen in 44% of the patients in one series (Changchien et al. 2002). Although highly specific, gas formation is present only in a minority of cases (Chang et al. 2006). On CECT, an abscess is typically hypodense, with rim enhancement after intravenous contrast, and may be well defined but is often irregular (Figs. 12, 13).

2.3.3 Differentials

The differential diagnosis for focal nodular lesions includes granulomas, lymphoma, metastatic disease, fungal infections, and sarcoid.

In the case of an abscess, the differential diagnosis includes splenic cysts, both "true" cysts and pseudocysts, hydatid cysts, and necrotic tumors (lymphoma).

2.4 Splenomegaly

2.4.1 Terminology and Clinical Issues

There are many recognized causes of splenomegaly, including congestive disease (portal hypertension), hematologic disease (thalassemia), neoplasm (lymphoma), storage disease (Gaucher's), infection (mononucleosis), and autoimmune disorders (sarcoid). The clinical findings are highly variable, with specific symptoms occurring only in a minority of patients.

2.4.2 Imaging

The normal size and weight of the spleen vary with patient age, sex, body length, and weight. Although the dimensions of a normal spleen are difficult to exactly quantify, publications suggest an upper limit for splenic length of 11–13 cm, a width of 7 cm, and a thickness of 5 cm. These values can be used for both US and CT (Figs. 14, 15). Nonetheless, there are no strict criteria to establish the diagnosis of splenomegaly; rather, it is generally based on a splenic length >15 cm in the craniocaudal dimension.

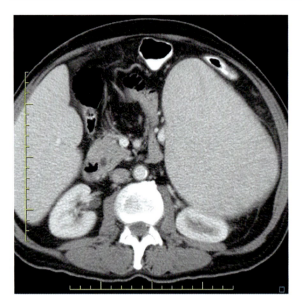

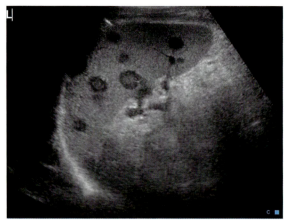

Fig. 16 Non-Hodgkin lymphoma as seen on US. Multiple solid nodules are present in the spleen of this 50-year-old male

Fig. 15 Splenomegaly as seen on CECT, portal-venous phase, axial view, in a patient with myelofibrosis

Diagnostic imaging is helpful to determine whether splenomegaly is caused by diffuse enlargement or by a focal lesion or lesions. One should also look for other signs, such as portal hypertension, portal vein and splenic vein thrombosis, and lymphadenopathy.

Splenic texture is often normal on US and CT, leaving the size of the spleen as the only abnormality.

2.4.3 Differentials
None.

2.5 Focal Lesions

2.5.1 Solid Lesions

2.5.1.1 Terminology and Clinical Issues
Focal masses or cysts are not infrequently encountered during imaging of the abdomen for other causes (Abbott et al. 2004; Bert et al. 2010).

2.5.1.2 Imaging
Unfortunately, it is often difficult to definitively characterize a focal solid splenic lesion based on imaging findings. Contrary to liver lesions, characteristic imaging features of focal splenic lesions have not been established as they depend on the underlying pathology

and range from well defined to ill-defined, solitary to multifocal, and solid, cystic, or complex cystic. The lesions may be vascular or hypovascular. Thus, to provide an accurate differential diagnosis and guide further management, one should look carefully for associated findings such as lymphadenopathy and liver lesions.

Lymphoma is one of the main considerations when a splenic mass is encountered. The most classic appearance is splenomegaly, with a solid hypovascular splenic mass or masses and lymphadenopathy. Splenic metastases (melanoma) are relatively rare and usually encountered during widespread metastatic disease. Primary splenic malignancies (angiosarcoma) are very rare, but often hypervascular.

On US, many focal solid lesions are hypoechoic, sometimes demonstrating internal flow on color imaging (Fig. 16). Hyperechoic lesions are more likely to be benign and may represent hemangiomas (Bert et al. 2010).

On CECT, most lesions are best visualized during the portal-venous phase (Fig. 17), although arterial and delayed images may help in further characterization.

2.5.1.3 Differentials
The differential diagnosis of focal solid splenic lesions is broad and most commonly includes malignant lesions (lymphoma, metastases (rare), primary splenic malignancies (very rare), benign lesions (hemangiomas, hamartomas, atypical infarcts), and infections (tuberculosis) (Abbott et al. 2004; Bert et al. 2010)).

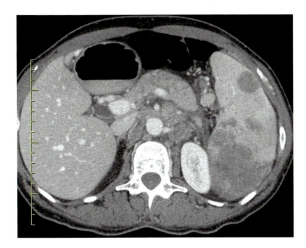

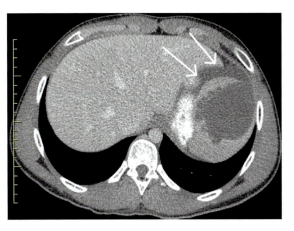

Fig. 17 B-cell lymphoma as seen on CECT, portal-venous phase, axial view. This 62-year-old female presented with upper abdominal pain. Imaging revealed marked splenomegaly with multiple splenic masses. Extensive retroperitoneal lymphadenopathy was also noted

Fig. 18 Ruptured non-traumatic splenic cyst as seen on CECT, portal-venous phase, axial view in a 19-year-old male. A large, slightly irregular splenic cyst and perisplenic fluid (*arrows*) are seen

2.5.2 Cystic Lesions

2.5.2.1 Terminology and Clinical Issues

Most common splenic cystic lesions in the Western world are true cysts (primary, true, mesothelial) or pseudocysts. Imaging is typically not helpful in differentiating one from the other, nor is this differentiation likely to be clinically significant (Morgenstern 2002). Rarely, a cyst may be symptomatic, due to a mass effect on surrounding structures or subsequent to rupture (Fig. 18). If symptomatic, percutaneous treatment (cyst ablation) or surgical management (splenectomy, fenestration) should be considered.

Splenic cyst should be differentiated from parasitic cyst. Hydatid (echinococcus) disease is the most common cause of splenic cysts in endemic areas, and knowledge of regional background as well as serology is paramount (Adas et al. 2009). Isolated hydatid splenic involvement without liver and peritoneal disease is very rare.

2.5.2.2 Imaging

Splenic cysts have the same imaging appearance as any other cyst in the body. On US and CECT, cystic lesions are usually well visualized. They may be simple or demonstrate complex features such as septations, calcifications, or debris (Figs. 19, 20). If a

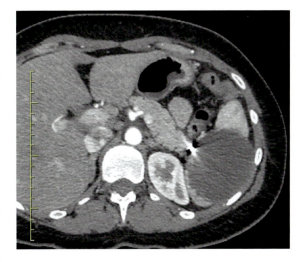

Fig. 19 Six months after embolization of a splenic artery aneurysm, this 47-year-old female presented with a round, 7-cm splenic cyst that had developed centrally in the spleen, consistent with a pseudocyst. CECT, portal-venous phase, axial view; same patient as in Fig. 8

solid or enhancing component is present, another pathology should be considered.

The appearance of hydatid cyst depends on the stage of the disease and varies from simple to complex with daughter cysts to partially solid, calcified lesions. Typically, there are associated liver and peritoneal findings.

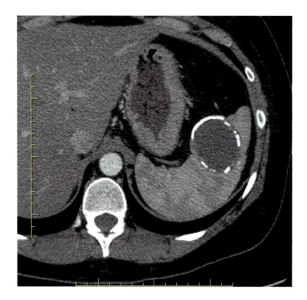

Fig. 20 A splenic pseudocyst, with a calcified rim (likely post-infarct or old trauma) was incidentally found in this 33-year-old female, CECT, arterial phase, axial view

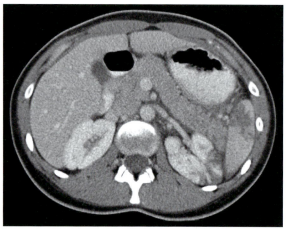

Fig. 21 Multiple, traumatic injuries to the spleen, tail of the pancreas, and the left kidney. CECT, portal-venous phase, axial view

2.5.2.3 Differentials

Rare presentations of cystic splenic lesions include cystic lymphangiomas and hamartomas, peliosis, and other rare primary splenic neoplasms. Cystic neoplasms are usually complex and often have a solid or enhancing component.

In some cases it can be difficult to differentiate a cystic lesion from a solid mass on US. Abscess, cystic metastasis, and necrotic tumors (lymphoma) may have a similar appearance on imaging.

3 Trauma

3.1 Terminology and Clinical Issues

The spleen is the most frequently affected organ in patients with abdominal organ injury after blunt trauma (Shanmuganathan and Killeen 2003). Traumatic injury of the spleen is associated with left-sided lower rib fractures and injuries to adjacent structures of the left upper abdomen: the left hemi-diaphragm, left liver lobe, left kidney, left adrenal gland, and the tail of the pancreas (Ledbetter and Smithuis 2007). These injuries may be visible on CT but most frequently do not need laparotomy (Fig. 21) (Miller et al. 2002).

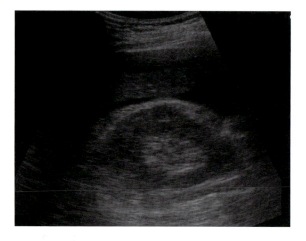

Fig. 22 Ultrasound of the right upper quadrant shows free fluid in Morrison's pouch in a patient with isolated splenic injury

3.2 Imaging

3.2.1 Ultrasound

In the evaluation of most trauma patients, the first imaging modality will be US. Hemodynamically unstable patients can be examined according to the FAST protocol, to select those requiring urgent laparotomy (Farahmand et al. 2005).

Free fluid originating from the splenic injury may be distributed diffusely throughout the abdomen or localized, either subphrenic, around the spleen, or in

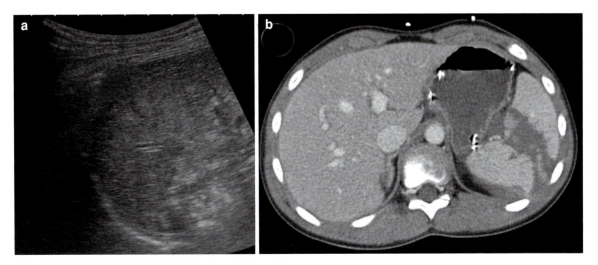

Fig. 23 Parenchymal and subcapsular hematomas. **a** US shows the inhomogeneous echo texture of the spleen, suspicious for traumatic injury. **b** Corresponding CECT image, portal-venous phase, axial view, through the upper abdomen in the same patient reveals a large parenchymal hematoma and a small subcapsular hematoma

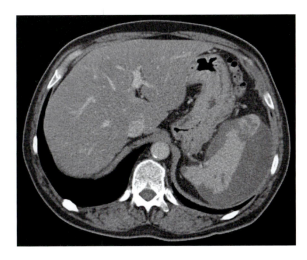

Fig. 24 After a motor vehicle collision, this patient was hemodynamically stable and complained of abdominal pain. No free fluid was seen on the FAST scan. CECT (portal-venous phase, axial view) demonstrates substantial splenic injury including a large subcapsular hematoma and multiple lacerations

Morrison's pouch (Fig. 22). Although parenchymal injury is often subtle, in many instances it can be visualized during a thorough investigation of the spleen on a formal abdominal US. A disrupted architecture or heterogeneous echotexture of the spleen and the presence of subcapsular fluid are direct sonographic signs of splenic injury (Fig. 23). On US,

(subcapsular) hematomas are often hypoechoic or heterogeneous compared to the splenic parenchyma, but they can be isoechoic and difficult to identify.

3.2.2 CECT

In hemodynamically stable patients, free fluid on FAST is an indication for CECT, in order to evaluate the intraperitoneal organs for evidence of a hemorrhagic focus. Unfortunately, in up to 34% of patients with abdominal organ injury, free intraperitoneal fluid is not present; therefore, the absence of free fluid on a FAST examination does not exclude splenic injury (Shanmuganathan et al. 1999; Poletti et al. 2003). Suspicious clinical signs, the presence of extra-abdominal distracting injuries, or an unreliable physical examination should mandate further evaluation with CECT (Deunk et al. 2010).

Splenic injury can have several appearances on CECT (Shanmuganathan and Killeen 2003; Clark et al. 2011). The sentinel clot sign, described as higher-attenuating free fluid near an injured organ, will often help to localize the bleeding site (Lubner et al. 2007).

3.2.2.1 Parenchymal Injury

Subcapsular hematomas usually demonstrate a concave rim at the periphery of the parenchyma and obtain a more lentiform shape when the hematoma indents the parenchyma. This contour change makes it possible to differentiate small amounts of perisplenic

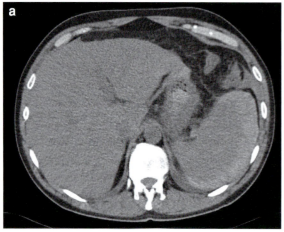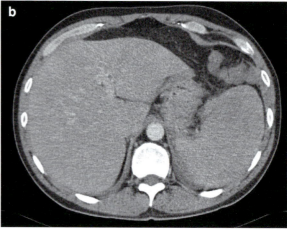

Fig. 25 Subcapsular hematoma, potential pitfall. **a** On axial NECT, the subcapsular hematoma is hyperdense compared to the splenic parenchyma. **b** On CECT, portal-venous phase, axial view, the hematoma is almost isodense compared to the splenic parenchyma

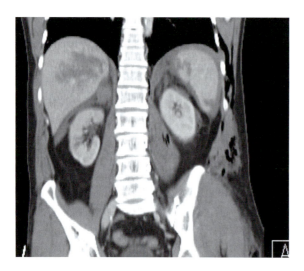

Fig. 26 Lacerations in the spleen as seen on CECT, portal-venous phase, coronal view. This patient also suffered a hemoperitoneum and liver and adrenal injuries after a fall from height

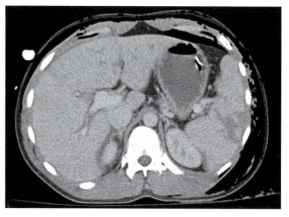

Fig. 27 Intrasplenic hematoma in a patient involved in a high-speed vehicle collision. The CT image obtained in portal-venous phase, axial view, shows an irregularly shaped, well-delineated low-attenuating area consistent with an intrasplenic hematoma

fluid from subcapsular hematomas. The appearance of a hematoma on CT depends on the stage. On non-enhanced CT (NECT), subcapsular hematomas can be hypodense, isodense or hyperdense compared to the splenic parenchyma. On CECT, hematomas are usually hypodense but can be isodense (Figs. 24, 25a, b).

Lacerations are linear or radial areas of decreased attenuation (Fig. 26).

Parenchymal hematoma presents as a low-attenuation mass, often well-delineated, that may expand the spleen (Figs. 27, 28). Parenchymal contusion is an area with diminished enhancement, often ill defined (Fig. 29). The differentiation between parenchymal hematoma and contusion is of no to little clinical relevance.

A splenic fracture is a laceration or hematoma involving the full width of the parenchyma, extending from the outer surface of the spleen to the hilum (see Fig. 23).

Infrequently, post-traumatic splenic infarcts occur. These are usually seen as well-defined wedge-shaped

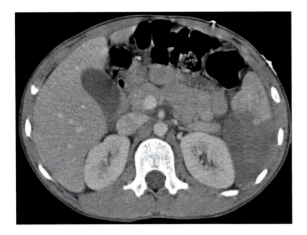

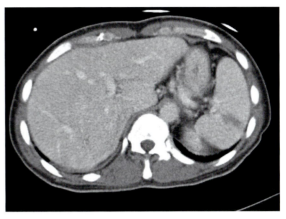

Fig. 28 Parenchymal hematoma in a patient who fell from a horse. CECT, portal-venous phase, axial view, shows a well-delineated low-attenuating area that expands the contours of the spleen

Fig. 29 This pedestrian was hit by a car. CECT, portal-venous phase, axial view, shows a not quite well-delineated low attenuating area consistent with a contusion

areas of decreased contrast enhancement with a broad base at the outer surface of the spleen and the apex pointing to the hilum (Miller et al. 2004).

3.2.2.2 Vascular Injury

Vascular injuries of the spleen include arterial and venous rupture, pseudo-aneurysm, arterio-venous (AV) fistula, and arterial and/or venous thrombosis. On CT, splenic artery rupture usually presents as active contrast extravasation and is typically seen as a linear or irregular "puff-of-smoke" deposit of contrast that increases in size with time and has a high attenuation, identical to or higher than that of arteries (Fig. 30) (Shanmuganathan et al. 1993). Although contrast extravasation typically arises from an artery, the origin is often not easily recognized.

If CECT is only performed in the venous phase, venous contrast extravasation can have an identical appearance. However, on CECT, the majority of venous hemorrhages show a hematoma without contrast extravasation.

An avulsed artery can also appear as an abrupt discontinuation of the involved artery or branch, i.e., the "cut off" sign, without contrast extravasation. This injury is often more difficult to appreciate.

A pseudo-aneurysm is a well-defined, round or oval contrast deposit originating from an artery with the same density as the arteries in all contrast phases and it does not change in shape or size (Fig. 31). An AV fistula also presents as a round or oval contrast

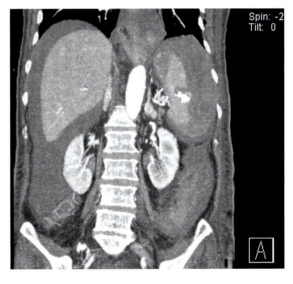

Fig. 30 Hemodynamically unstable patient involved in a motor vehicle accident, who transiently responded to infusion therapy. A large hemoperitoneum as well as parenchymal and subcapsular hematomas of the spleen with active contrast extravasation from its lateral portion. CECT, arterial phase, coronal view

deposit; on CECT, it can often not be distinguished from a pseudo-aneurysm. On angiography, AV fistula shows premature enhancement of the veins. Pseudo-aneurysms and AV fistulae are best seen in the arterial phase; however, as long as the arteries can be distinguished from the parenchyma, pseudo-aneurysms and AV fistulae will be visible.

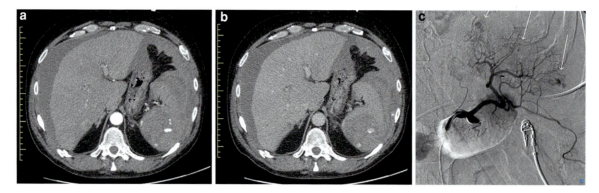

Fig. 31 Pseudo-aneurysm as seen on CECT, axial views in **a** arterial phase and **b** portal-venous phase, and **c** on DSA. This 52-year-old male was involved in a motor vehicle collision, resulting in hemoperitoneum, perisplenic hematoma, and multiple pseudo-aneurysms best seen in arterial phase and on angiography pre-embolization

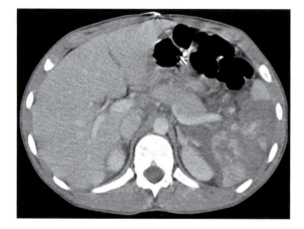

Fig. 32 Completely shattered spleen as seen on CECT, portal-venous phase, axial view

When a single-phase CECT is performed in the portal-venous phase, it can be difficult to differentiate contrast extravasation from a pseudo-aneurysm or AV fistula. In these cases, an additional delayed CT scan or the use of angiography with or without embolization should be considered (Fig. 31c). Identical to the arteries that feed them, pseudo-aneurysms and AV fistula will decrease in density in delayed phases, making it impossible to delineate them from the surrounding parenchyma, while contrast extravasation will remain at its high initial density (Anderson et al. 2007).

Pseudo-aneurysms, AV fistulas, and cut-off arteries are not actively bleeding but hemorrhage can start at a later stage, giving rise to "delayed" splenic hemorrhage or rupture.

3.3 Grading Systems

Of the several systems used to grade splenic injury, those of the American Association Surgery Trauma (AAST) Organ Injury Severity score (OIS) and the Baltimore CT-based classification are the most often used (Tables 1, 2) (Moore et al. 1995; Marmery et al. 2007).

One of the complications of splenectomy is the risk of a rapidly developing, potentially lethal sepsis (overwhelming post-splenectomy infection, OPSI) caused by encapsulated bacteria (de Porto et al. 2010). Unfortunately, this cannot be prevented by vaccination in all patients and, together with other contraindications to surgery, has contributed to the preference for non-operative therapeutic management of traumatic splenic injury. However, hemodynamically unstable patients require urgent intervention, either surgical or by means of arterial embolization. In addition, the non-operative management, by clinical observation alone, of initially hemodynamically stable patients reportedly has a high failure rate, especially in patients with high-grade injuries (van der Vlies et al. 2010). Thus, the challenge for grading systems is to differentiate those patients who require surgical management or embolization from those who do not.

The AAST OIS was last revised in 1994 and was traditionally used to grade injuries based on anatomic findings at surgery; however, it is now also used to grade injuries as determined on CECT in patients not undergoing surgery (Moore et al. 1995; Moore et al. 1989). Contrast extravasation on CECT, as an

Table 1 American Association Surgery Trauma (AAST) Organ Injury Severity (OIS) score of the spleen [from (Moore et al. 1995)]

Injury grade[a]	Type	Description
I	Hematoma	Subcapsular, <10% surface area
	Laceration	Capsular tear, <1 cm parenchymal depth
II	Hematoma	Subcapsular, 10–50% surface area
		Intraparenchymal, <5 cm in diameter
	Laceration	1–3 cm parenchymal depth; which does not involve a trabecular vessel
III	Hematoma	Subcapsular, >50% surface area or expanding;
		Ruptured subcapsular or parenchymal hematoma
		Intraparenchymal hematoma >5 cm or expanding
	Laceration	>3 cm parenchymal depth or involving trabecular vessels
IV	Laceration	Laceration involving segmental or hilar vessels producing major devascularization (>25% of spleen)
V	Laceration	Completely shattered spleen (Fig. 32)
	Vascular	Hilar vascular injury which devascularizes spleen

[a] Advance one grade for multiple injuries up to grade III

Table 2 Baltimore MDCT grading system [from (Marmery et al. 2007)]

Grade	Criteria
1	Subcapsular hematoma <1 cm thick
	Laceration <1 cm parenchymal depth
	Parenchymal hematoma <1 cm diameter
2	Subcapsular hematoma 1–3 cm thick
	Laceration 1–3 cm in parenchymal depth
	Parenchymal hematoma 1–3 cm in diameter
3	Splenic capsular disruption
	Subcapsular hematoma >3 cm thick
	Laceration >3 cm in parenchymal depth
	Parenchymal hematoma >3 cm in diameter
4a	Active intraparenchymal and subcapsular splenic bleeding
	Splenic vascular injury (pseudo-aneurysm or arteriovenous fistula)
	Shattered spleen
4b	Active intraperitoneal bleeding

indicator of active bleeding, is not part of the AAST OIS classification, nor are vascular injuries as potential bleeding sites, such as pseudo-aneurysm, AV fistulas, and avulsed arteries, mentioned. Vascular injury is only included in the AAST grading system in case of devascularization of the spleen. However, it has been shown that contrast extravasation and vascular injuries detected on CECT are important prognostic factors (van der Vlies et al. 2010). Embolization of these injuries can improve the success rate of non-operative management and reduces the number of necessary laparotomies, particularly in high-grade injuries. By contrast, successful non-operative management of AV fistulae is limited even after embolization (Haan et al. 2005; Jeremitsky et al. 2011; Wei et al. 2008). Accordingly, the AAST classification may be of limited prognostic value and as an independent grading system cannot be used to select patients for surgery vs. non-operative management (van der Vlies et al. 2010).

In the more recently published Baltimore CT-based classification system, contrast extravasation and vascular injury are included. This addition to the AAST was retrospectively evaluated by (Marmery et al. 2007). In that study, all patients with high-grade injuries, according to the AAST, and all patients with low-grade injuries with contrast extravasation or vascular injuries were treated with embolization or surgery (splenectomy or splenorrhaphy). The failure rate of non-operative management was only 5% (Marmery ct al. 2007). In the Baltimore CT grading system, patients with contrast extravasation or vascular injuries on CT were classified as grade 4 and the chance that patients were correctly triaged for surgery, embolization, or observation exceeded 80%. Therefore, this classification seems to be a better than the AAST OIS at predicting outcome (Marmery et al. 2007).

The influence of both the presence of a large hemoperitoneum and the age of the patient on the expected success rate of non-operative management with or without embolization is debated in the literature; neither of these parameters is included in the AAST or Baltimore classification (Haan et al. 2005; Velmahos et al. 2003; Thompson et al. 2006; Sharma et al. 2005; Peitzman et al. 2000; Haan et al. 2004; Omert et al. 2001).

The most frequent complications of embolization are infarcts (van der Vlies 2010). While in most patients infarcts are asymptomatic, in 5–12% recurrent bleeding requires re-embolization or a splenectomy (Marmery et al. 2007; Haan et al. 2005; Peitzman et al. 2000; Schnüriger et al. 2011). Abscesses occur in 4% and can usually be treated percutaneously (van der Vlies et al. 2010; Haan et al. 2004). However, the presence of air in the spleen is a normal phenomenon after splenic embolization and in this context should not be considered a sign of infection (van der Vlies 2010)

The embolization of splenic injuries is associated with fewer major abdominal complications than following surgery (Wei et al. 2008), but pancreatitis and systemic complications such as ARDS are more frequent after splenic embolization (Madoff et al. 2005; Duchesne et al. 2008). In addition, elderly patients tend to have more complications, including more frequent failure, when non-operatively managed (Wu et al. 2011; Renzulli et al. 2010).

Most studies on the benefits of embolizing splenic injuries and on the ensuing complications are retrospective and there is no consensus whether all vascular injuries require embolization. Prospective randomized or observational studies are needed (van der Vlies et al. 2010; Omert et al. 2001; Duchesne et al. 2008; Nwomeh et al. 2004).

3.4 Differentials

Traumatic splenic lacerations must be differentiated from persistent fetal lobulation, congenital clefts, and humps, all of which have smooth edges, unlike lacerations.

On CECT, lacerations can be difficult to distinguish from beam-hardening artifacts, which if present are often due to positioning of the arms of the patient next to the body (Brink et al. 2008; Karlo et al. 2011).

Without the context of trauma, splenic parenchymal contusion and hematomas should be differentiated from benign and malignant tumors.

References

Abbas MA, Stone WM, Fowl RJ et al (2002) Splenic artery aneurysms: two decades experience at Mayo clinic. Ann Vasc Surg 16:442–449

Abbott RM, Levy AD, Aguilera NS et al (2004) From the archives of the AFIP: primary vascular neoplasms of the spleen: radiologic-pathologic correlation. Radiographics 24:1137–1163

Adas G, Karatepe O, Altiok M et al (2009) Diagnostic problems with parasitic and non-parasitic splenic cysts. BMC Surg. 29;9:9. doi:10.1186/1471-2482-9-9 http://www.biomed central.com/1471-2482/9/9

Agrawal GA, Johnson PT, Fishman EK (2007) Splenic artery aneurysms and pseudoaneurysms: clinical distinctions and CT appearances. AJR Am J Roentgenol 188:992–999

Al-Habbal Y, Christophi C, Muralidharan V (2010) Aneurysms of the splenic artery–a review. Surgeon 8:223–231

Anderson SW, Varghese JC, Lucey BC et al (2007) Blunt splenic trauma: delayed-phase CT for differentiation of active hemorrhage from contained vascular injury in patients. Radiology 243:88–95

Antopolsky M, Hiller N, Salameh S et al (2009) Splenic infarction: 10 years of experience. Am J Emerg Med 27:262–265

Ben Ely A, Zissin R, Copel L et al (2006) The wandering spleen: CT findings and possible pitfalls in diagnosis. Clin Radiol 61:954–958

Bert T, Tebbe J, Görg C (2010) What should be done with echoic splenic tumors incidentally found by ultrasound? Z Gastroenterol 48(4):465–471

Braat MN, Hueting WE, Hazebroek EJ (2009) Pneumoperitoneum secondary to a ruptured splenic abscess. Intern Emerg Med 4:349–351

Brink M, de Lange F, Oostveen LJ et al (2008) Arm raising at exposure-controlled multidetector trauma CT of thoracoabdominal region: higher image quality, lower radiation dose. Radiology 249:661–670

Casadei R, Antonacci N, Calculli L et al (2007) Thrombosed splenic artery aneurysm simulating a pancreatic body mass: can two entities be distinguished preoperatively thus avoiding diagnostic and therapeutic mistakes? JOP 8(2):235–239

Chang KC, Chuah SK, Changchien CS et al (2006) Clinical characteristics and prognostic factors of splenic abscess: a review of 67 cases in a single medical center of Taiwan. World J Gastroenterol 12:460–464

Changchien CS, Tsai TL, Hu TH et al (2002) Sonographic patterns of splenic abscess: an analysis of 34 proven cases. Abdom Imaging 27:739–745

Clark TJ, Cardoza S, Kanth N (2011) Splenic trauma: pictorial review of contrast-enhanced CT findings. Emerg Radiol 18:227–234

de Porto APNA, Lammers AJJ, Bennink RJ et al (2010) Assessment of splenic function. Eur J Clin Microbiol Infect Dis 29:1465–1473

Deunk J, Brink M et al (2010) Predictors for the selection of patients for abdominal CT after blunt trauma: a proposal for a diagnostic algorithm. Ann Surg 251:512–520

Donnelly LF, Foss JN, Frush DP et al (1999) Heterogeneous splenic enhancement patterns on spiral CT images in children: minimizing misinterpretation. Radiology 210:493–497

Duchesne JC, Simmons JD, Schmieg RE Jr et al (2008) Proximal splenic angioembolization does not improve outcomes in treating blunt splenic injuries compared with splenectomy: a cohort analysis. J Trauma 65:1346–1351

Farahmand N, Sirlin CB, Brown MA et al (2005) Hypotensive patients with blunt abdominal trauma: performance of screening US. Radiology 235:436–443

Fotiadis C, Lavranos G, Patapis P et al (2008) Abscesses of the spleen: report of three cases. World J Gastroenterol 14:3088–3091

Giagounidis AA, Burk M, Meckenstock G et al (1996) Pathologic rupture of the spleen in hematologic malignancies: two additional cases. Ann Hematol 73:297–302

Goerg C, Schwerk WB (1990) Splenic infarction: sonographic patterns, diagnosis, follow-up, and complications. Radiology 174:803–807

Ha JF, Phillips M, Faulkner K (2009) Splenic artery aneurysm rupture in pregnancy. Eur J Obstet Gynecol Reprod Biol 146:133–137

Haan JM, Biffl W, Knudson MM et al (2004) Splenic embolization revisited: a multicenter review. J Trauma 56:542–547

Haan JM, Bochicchio GV, Kramer N et al (2005) Nonoperative management of blunt splenic injury: a 5-year experience. J Trauma 58:492–498

Imbert P, Rapp C, Buffet PA (2009) Pathological rupture of the spleen in malaria: analysis of 55 cases (1958–2008). Travel Med Infect Dis 7(3):147–159

Jeremitsky E, Kao A, Carlton C et al (2011) Does splenic embolization and grade of splenic injury impact nonoperative management in patients sustaining blunt splenic trauma? Am Surg 77:215–220

Joazlina ZY, Wastie ML, Ariffin N (2006) Computed tomography of focal splenic lesions in patients presenting with fever. Singapore Med J 47:37–41

Karlo C, Gnannt R, Frauenfelder T et al (2011) Whole-body CT in polytrauma patients: effect of arm positioning on thoracic and abdominal image quality. Emerg Radiol 18:285–293

Krüger C, Malleyeck I, Naman N (2011) Amoebic abscess of the spleen and fatal colonic perforation. Pediatr Infect Dis J 30:91–92

Ledbetter S, Smithuis RH (2007) Abdominal trauma–role of CT. Radiology assistant. http://www.radiologyassistant.nl/en/466181ff61073#p4661853ae1bd1 Accessed 4 Aug 2011

Lubner M, Menias C, Rucker C et al (2007) Blood in the belly: CT findings of hemoperitoneum. Radiographics 27:109–125

Madoff DC, Denys A, Wallace MJ et al (2005) Splenic arterial interventions: anatomy, indications, technical considerations, and potential complications. Radiographics 25(1):S191–S211

Marmery H, Shanmuganathan K, Alexander MT et al (2007) Optimization of selection for nonoperative management of blunt splenic injury: comparison of MDCT grading systems. AJR Am J Roentgenol 189:1421–1427

Miller PR, Croce MA, Bee TK et al (2002) Associated injuries in blunt solid organ trauma: implications for missed injury in nonoperative management. J Trauma 53:238–242

Miller LA, Mirvis SE, Shanmuganathan K et al (2004) CT diagnosis of splenic infarction in blunt trauma: imaging features, clinical significance and complications. Clin Radiol 59:342–348

Moore EE, Shackford SR, Pachter HL et al (1989) Organ injury scaling: spleen, liver, and kidney. J Trauma 29(12):1664–1666

Moore EE, Cogbill TH, Jurkovich GJ et al (1995) Organ injury scale: spleen and liver (1994 revision). J Trauma 38:323–324

Morgenstern L (2002) Nonparasitic splenic cysts: pathogenesis, classification, and treatment. J Am Coll Surg 194(3):306–314

Ng CY, Leong EC, Chng HC (2008) Ten-year series of splenic abscesses in a general hospital in Singapore. Ann Acad Med Singapore 37:749–752

Nores M, Phillips EH, Morgenstern L et al (1998) The clinical spectrum of splenic infarction. Am Surg 64:182–188

Nwomeh BC, Nadler EP, Meza MP et al (2004) Contrast extravasation predicts the need for operative intervention in children with blunt splenic trauma. J Trauma 56:537–541

Omert LA, Salyer D, Dunham CM et al (2001) Implications of the "contrast blush" finding on computed tomographic scan of the spleen in trauma. J Trauma 51:272–277

Peitzman AB, Heil B, Rivera L et al (2000) Blunt splenic injury in adults: multi-institutional study of the eastern association for the surgery of trauma. J Trauma 49:177–178

Poletti PA, Kinkel K, Vermeulen B et al (2003) Blunt abdominal trauma: should US be used to detect both free fluid and organ injuries? Radiology 227(1):95–103

Renzulli P, Hostettler A, Schoepfer AM et al (2009) Systematic review of atraumatic splenic rupture. Br J Surg 96: 1114–1121

Renzulli P, Gross T, Schnüriger B et al (2010) Management of blunt injuries to the spleen. Br J Surg 97:1696–1703

Robertson F, Leander P, Ekberg O (2001) Radiology of the spleen. Eur Radiol 11:80–95

Safapor F, Aghajanzade M, Kohsari MR et al (2007) Spontaneous rupture of the spleen: a case report and review of the literature. Saudi J Gastroenterol 13:136–137

Schnüriger B, Inaba K, Konstantinidis A et al (2011) Outcomes of proximal versus distal splenic artery embolization after trauma: a systematic review and meta-analysis. J Trauma 70:252–260

Shanmuganathan K, Killeen KL (2003) Imaging of abdominal trauma. In: Mirvis SE, Shanmuganathan K (eds) Imaging in trauma and critical care, 2nd edn. Saunders, Philadephia, pp 387–417

Shanmuganathan K, Mirvis SE, Sover ER (1993) Value of contrast-enhanced CT in detecting active hemorrhage in patients with blunt abdominal or pelvic trauma. AJR 161: 65–69

Shanmuganathan K, Mirvis SE, Sherbourne CD et al (1999) Hemoperitoneum as the sole indicator of abdominal visceral injuries: a potential limitation of screening abdominal US for trauma. Radiology 212:423–430

Sharma OP, Oswanski MF, Singer D et al (2005) Assessment of nonoperative management of blunt spleen and liver trauma. Am Surg 71:379–386

Soleimani M, Mehrabi A, Kashfi A et al (2007) Surgical treatment of patients with wandering spleen: report of six cases with a review of the literature. Surg Today 37: 261–269

Testerman GM, Easparam S, Jacome F (2011) Western trauma association blunt splenic injury algorithm is useful in spontaneous rupture of a normal spleen. Am Surg 77(5): E85–E86

Thompson BE, Munera F, Cohen SM et al (2006) Computed tomography scan scoring system predicts the need for intervention after splenic injury. J Trauma 60:1083–1086

van der Vlies CH, van Delden OM, Punt BJ et al (2010) Literature review of the role of ultrasound, computed tomography, and transcatheter arterial embolization for the treatment of traumatic splenic injuries. Cardiovasc Intervent Radiol 33:1079–1087

Velmahos GC, Toutouzas KG, Radin R et al (2003) Nonoperative treatment of blunt injury to solid abdominal organs: a prospective study. Arch Surg 138:844–851

Wei B, Hemmila MR, Arbabi S et al (2008) Angioembolization reduces operative intervention for blunt splenic injury. J Trauma 64:1472–1477

Wu SC, Fu CY, Chen RJ et al (2011) Higher incidence of major complications after splenic embolization for blunt splenic injuries in elderly patients. Am J Emerg Med 29:135–140

Pancreas

Lucas L. Geyer and Ulrich Linsenmaier

Contents

L. L. Geyer (✉) · U. Linsenmaier
Department of Clinical Radiology,
University Hospital LMU Munich,
Nussbaumstrasse 20, 80336,
Munich, Germany
e-mail: lucas.geyer@med.uni-muenchen.de

Abstract

Pancreatic emergencies can be categorized as traumatic and non-traumatic, with the latter mainly caused by inflammation. Both acute pancreatitis (AP) and chronic pancreatitis (CP) can indicate the need for emergency imaging. As the detection of postoperative complications also requires immediate imaging, postoperative imaging findings are discussed in a separate section of this chapter.

1 Imaging

In general, multidetector computed tomography (MDCT) is the most important imaging modality for the diagnosis of pancreatic emergencies. However, several other imaging modalities are available as well: transabdominal ultrasound and endosonography, magnetic resonance imaging (MRI) and magnetic resonance cholangiopancreatography (MRCP), and endoscopic retrograde cholangiopancreatography (ERCP). Plain-film radiography of the abdomen is omitted in imaging pancreatic emergencies. The indications for pancreatic emergency imaging are listed in Table 1.

1.1 (Transabdominal) Ultrasound and Endosonography

The main limitations of transabdominal ultrasound (US) are superimposed bowel gas, patient size, and a strong dependency on the investigator's experience. Endosonography (EUS) is less affected by intestinal air and patient constitution. Therefore, it is more suitable than

M. Scaglione et al. (eds.), *Emergency Radiology of the Abdomen*,
Medical Radiology. Diagnostic Imaging,
DOI: 10.1007/174_2011_469, © Springer-Verlag Berlin Heidelberg 2012

Table 1 Indications for pancreatic emergency imaging

Aims of imaging
Confirmation of the diagnosis by visualization of pancreatic findings
Detection of concomitant diseases and/or complications
Assessment of the severity and the resulting prognosis
Identification or exclusion of the cause
Guiding interventional procedures

transabdominal ultrasound for interventional procedures, such as puncture or fine-needle biopsy, which may be indicated in suspected acute necrotic pancreatitis. However, the diagnostic value of EUS is restricted by its invasive character and limited availability.

1.2 Radiography

Chest radiographs might show concomitant pleural effusions or demonstrate pericardial effusion. Plain films of the abdomen should be avoided because they are of insufficient diagnostic value, despite their high specificity in the detection of calcifications.

1.3 MDCT

Since the introduction of MDCT and its rapid development in recent years, this modality has become the first-line imaging tool in AP, mainly due to its wide availability, non-invasiveness, the short duration of the examination, and its comprehensive depiction of the pancreas and adjacent organs. Healthy pancreatic tissue has an average density of 30–60 HU on non-enhanced CT (NECT) and a peak enhancement of 80–150 HU on contrast-enhanced CT (CECT) and is best visualized in the late-arterial pancreatic parenchymal phase (Table 2). Age-dependent involution decreases the density of the pancreas.

1.4 MRI/MRCP

In the diagnosis of pancreatic emergencies, MRI is a sophisticated second-line imaging tool. It also offers MRCP as non-invasive alternative to ERCP in the evaluation of the biliary and pancreatic duct systems (Table 3).

Table 2 MDCT scan protocol for pancreatic emergencies

Parameters	
Oral CM	If applicable: 1000–1500 mL water or positive CM
Patient's position	Supine with elevated arms
Scan field	Entire abdomen and pelvis (portal venous phase)
Hounsfield window (w/c)	NECT: 350/40
	CECT: 400/60
Injection protocol (mL CM/mL saline chaser)	150/50
Flow rate (mL/s)	4–5
Delay	
Arterial phase	20 s after bolus tracking[a]
Parenchymal phase	35–40 s after bolus tracking[a]
Porto venous phase	60–70 s after bolus tracking[a]
Unenhanced scan	Optional
Slice thickness (mm)	
Axial	5
MPR: sagittal/coronal	3/3

CM Contrast material, *MPR* multiplanar reconstruction
A monophasic scan is sufficient for most cases (recommended: porto venous phase); if a multiphasic scan is required, the scan field can be limited to the pancreatic area for the arterial and parenchymal phases
[a] Bolus tracking in the abdominal aorta (threshold 100 HU, level of lumbar vertebrae I/II)

Table 3 MRI protocol

Standard MRI protocol
T1w GRE sequences with fat-saturation
T2w sequences without fat saturation, e.g. "single shot" TSE sequences
T2w sequences with fat saturation (T2 TSE fat-saturated)
Recommended: parallel imaging
Contrast-enhanced T1w 3D-GRE sequences (timing: arterial, venous, late venous)
Optional: MRCP sequences

T1w, T2w T1-, T2-weighted, *GRE* gradient echo imaging, *TSE* turbo spin echo, *MRCP* magnetic resonance cholangiopancreatography

1.5 ERCP

As an adjunct to non-invasive radiological imaging of the pancreas, ERCP is today mostly used as a therapeutic procedure to drain the pancreatic and or biliary ducts or to remove concretions. The reader is referred to the literature describing ERCP findings.

2 Non-Traumatic Emergencies

2.1 Acute Pancreatitis

2.1.1 Terminology and Clinical Issues

Acute pancreatitis may be diagnosed if two of the following three criteria are met: abdominal pain strongly indicative of AP, elevation of amylase or lipase to three times the normal value, and pathologic findings on US or CECT.

2.1.1.1 Overview and Etiology

Acute pancreatitis is an acute inflammation of the pancreas and an important cause of clinical acute abdomen. It accounts for more than 200,000 hospital admissions in the USA each year (Whitcomb 2006), and the overall incidence has increased in Western countries over time. Over the last few decades, several classifications and scoring systems have been developed for risk stratification and prediction of outcome. In 1992, the Atlanta classification system was introduced and served as the basis for subsequent classifications (Table 4). The severity of AP is categorized as mild or severe based on morphologic abnormalities of the pancreas, identified in CT images: Mild AP, so-called interstitial edematous pancreatitis (IEOP), is associated without or with minimal organ failure and an uneventful recovery. In severe AP, so-called necrotizing pancreatitis (NP), there is organ failure and complications (Bradley 1993). The majority (about 80%) of AP cases can be classified as mild and self-limiting; however, about 20% of these patients develop a severe and life-threatening clinical course associated with significant morbidity and mortality. Gallstone obstruction (Fig. 1) and alcohol abuse are the most common causes of AP (80% of cases). Rare causes comprise drugs, heredity, infection, metabolic dysfunction, and abdominal trauma, surgery or other intervention, such as ERCP (Frossard et al. 2008).

2.1.1.2 Clinical Featuress

Acute onset of severe pain in the upper abdomen with band-like radiation into the back is the cardinal symptom and might last for several days. It is often accompanied by several unspecific disorders, such as nausea, vomiting, and fever. Severe AP is indicated by serious symptoms and complications, such as hypotension, tachycardia, respiratory insufficiency, signs of peritonitis, shock, and multi-organ failure (MOF). In addition, both clinical Grey-Turner's signs (ecchymotic staining of the lateral abdominal wall) and Cullen's sign (bruising of the peri-umbilical area) are rare and unspecific physical findings, but indicate severe disease and impaired prognosis.

2.1.1.3 Laboratory Findings

Elevated blood levels of pancreatic enzymes (amylase, lipase), non-enzymatic products of pancreatic secretion, and unspecific markers of inflammation are usually diagnostic of AP. A more than threefold elevated serum level of amylase is characteristic and can confirm the clinically suspected diagnosis. Nevertheless, false-negative and false-positive serum concentrations can occur. Elevated concentrations of lipase in serum might also be measured. In contrast to amylase, serum lipase levels remain raised for a longer period of time (>3–5 days), although neither parameter correlates with outcome (Balthazar 2002). Serial enzyme measurements can, however, help to clinically monitor the extent of traumatic and non-traumatic pancreatic disease.

2.1.1.4 Grading of AP

Since the early 1970s, several multidisciplinary (clinical, biochemical, radiological) scoring systems have been developed. The two most widely used clinical scores are Ranson's criteria and the Acute Physiology and Chronic Health Evaluation (APACHE II). The CT severity index was developed by Balthazar et al. as a radiological score and it is based on the presence and degree of pancreatic inflammation and necrosis (Balthazar 2002). Although the index is predictive of the patient's prognosis, the original score does not take into account organ failure and extrapancreatic complications. In light of these shortcomings, Mortele et al. developed the modified CT severity index (Table 5), which showed an improved correlation with the patient's outcome. The modified index distinguishes between mild (0–2 points), moderate (4–6 points), and severe (8–10 points) degrees of AP (Mortele et al. 2004).

2.1.2 Imaging

2.1.2.1 Ultrasound

Acute pancreatitis leads to an enlargement of the organ, with a diffuse hypoechogenicity or focal hypoechogenic spots on US and hyodensities and edema

Table 4 Summary of the 1992 Atlanta classification

Entities	Description
AP	An acute inflammatory process of the pancreas with variable involvement of other regional tissues or remote organ systems associated with raised pancreatic enzyme levels in blood and/or urine
Severity	
Mild AP	Associated with minimal organ dysfunction and an uneventful recovery; lacks the features of severe AP. Usually normal enhancement of pancreatic parenchyma on CECT
Severe AP	Associated with organ failure and/or local complications such as necrosis, abscess or pseudocyst
Predicted severity	Ranson score $\geq$ 3 or APACHE II score $\geq$ 8
Organ failure and systemic complications, multi-organ failure (MOF)	
Shock	Systolic blood pressure < 90 mmHg
Pulmonary insufficiency	PaO_2 $\leq$60 mmHg
Renal failure	Creatinine $\geq$ 177 µmol/l or $\leq$ 2 mg/dl after rehydration
Gastrointestinal bleeding	500 ml in 24 h
Disseminated intravascular coagulations	Platelets $\leq$ 100, 000/mm^3, fibrinogen < 1.0 g/l and fibrin-split products > 80 µg/l
Severe metabolic disturbance	Calcium $\leq$ 1.87 mmol/l or $\leq$ 7.5 mg/dl
Local complications	
Acute fluid collections	Occur early in the course of AP, are located in or near the pancreas and always lack a of a fibrous wall of granulation tissue. In about half of patients, spontaneous regression occurs. In the other half, an acute fluid collection develops into a pancreatic abscess or pseudocysts.
Pancreatic necrosis	Diffuse or focal area(s) of non-viable pancreatic parenchyma, typically associated with peripancreatic fat necrosis non-enhanced pancreatic parenchyma >3 cm or involving >30% of the area of the pancreas
Acute pseudocyst	Collection of pancreatic fluid enclosed by a wall of fibrous or granulation tissue, which arises as a result of acute or chronic pancreatitis or pancreatic trauma, occurring at least 4 weeks after onset of symptoms; it is round or ovoid and most often sterile; when pus is present, lesion is termed a "pancreatic abscess."
Pancreatic abscess	Circumscribed, intra-abdominal collection of pus, usually in proximity to the pancreas, containing little or no pancreatic necrosis, which arises as a consequence of AP or pancreatic trauma often $\geq$4 weeks after onset. Pancreatic abscess and infected pancreatic necrosis differ in clinical expression and extent of associated necrosis.

on CT. In addition, US can detect gallstones in the gallbladder, cholestasis, free intra-abdominal fluid, and pleural effusion. Gallstones within the common bile duct can be detected by endosonography. Recent studies suggest that contrast enhanced US is able to display pancreatic necrosis. As US provides only limited information, it plays a minor role in the initial diagnosis of AP in adults, but might be preferable in children and for follow-up studies because of both the absence of radiation exposure and its beside availability.

2.1.2.2 MRI/MRCP

In AP, MRI is of minor importance but can be indicated in equivocal CT findings, contraindications to IV iodinated contrast material, or to differentiate between fluid and necrotic areas. Subtle, early findings might be demonstrated more sensitively. Edematous organ swelling and/or exudation increase the intra- and/or peripancreatic signal intensity in T2w imaging. MRCP is increasingly being used to avoid ERCP in the acute inflammatory phase for the detection of gallstones (see also Chronic Pancreatitis).

Table 5 Modified CT severity index

Prognostic indicator	Points
Pancreatic inflammation	
Normal pancreas	0
Intrinsic pancreatic abnormalities with/without inflammatory changes in peripancreatic fat	2
Pancreatic or peripancreatic fluid collection or peripancreatic fat necrosis	4
Pancreatic necrosis	
0	0
≤30	2
>30	4
Extrapancreatic complications (one or more of pleural effusion, ascites, vascular complications, parenchymal complications, or gastrointestinal tract involvement)	2

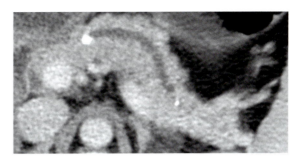

Fig. 1 Intraductal calculus with enlarged pancreatic duct

2.1.2.3 MDCT

Indications of an initial MDCT scan are: (a) Equivocal clinical and biochemical diagnosis (within 48 h after onset of symptoms); (b) therapy-refractory AP (within 72 h after beginning of therapy; (c) suspicion of NP; (d) a sudden change in the patient's condition.

In 30% of the patients, the pancreatic parenchyma is normal on MDCT despite a clinical and biochemical diagnosis of AP; particularly early CECT, may fail to detect morphologic changes in patients with clinical severe AP. Thus, severe AP with parenchymal necrosis cannot be excluded within the first 48–72 h (Bollen et al. 2007a).

Interstitial edematous pancreatitis (Fig. 2). This condition is marked by a focal or diffuse swelling of the pancreatic parenchyma. The affected parts of the organ are hypodense on NECT and show a mild, inhomogeneous enhancement without perfusion defects on CECT. The organ's contour becomes blurred, and Gerota's capsule thickened. The adjacent fat-tissue can be normal or shows peripancreatic stranding and varying amounts of non-enhanced, hypodense (<15 HU) fluid collections (serous-exudative pancreatitis). Inflammatory peripancreatic exudation may have a diffuse appearance, whereas the necrotic peripancreatic fat tissue is typically better delineated and slightly increased in density due to debris (>25 HU). Nevertheless, inflammatory peripancreatic exudation and necrotic peripancreatic fat tissue might coexist and difficult to distinguish.

Necrotizing pancreatitis (Figs. 3, 4). There is an obvious alteration of the organ's contour and internal structure. The pancreatic gland appears inhomogeneous, enlarged, and unclearly demarcated. The presence of hypodense, necrotic diffuse, or focal areas is prominent at this stage. Unaffected parenchyma is isodense, and hemorrhage hyperdense on NECT. Necrotic tissue (unenhanced) can be distinguished from vital parenchyma (contrast-enhanced) on CECT. The extent of peripancreatic exudation and/or necrosis of fat tissue is significantly larger than in IOP. The early identification of necrotic areas is crucial; whereas the mortality rate of IOP is <1%, it increases dramatically, up to 23%, in NP (Balthazar 2002).

2.1.3 Complications of Acute Pancreatitis

2.1.3.1 Pathophysiology and Anatomical Routes of Inflammatory Expansion

The broadening of inflammation usually follows the anatomically preformed pathways: (a) retroperitoneal expansion into the anterior pararenal space along Gerota's capsule, the parietal peritoneum, the mesenterium, and the gastrohepatic, gastrosplenic, and along the gastrocolic ligaments; (b) penetration into the intraperitoneal and perirenal spaces and the mediastinum after enzymatic destruction of the anatomic fascial borders. The exudative phase is followed by the resorptive phase, according to the pathophysiology of the inflammation (duration: weeks–months). Granulation tissue might occur at the periphery of the necrosis, with the formation of pseudocysts by encapsulation (duration: at least 4 weeks).

2.1.3.2 Local and Systemic Complications

The complications of AP can be grouped as local and systemic; the former can be further subdivided into

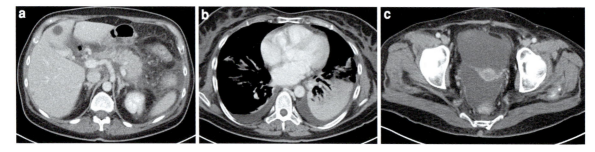

Fig. 2 Interstitial edematous pancreatitis. **a** Pancreatic enlargement, peripancreatic fluid collections; **b** pleural effusion; **c** intra-abdominal fluid in the pouch of douglas

early (acute fluid collection, vascular complications, infected necrosis) and late (pseudocysts, pancreatic / peripancreatic abscess) sequelae.

Acute fluid collection occur depending on the inflammatory expansion and comprise ascites and pleural and pericardial effusions. However, the activity of digestive enzymes also plays an important role regarding the peripancreatic vessels. Small erosions can lead to bleeding. Over time, pseudoaneurysms, especially involving the splenic artery, are also detected in up to 10% of patients with AP. Thrombotic occlusions affect the venous system, particularly the splenic vein. Following bacterial contamination, pancreatic necrosis can progress to an infected necrosis, which can be detected as a non-enhanced area on CECT. The majority of these cases develop during the second and third week (Bollen et al. 2007a). The distinction between an infected and uninfected necrotic area is often impossible by imaging, but the distinction is essential because infected necrosis, if untreated, is fatal. An intranecrotic air collection strongly supports the suspicion of secondary infection, but can also be caused by an evolved fistula or iatrogenically. Pseudocysts are collections of pancreatic secretion enclosed by a non-epithelialized wall; they are seen as spherical-shaped semi-liquid fluid collections (0–25 HU) with a contrast-enhanced margin (granulation tissue). A pseudocyst that contains pus is defined as a pancreatic abscess, which has a (semi-) liquid center and a contrast-enhanced wall, neither of which is seen in infected necrosis. Intracystic air might also indicate secondary infection. In contrast to infected necrosis, a pancreatic abscess contains little or no necrotic areas. The reliability of imaging modalities in diagnosing these infections is poor and microbiological testing is thus required. Moreover, further signs of an acute inflammation, such as peripancreatic stranding

Table 6 Differential diagnosis

Differential diagnosis: pancreatic mass and/or fat tissue infiltration
Pancreatitis
Pancreatic neoplasm
Perforation of a duodenal ulcer

or exudation, have usually decayed by the time an abscess appears. Whereas sterile fluid collections, pseudocysts, and necroses can be treated conservatively, US- or CT-guided drainage is a proper diagnostic and even therapeutic concept in case of infection.

Systemic complications such as sepsis, acute renal failure, and diabetes cannot be visualized by radiological imaging. The involvement of the adjacent gastrointestinal tract might cause peritonitis or paralytic ileus, which might show indirect signs, such as ascites, affected bowel loops, and/or pathological intestinal fluid levels.

2.1.4 Differentials

Most differential diagnoses of AP are based on its cardinal symptom "pain" and are summarized as the "acute abdomen," discussed extensively in this volume. The main differentials in imaging are: (a) inflammatory processes involving the adjacent organs, in particular the duodenum or stomach, which cause unspecific changes in fat tissue; (b) perforation of a duodenal or gastric ulcer, which might show extra luminal fluid collections; and (c) pancreatic neoplasms and attacks of chronic pancreatitis (Table 6).

2.1.4.1 Hemorrhagic Pancreatitis

An extremely rare variety of severe AP is hemorrhagic pancreatitis, which while characterized by intraparenchymal hemorrhage, lacks a uniform definition. Only a

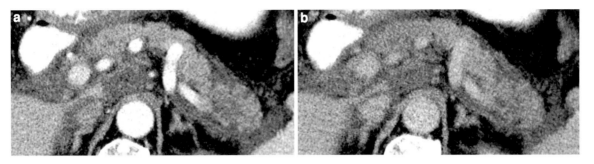

Fig. 3 Acute pancreatitis: severe AP with necrosis in the pancreatic tail; in a biphasic CT scan (**a** arterial phase, **b** venous phase), arterial phase better delineates the hypodense necrosis

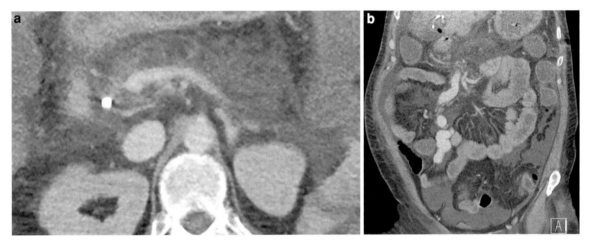

Fig. 4 Acute pancreatitis. **a** Severe necrotizing AP affecting >50% of the parenchyma. **b** A large-volume of intra-abdominal fluid collection

few, predominantly post-mortem cases have been reported in the literature (Bollen et al. 2007b). According to the Atlanta Classification, the term "hemorrhagic pancreatitis" should be restricted to descriptions of the operative or post-mortem appearance of the gland (Bradley et al. 1998).

2.2 Chronic Pancreatitis

2.2.1 Terminology and Clinical Issues

2.2.1.1 Overview and Etiology

Chronic pancreatitis is a recurrent, progressive inflammation of the pancreatic gland with morphological destruction and the replacement of the parenchyma by fibrosis, which can lead to failure of the pancreas' exocrine and endocrine functions.

While chronic alcoholism is the most common cause, 30–40% of all cases are considered to be idiopathic in origin (Steer et al. 1995); together these two etiologies account for 90–95% of all cases (Braganza et al. 2011). The various other causes are rare and include exposure to toxic substances such as cigarette smoke, hypocalcemia, hyperlipidemia, infections (e.g., HIV), hereditary disease (e.g., cystic fibrosis), autoimmunity, post-transplantation, vascular alterations, and structural changes of the pancreatic duct. However, the pathogenesis underlying these triggers is unclear. The mortality rate of patients with CP is up to 50% within 20–25 years after disease onset (Braganza et al. 2011); moreover, there is an elevated risk of pancreatic cancer (Lowenfels et al. 1993). Pathohistological findings are chronic inflammation, parenchymal fibrosis with ductal strictures, dilatation, calculi, and atrophy of the acinar and islet tissues.

The main challenge in the diagnosis of CP is the reliable identification at an early stage, as the macroscopic changes are subtle and thus not always visible in radiological imaging. Since the early changes are distributed in patches, needle biopsy might lead to false-negative results (Braganza et al. 2011).

2.2.1.2 Clinical Features

Alcohol-induced CP has its epidemiological peak in men between the ages of 40–50 years (Braganza et al. 2011). Recurrent epigastric pain, which occurs suddenly or evolves continuously, is the chief complaint. The pain sometimes mimics that reported by AP patients; however, a history of previous episodes of abdominal pain and alcoholism suggest the diagnosis of a chronic pancreatic inflammation. In some 10–15% of CP patients, especially those with idiopathic or autoimmune diseases, symptoms other than pain, including steatorrhea, diabetes, and jaundice, are noted. Additionally, signs of malnutrition due to pancreatic dysfunction as well as clinical signs due to acute complications are reported (Braganza et al. 2011).

2.2.1.3 Laboratory Findings

In addition to laboratory tests of endocrine or exocrine pancreatic failure and for etiological indicators, the pancreatic enzymes lipase and amylase are useful for the diagnosis of an acute, recurrent process. In contrast to AP, there is no generally accepted classification system that takes recent developments in imaging, such as MDCT, into account, because morphological changes have been difficult to correlate with pancreatic function. The international Cambridge Classification, drawing on ERCP findings, was developed in 1984 but its clinical relevance is limited as there is no clinical correlation. Recent classification systems are mainly based on clinical features and have been used to distinguish between an early stage, an intermediate stage with complications, and an end stage with fibrosis and loss of pancreatic function (Braganza et al. 2011).

2.2.2 Imaging

2.2.2.1 Ultrasound

Typical findings are pancreatic calculi, detected as disseminated hyperechoic foci with facultative acoustic shadowing in 40% of patients (Alpern et al. 1985). A late sign is a heterogeneous mixture of hyper- and hypoechoic pancreatic parenchyma, representing

fibrosis or calcifications and areas of inflammation, respectively. Up to 40% of patients will have a focal hypoechoic mass with an irregular, winding pancreatic duct; in such cases differentiation from pancreatic malignant tumor is difficult. Alternating constrictions and dilatations of the pancreatic duct can be caused by ductal strictures ("chain of lakes" sign) (Alpern et al. 1985). Pancreatic pseudocysts are reported in 25–40% of all cases (Alpern et al. 1985). Vascular changes can be identified using Doppler sonography.

On EUS, discreet signs of early CP can be identified that are often missed by transabdominal ultrasound or CT. These include heterogenous parenchymal echogenicity with subtle globularity of the pancreatic margin, slight cystic changes of the parenchyma, fibrotic interlobular septa (hyperechoic reticulation), ductal changes (hyperechoic margins, ectatic side-branches, intraductal calcifications, ductal dilatation >3 mm, and irregularity) (Wallace and Hawes 2001). The main limitations of EUS, however, are the examiner's dependency and a potential overestimation of the changes, with subsequent false-positive results.

2.2.2.2 MRI, MRCP, and ERCP

Magnetic resonance technology is increasingly being used in the imaging of CP due to recent advances and the proven diagnostic value of MRCP for the pancreatic duct system. Due to its excellent soft-tissue contrast, MRI has superior sensitivity, with signal alterations occurring at early stages of CP while the CT findings are still normal. These early MRI findings are: (a) loss of high signal intensity of the pancreatic parenchyma on T1w fat-suppressed images, (b) decreased, inhomogeneous contrast enhancement in the arterial phase, (c) augmented enhancement in delayed phases, and (d) dilated side branches (Miller et al. 2004). Late MRI findings include atrophy or enlargement, pseudocysts, and parenchymal calcifications (Miller et al. 2004). Even if CT detects calcifications more sensitively, MRI allows for a better distinction of intraductal and intraparenchymal calculi.

In addition, MRCP provides excellently depicts the pancreatic and common bile ducts. The typical sign is a dilated, irregular pancreatic duct and its side branches both of which often contain calcifications and appear as signal-void filling defects, while the pancreatic secretions are hyperintense. Similar to US, the alternating areas of constriction and dilatation of the pancreatic duct manifest as the "chain of lakes"

Fig. 5 Complicated chronic pancreatitis. Parenchymal calcifications as a sign of CP; acute inflammation of the pancreatic head, with blurry margins and peripancreatic exudation caused by an intraductal calculi (detected by MRCP as a flow void)

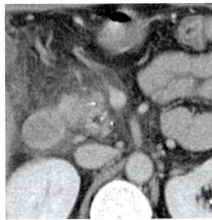 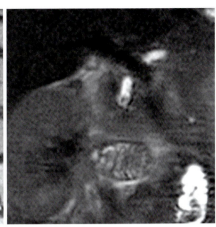

sign (Miller et al. 2004). Other findings include pseudocyst, fistulas, and strictures or ductal obstructions, with resulting congestion of the bile duct (Leyendecker et al. 2002). Intravenous administration of secretin can in some cases improve visualization of the duct system by increasing the tonus of the sphincter of Oddi, thus allowing a non-invasive evaluation of exocrine pancreatic function (Fukukura et al. 2002). Nevertheless, ERCP is considered the gold standard for the detection of pancreatic duct system abnormalities. Invasiveness and an association with acute, post-interventional pancreatitis in up to 4% of patients (Mitchell et al. 2003) have triggered the increasing replacement of ERCP by MRCP, which also has been shown to be superior to ERCP in the identification of the main pancreatic duct, with an overall sensitivity and specificity for delineating pathologic pancreatic alterations of 88% and 98%, respectively (Tamura et al. 2006).

MRI has a superior sensitivity for the detection and characterization of post-pancreatitis pseudocysts. Complex pseudocysts with hemorrhagic or pertinacious content show a hyperintense signal on T1w images. Within a single MRI examination, vascular complications, including splenic artery pseudoaneurysms and splenic or portal vein thrombosis, can be detected.

2.2.2.3 MDCT

In patients with CP, the detection of acute complications and/or signs of long-standing CP is readily accomplished by CT. However, early changes can remain undetected since, at this stage, in 10% of patients the morphology of the pancreas is normal. Typical findings of CP are an irregular, dilated pancreatic duct and an atrophic pancreatic gland,

occurring in 68 and 54% of all cases, respectively. In contrast, age-depending pancreatic involution is usually not associated with ductal alterations. The chronic inflammatory process might cause intra-/periductal calcifications, which are considered as most specific (50% of patients), or a focal inflammatory mass (30% of patients) (Luetmer et al. 1989).

2.2.3 Complications of Chronic Pancreatitis

An acute exacerbation of CP can cause the same local and systemic complications as AP, with its typical findings of pancreatic enlargement, contrast enhancement, or peripancreatic stranding. Intra- or extrapancreatic pseudocysts occur in about 30% of all patients with CP and usually resolve spontaneously, but may also cause further complications: infection (abscess), hemorrhage, gastric or biliary obstruction, or fistulae formation. In general, pancreatic fistula is a rare complication and originates from a ruptured pancreatic duct. Besides abdominal inflammation, the fistula can affect the mediastinal or pleural space by spreading through the aortic or esophageal hiatus or the diaphragm.

2.2.4 Differentials

2.2.4.1 Pancreatic Inammatory Mass and Pancreatic Cancer

Chronic pancreatitis and pancreatic neoplasms, such as pancreatic or ampullary carcinoma or cholangiocarcinoma, can present similar clinical symptoms as well as imaging features. Chronic inflammatory mass of the pancreatic head can mimic pancreatic adenocarcinoma, especially if non-calcified. Both entities may be hypointense on MRI and hypodense on CT,

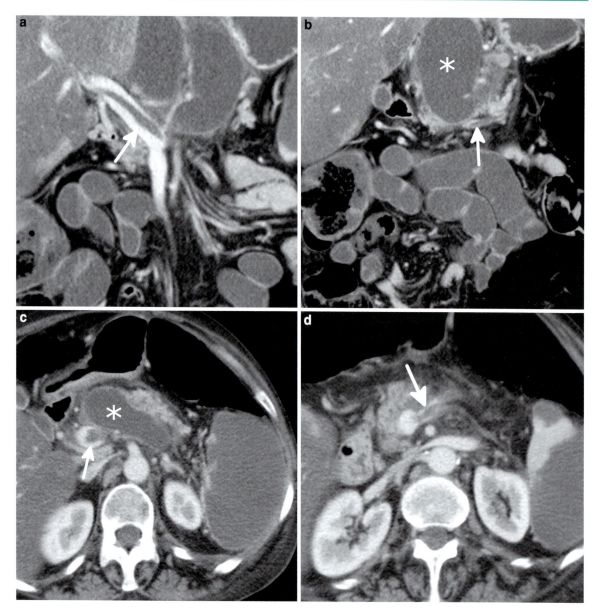

Fig. 6 Complications of chronic pancreatitis. Thrombosis of the splenic and portal veins (*white arrows*); non-homogeneous liver parenchyma due to perfusion deficits; hypodense lesions within the pancreas (pseudocysts; *asterixis*); cystic transformation of the spleen, probably secondary to splenic infarction

with dilatation of both the common bile duct and the pancreatic duct ("double duct" sign) (Table 7). Further similarities include ductal strictures, infiltration of the peripancreatic fat tissue, arterial wrapping, and venous obstruction. The "duct-penetrating" sign (non-dilated, funneling ducts running through the mass), an irregular pancreatic duct, and calculi are considered to be specific findings for a benign inflammatory mass (Ichikawa et al. 2001). In contrast, a prompt interruption of the duct is associated with malignancy. The distinction between CP and pancreatic cancer is further complicated by the fact that the two can occur simultaneously, so that malignancy cannot be ruled out safely based on imaging findings alone. PET/CT can be helpful to rule out malignancies if the diagnosis remains unclear. CT- or EUS-guided biopsy can aid in the histological evaluation.

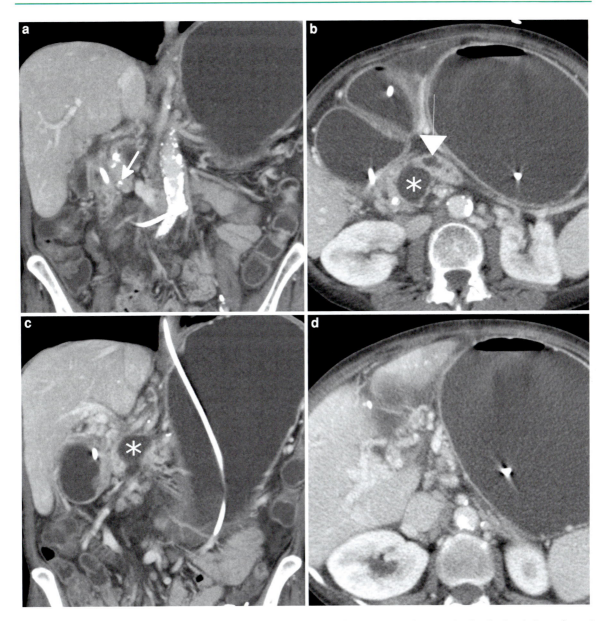

Fig. 7 Complications of chronic pancreatitis. **a** Parenchymal calcifications as a typical finding in CP (*arrow*); **b, c** formation of an pseudocyst (*asterixis*); dilatation of the pancreatic duct (*arrow head*); duodenal stenosis with resulting gastric dilatation, treatment via gastroduodenal tube; **d** signs of portal vein thrombosis: missing CM enhancement at the hepatic hilum and extensive venous bypassing (cavernous transformation)

Table 7 Differential diagnosis of benign and malignant alterations of the pancreatic duct system on MRI

	CP with inflammatory mass	Neoplasm, e.g. adenocarcinoma, intraductal mucinous tumor
"Double-duct" sign	(+)	+
"Duct-penetrating" sign	+	–
Ductal morphology	Gradual funneling, strictures	Abrupt interruption

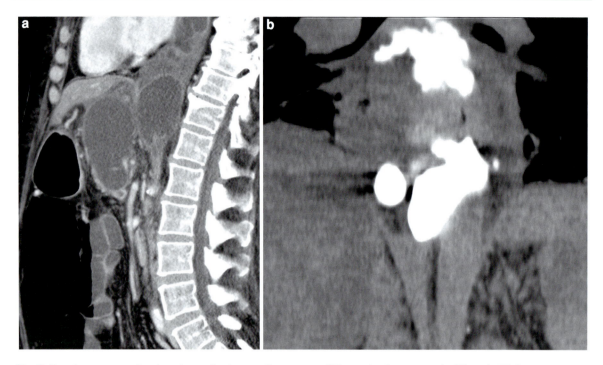

Fig. 8 Pseudocysts expanding into the mediastinum. **a** Portovenous CT scan; **b** after retrograde filling via ERCP

2.2.4.2 Autoimmune Pancreatitis

In this form of pancreatitis, there is autoimmune inflammation with an infiltration of lymphoplasmatic cells and fibrosis. Autoimmune pancreatitis can resemble CP but without the latter's typical attacks of pain. It is often associated with other autoimmune diseases, e.g. sclerosing cholangitis or primary biliary cirrhosis. Laboratory findings show elevated immune markers and there is marked response to steroids. Typical CT findings are a diffuse parenchymal enlargement with homogeneous iso- or hypoattenuation and loss of lobular architecture ("sausage" shape). The pancreatic duct can be non-dilated or diffusely narrowed and the margins show hypoattenuation with delayed enhancement. The extent of fibrosis and lymphocytic infiltration is variable. Peripancreatic stranding, regional lymphadenopathy, or a pancreatic inflammatory mass make it difficult to distinguish autoimmune pancreatitis from other types of pancreatitis or pancreatic neoplasms sometimes. In contrast to the typical appearance of CP, calculi, pseudocysts formation, and vascular sheathing are uncommon (Shanbhogue et al. 2009).

3 Traumatic Emergencies: Pancreatic Trauma Trauma

3.1 Terminology and Clinical Issues

3.1.1 Overview and Etiology

Blunt pancreatic trauma accounts for <2% of all abdominal injuries. In most cases (50–98%), there are concomitant injuries, especially those involving the liver (46.8% of cases), but gastric (42.3%), major vascular (41.3%), splenic (28.0%), renal (23.4%), and duodenal (19.3%) injuries are also frequently noted. Isolated injury of the pancreas is seldom because of the high-energy mechanism of trauma and the central location of the pancreas (Linsenmaier et al. 2008). In addition to coexisting injuries, the main influencing factors of patients' outcome are the mechanism of trauma, the time to diagnosis, and the presence or absence of major ductal injury. As imaging findings are subtle, the correct diagnosis might be deferred. The resulting delays in diagnosis, missed findings, an incorrect classification of the injury, and/or delays in treatment can increase morbidity and mortality

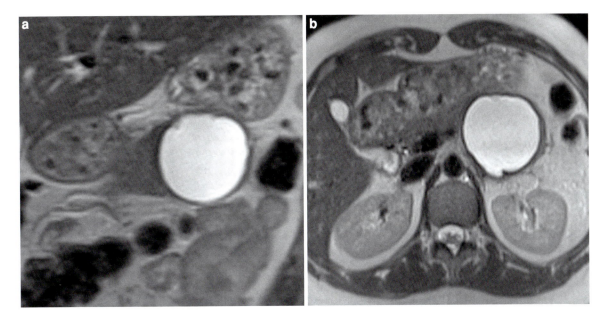

Fig. 9 Typical MRI appearance of a (post-traumatic) pseudocyst

considerably (Jurkovich 2000). Indeed, a delay of the correct diagnosis for more than 24 h is a risk factor for death in up to 40% of patients, as opposed to 11% of those patients who undergo surgery within 24 h (Lucas and Ledgerwood 1975; Heitsch et al. 1976; Smego et al. 1985). In general, morbidity and mortality after pancreatic trauma are notably high; with mortality ranging from 9 to 34%, although in only 5% of these cases is the pancreatic injury directly related to the fatal outcome. Morbidity ranges between 11 and 62%, covering the entire spectrum of complications. Post-traumatic complications occur in 30–60% of all cases.

The first 48 h after pancreatic injury (early phase) are crucial in terms of the clinical course, because hemorrhage from splenic, hepatic, or vascular injuries is to be expected in most patients (Linsenmaier et al. 2008; Gupta et al. 2004). Fatal hemorrhage and substantial coexisting injuries are responsible for deaths during the early phase, and infections and MOF during the subsequent period. About one-third of the early-phase survivors suffer from post-traumatic complications, such as pancreatitis, pseudocysts, fistulas, and intra-abdominal abscesses. Moreover, pneumonia and anastomotic insufficiency after additional duodenal injury are commonly reported and can also lead to MOF and septicemia. About one-third of the late deaths are directly attributable to the pancreatic trauma and usually occur during the first 3 weeks or later.

3.1.2 Mechanisms of Injury

The pancreas is naturally protected due to its retroperitoneal location within surrounding fat tissue. Children are at risk because the peripancreatic fat is thinner. Usually, a severe compression trauma against the spinal column is necessary to cause pancreatic injuries. The typical situation is a traffic accident, in which there is a direct impact of the steering wheel or handlebar on the upper abdomen, seat-belt-related injuries, or deceleration trauma. Sports injuries, falls, and blows to the upper abdomen are less common as mechanisms of injury. The pancreatic body is most often affected in blunt trauma (>65%). If the pancreatic head or uncinate process is involved, there is likely to also be injuries to the descending and transverse portions of the duodenum, or to the liver, bile duct, gallbladder, right kidney, or ascending colon. Force exerted on the left upper quadrant results mainly in injuries to the pancreatic body or tail. Coexisting injuries can affect the transverse and ascending portions of the duodenum, the spleen, stomach, and left kidney.

3.1.3 Clinical Features

As pancreatic trauma occurs regularly in multiple-injured patients, the clinical presentation might be confused by the symptoms of the concomitant injuries. The pain may be variable, non-specific, or sometimes absent. Even major pancreatic injuries can occur with initially minimal epigastric symptoms. A reliable history is desirable, but difficult to obtain in an emergency situation (Venkatesh and Wan 2008).

3.1.4 Laboratory Findings

Besides upper abdominal pain, leukocytosis and raised serum amylase activity complete the clinical triad, but these findings may be absent within the first few days. The analysis of serum amylase activity provides vital information, if it is raised, since it typically remains normal for 2–48 h after an injury in up to 40% of cases, a retest is recommended and serial testing can monitor the course of injury. As amylase is also secreted from other salivary glands, it is considered non-specific for pancreatic injury, as is the activity of serum lipase. The accuracy of trypsinogen-activating peptide levels has not been fully evaluated so far (Bradley et al. 1998; Greenlee and Murphy 1984; White and Benfield 1972).

3.1.5 Grading of Pancreatic Injuries

The most widely accepted classification system was published by the American Association for the Surgery of Trauma (AAST) and offers five grades (I–V) for assessing hematomas, contusions, lacerations with and without ductal involvement, and complete disruption of the organ as well as the site of the injuries (Table 8) (Moore et al. 1990). Major variables for pancreatic injury are anatomic site (proximal vs. distal); the type of injury, such as hematoma, laceration, or transection; and the state of the main pancreatic duct. The grading of pancreatic injuries aims to standardize CT diagnoses and to serve as a rationale for objective management. The grading system correlates with patient outcome: the mean morbidity in patients with pancreatic trauma is 36%, with a mortality for injuries graded I and II of around 7%. However, mortality increases dramatically with grade III and IV injuries, to about 29% (Linsenmaier et al. 2008; Venkatesh and Wan 2008).

3.2 Imaging

3.2.1 Ultrasound

The pancreatic region is routinely not included in the FAST (focused assessment with sonography for trauma) examination. Furthermore, subtle injuries such as a contusion or a small rupture are frequently overlooked. In general, there is little evidence supporting the diagnostic accuracy of US in the detection of pancreatic injuries: sensitivity is unacceptably low at 44–71%, whereas specificity can reach 100% (Körner et al. 2008).

3.2.2 ERCP and MRCP

There are no general recommendations regarding the use of ERCP or MRCP in the diagnostic workup of pancreatic or biliary duct injury. ERCP, however, allows the placement of pancreatic duct stents. It has also been used postoperatively after laparotomy in cases of persistent leakage of pancreatic fluid and in those in which there is posttraumatic strictures of the pancreatic duct. Clinically stable conditions are usually required for MRCP and ERCP, but NECT can be performed optionally after ERCP to demonstrate duct injuries in unclear cases (Linsenmaier et al. 2008; Soto et al. 2001).

3.2.3 MDCT

Computed tomography is the first-line imaging tool in patients with pancreatic and concomitant injuries, as it is the safest and most comprehensive means of diagnosis. Combined scans with a standard portal-venous phase of the abdomen and CT angiography of the thorax and upper abdomen are routinely used in whole-body CT of multiple-injured patients. An additional pancreatic parenchymal phase is recommended for follow-up CT or in cases of equivocal initial CT findings. The administration of contrast material, with a resulting optimal enhancement, can increase the sensitivity of CT in the detection of subtle parenchymal injuries. An optional delayed phase after 2–3 min is recommended in cases of suspected active abdominal bleeding, such as pancreatic hemorrhage. In general, the use of multiplanar reformation, thin-slice axial images, or pancreatic parenchymal phase can improve diagnostic confidence (Linsenmaier et al. 2008).

3.2.3.1 CT Findings in Pancreatic Injury

The correct and early diagnosis of pancreatic trauma is essential for injured patients because of the influence on prognosis. The initial CT scan of 20–40% patients with pancreatic injuries may be without pathological findings within the first 12 h after the injury. Diagnostic sensitivity and specificity are reported to be around 80% with spiral CT. In general,

Table 8 AAST injury grading

Grade	Injury	Description
I	Hematoma	Minor contusion without duct injury
	Laceration	Superficial laceration without duct injury
II	Hematoma	Major contusion without ductal injury
	Laceration	Major laceration without ductal injury or tissue loss
III	Laceration	Distal transection or parenchymal injury with duct injury
IV	Laceration	Proximal transection or parenchymal injury involving ampulla
V	Laceration	Massive disruption of pancreatic head

CT tends to underestimate the grade of injury, while modern MDCT has been shown, in a few reports, to be superior, with improved diagnostic characteristics (Linsenmaier et al. 2008; Venkatesh and Wan 2008; Rekhi et al. 2010).

A normal appearance of the pancreas does not exclude pancreatic trauma as CT findings may be subtle or slow to develop. A thin layer of peripancreatic fat tissue adversely affects the detection of pancreatic injuries by CT, as it can obscure pathologic alterations of the surrounding tissue that might provide diagnostic clues.

There are a few specific signs of pancreatic trauma: fractures or lacerations of the pancreatic tissue, the presence of parenchymal edema or hematoma active bleeding, and blood collections between the parenchyma and the splenic vein. Pancreatic fractures or lacerations appear as hypoattenuating linear findings, ideally with separated structures, whereas pancreatic contusions are visualized as a diffuse or localized hypoattenuating area within the normal parenchyma. Complete disruption of the pancreas can result in extended hypoperfusion of the entire organ. Areas of mixed or slightly increased attenuation within the pancreatic gland or adjacent tissue are signs of a pancreatic hematoma; in up to 90% of cases, focal fluid collections can be found in the space between the pancreas and the splenic vein.

The integrity of the pancreatic duct is the most crucial parameter in the decision whether surgery is required. Ductal injuries can be detected by MDCT with a sensitivity of up to 91%; in particular, in case of severe pancreatic laceration involving more than half of the organ's diameter, ductal injury has to be suspected. Extravasation of contrast material from the pancreatic duct can be shown by curved-plane reformation along the pancreatic duct and NECT after

Table 9 Differential diagnosis of cystic pancreatic lesions

Pancreatic pseudocyst

Pancreatic neoplasm (serous cystadenoma, mucinous cystic tumor, intraductal papillary mucinous tumor)

Congenital cyst

ERCP. As a second-line diagnostic tool, MRI can be used in combination with MRCP and ERCP in order to ascertain ductal integrity.

3.3 Complications of Pancreatic Trauma

Pancreatic fistulas (23%), post-traumatic pancreatitis (10%), and the formation of pseudocysts (5%) account for the most common post-traumatic complications. Post-traumatic internal pancreatic fistulas can be formed between the pancreas and adjacent organs or spaces and structures. They are defined as extra-anatomic connections with a continuing leakage of pancreatic secretions from disrupted pancreatic ducts. Post-traumatic pancreatitis as well as post-traumatic pancreatic pseudocysts cannot be differentiated from non-traumatic inflammation and pseudocysts, respectively, based on imaging features (Table 9).

4 Postoperative Changes: Pancreatic Resection

Pancreatic surgery is usually indicated in patients with pancreatic cancer, and less frequently in those with CP, pancreatic trauma or periampullary tumors. Depending on the indication, surgery may consist of partial or full resection of the pancreatic gland, perhaps accompanied

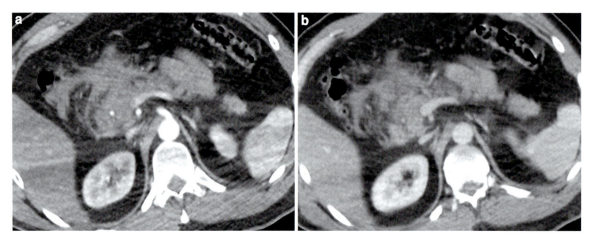

Fig. 10 Pancreatic trauma grade I: initial whole-body CT scan shows contusion of the pancreatic head and body; **a** arterial phase, **b** venous phase

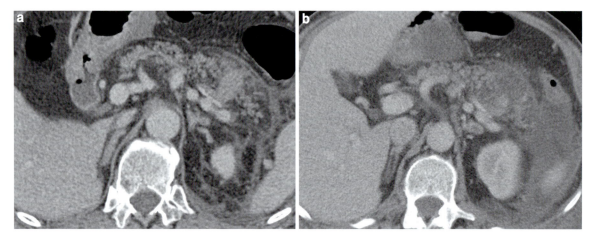

Fig. 11 Pancreatic trauma grade I. **a** Initial whole-body CT scan shows a parenchymal hematoma of the pancreatic tail; **b** follow-up scan 5 days later demonstrates the progressive hematoma

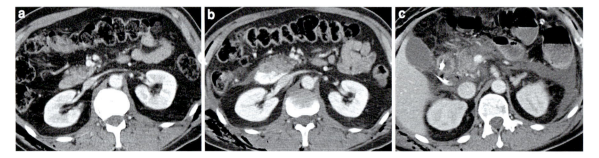

Fig. 12 Pancreatic trauma grade II. **a** Initial whole-body CT scan without signs of pancreatic injury; **b** follow-up scan after 4.5 h shows active contrast extravasation; **c** follow-up scan 4 days later demonstrates post-traumatic pancreatitis

by resection of adjacent organs and resulting in the construction of anastomoses. Pancreatico-duodenectomy ("Whipple procedure") is the standard procedure for malignancy of the pancreatic head and carcinoma of the periampullary region. The classic Whipple procedure involves resection of the pancreatic head

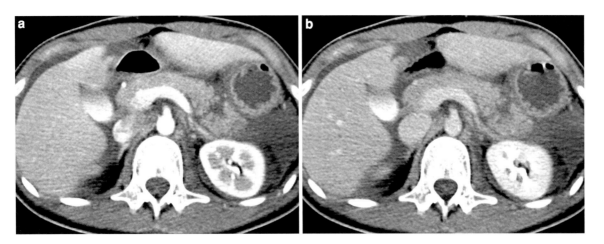

Fig. 13 Pancreatic trauma grade III. Initial whole-body CT scan shows distal parenchymal injury with duct injury (**a** arterial phase, **b** venous phase)

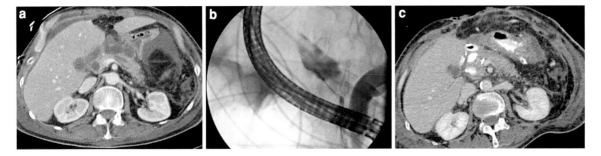

Fig. 14 Pancreatic trauma grade IV. **a** Initial whole-body CT scan shows proximal parenchymal injury with duct injury; **b** ERCP reveals extravasation from the pancreatic duct; **c** follow-up scan after stenting of the pancreatic duct

including the distal common bile duct, and of the duodenum, gallbladder, distal stomach, and local lymph nodes followed by a hepatico-jejunostomy, a pancreatico-jejunostomy, and a gastro-jejunostomy. The pylorus-preserving pancreatico-duodenectomy according to the Traverso-Longmire approach is a variant of the pancreatico-duodenectomy; it preserves the pylorus and the first 2 cm of the duodenum. Distal pancreatectomy is indicated for the resection of tumors of the left pancreatic body or tail and usually involves a splenectomy as well. A central pancreatectomy implies a Roux-en-Y pancreatico-jejunostomy, but there is no standard procedure. Total pancreaticotomy is another option for tumors of the pancreatic head. In contrast to the classic Whipple procedure, the entire pancreatic gland is removed. In general, imaging is indicated to detect postoperative complications or the local recurrence of the underlying disease.

US might detect indirect, but unspecific signs of postoperative complications, such as free intra-abdominal fluid or abscesses. Under ideal conditions, it may be able to identify a local recurrence or liver metastases.

The imaging modality of choice after pancreatic surgery is CT. Since the most common operation in patients requiring pancreatic cancer is the Whipple procedure, the associated postoperative changes have been well-documented.

The reliable identification of each anastomosis is the basis for image interpretation. Surgical clips can impair the diagnostic image quality by obscuring the surgical bed (Scialpi et al. 2005). Importantly, physiological CT features have to be distinguished from initial complications in the early postsurgical phase (Scialpi et al. 2005; Mortele et al. 2000). Pneumobilia or air in the biliary tree is detected in 67–80% of the patients postoperatively and helps to identify the hepatico-jejunostomy. Transient fluid collections,

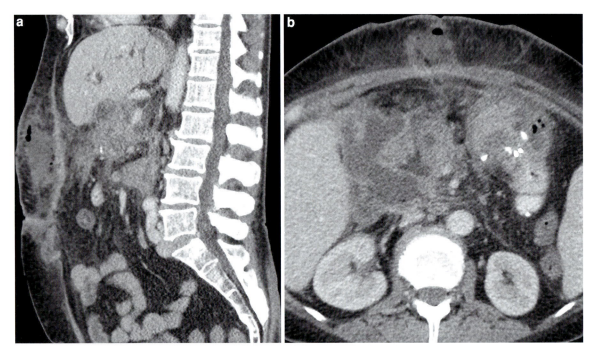

Fig. 15 Complications following a whipple procedure. **a** Abscess formation in the abdominal wall with consolidation and intralesional air. **b** Indirect signs of anastomotic leakage with perianastomic fluid and air collection; the gastro-jejunostomy can be safely identified by metallic surgical clips

defined as thin-walled or poorly delineated fluid collections, or perivascular cuffing, defined as hyperattenuating perivascular fat tissue, are present in about one-third and two-thirds of the patients, respectively. Reactive lymphadenopathy or dilated bile ducts are seen in about 30% of patients. In addition, there may be free abdominal air and edema of the fresh anastomosis. All these findings can be judged as changes within normal limits depending on the patient's clinical presentation, but should also regress continuously. An atrophic remnant of the pancreatic gland may develop after some time.

The early postoperative phase is defined as the first 30 days. During this period, patients are likely to undergo a CT examination because of persisting fever or hyperbilirubinemia (Scialpi et al. 2005). Typical CT findings are leakage of the anastomosis, intra-abdominal abscess, pancreatico-jejunal fistula, intra-abdominal bleeding, or remnant pancreatitis. Vascular complications, such as aneurysms or portal vein thrombosis, occur rarely. Anastomotic insufficiency should be suspected especially within the first 1–2 weeks; extraintestinal collocations of (positive)

oral contrast material is considered as a direct sign; indirect signs are perianastomotic fluid collections or pathologic extraintestinal air. Pancreatico-jejunal fistula is suspected clinically if the concentrations of pancreatic enzymes (amylase, lipase) in the drainage fluid exceed the serum concentration by at least a factor of three and the drainage volume is >10 mL 3 days after surgery. MRCP or ERCP can be used to visualize internal fistulae, and direct fistulography to confirm a pancreatico-cutaneous fistula. In contrast, MDCT may show inflammatory thickening along the fistula. Acute hemorrhage, such as due to (hepatic) artery injury, will be reflected in laboratory findings. In NECT, fresh blood is seen as a hyperdense fluid collection but its origin should be examined on biphasic CECT: in the arterial phase, the extravasation of contrast material is a direct sign of active bleeding whereas extra-anatomical pooling will be seen in the venous phase. Besides local infection of the surgical sutures, abdominal abscesses, peritonitis, and pancreatitis are reasons for postoperative inflammation. Typical locations of postsurgical abscesses are the surgical bed in the retroperitoneum, the liver, the abdominal wall, and the abdominal cavity. The differentiation between

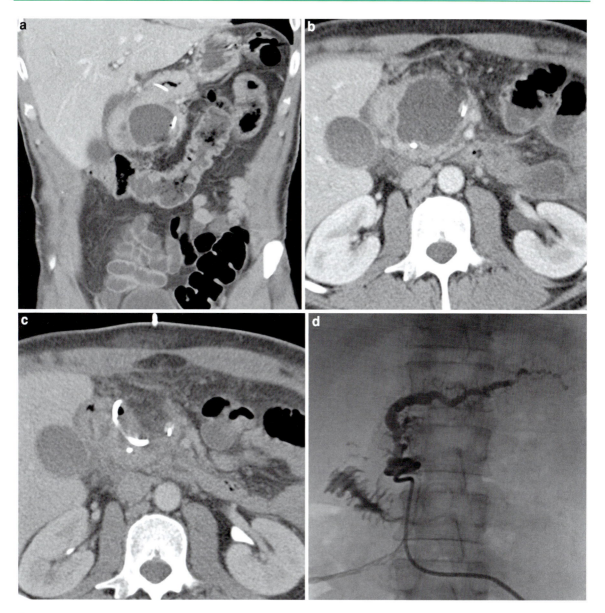

Fig. 16 Complications following pylorus-preserving pancreatico-duodenectomy: **a, b** Pseudocyst in the surgical bed; clinical suspicion of fistula; **c** successful CT-guided drainage and aspiration of a turbid secretion; **d** retrograde fistulography with depiction of the pancreatic duct and opacification of the intestinal tract

an initial stage of abscess formation and harmless postoperative fluid collections is challenging and might require microbiological testing after puncturing the site of the suspected abscess. The administration of positive oral contrast material might improve the detection of a hypodense abscess. Peritonitis appears as a thickening and hyperattenuation of the peritoneum and intra-abdominal fasciae accompanied by non-specific imbibition by fat tissue and by ascites. Postoperative pancreatitis shows the typical CT findings described in this chapter. Moreover, constricting anastomoses or scarred stenoses can evolve during the early and late phases. Typical CT findings are the dilatation of bowel loops or the distal stomach proximal to the gastrointestinal anastomosis or a dilated biliary tree if the hepatico-jejunostomy is affected. Late

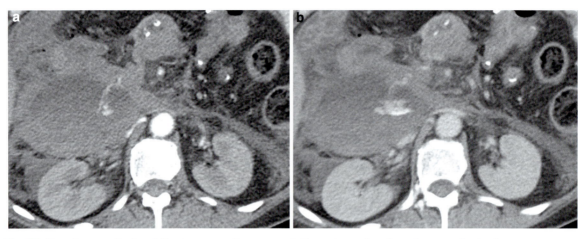

Fig. 17 Vascular complication following pancreatic surgery. Active extravasation from the gastroduodenal artery is seen on arterial phase (**a**) and increased extravasal volume on venous phase (**b**)

complications comprise chronic fistula, anastomotic stenosis, peri-anastomotic ulcers, bilioma, abscess, and aneurysms (Scialpi et al. 2005).

References

Alpern MB, Sandler MA, Kellman GM et al (1985) Chronic pancreatitis: ultrasonic features. Radiology 155(1):215–219

Balthazar EJ (2002) Acute pancreatitis: assessment of severity with clinical and CT evaluation. Radiology 223(3):603–613

Bollen TL, van Santvoort HC, Besseling MGH et al (2007a) Update on acute pancreatitis: ultrasound, computed tomography, and magnetic resonance imaging features. Semin Ultrasound CT MR 28(5):371–383

Bollen TL, Besselink MG, van Santvoort HC et al (2007b) Toward an update of the atlanta classification on acute pancreatitis: review of new and abandoned terms. Pancreas 35(2):107–113

Bradley EL, 3rd (1993) A clinically based classification system for acute pancreatitis. In: Summary of the international symposium on acute pancreatitis, Atlanta, Ga, 11–13 Sept 1992. Arch Surg 128(5): 586–590

Bradley EL 3rd, Young PR Jr, Chang MC et al (1998) Diagnosis and initial management of blunt pancreatic trauma: guidelines from a multiinstitutional review. Ann Surg 227(6):861–869

Braganza JM, Lee SH et al (2011) Chronic pancreatitis. Lancet 377(9772):1184–1197

Frossard JL, Steer ML et al (2008) Acute pancreatitis. Lancet 371(9607):143–152

Fukukura Y, Fujiyoshi F, Sasaki M et al (2002) Pancreatic duct: morphologic evaluation with MR cholangiopancreatography after secretin stimulation. Radiology 222(3):674–680

Greenlee T, Murphy K (1984) Amylase isoenzymes in the evaluation of trauma patients. Am Surg 50(12):637–640

Gupta A, Stuhlfaut JW, Fleming KW et al (2004) Blunt trauma of the pancreas and biliary tract: a multimodality imaging approach to diagnosis. Radiographics 24(5):1381–1395

Heitsch RC, Knutson CO, Fulton RL et al (1976) Delineation of critical factors in the treatment of pancreatic trauma. Surgery 80(4):523–529

Ichikawa T, Sou H, Araki T et al (2001) Duct-penetrating sign at MRCP: usefulness for differentiating inflammatory pancreatic mass from pancreatic carcinomas. Radiology 221(1):107–116

Jurkovich GJ (2000) Duodenum and pancreas. In: Mattox KL, Feliciano DV, Moore EE (eds) Trauma. McGraw-Hill, New York, pp 735–762

Körner M, Krötz MM, Degenhart C et al (2008) Current role of emergency US in patients with major trauma. Radiographics 28(1):225–242

Leyendecker JR, Elsayes KM, Gratz B, Brown JJ (2002) MR cholangiopancreatography: spectrum of pancreatic duct abnormalities. AJR Am J Roentgenol 179(6):1465–1471

Linsenmaier U, Wirth S, Reiser M et al (2008) Diagnosis and classification of pancreatic and duodenal injuries in emergency radiology. Radiographics 28(6):1591–1602

Lowenfels AB, Maisonneuve P, DiMagno EP et al (1993) Pancreatitis and the risk of pancreatic cancer. International Pancreatitis Study Group. N Engl J Med 328(20):1433–1437

Lucas CE, Ledgerwood AM (1975) Factors influencing outcome after blunt duodenal injury. J Trauma 15(10): 839–846

Luetmer PH, Stephens DH, Ward EM (1989) Chronic pancreatitis: reassessment with current CT. Radiology 171(2): 353–357

Miller FH, Keppke AL, Wadhwa A et al (2004) MRI of pancreatitis and its complications: part 2, chronic pancreatitis. AJR Am J Roentgenol 183(6):1645–1652

Mitchell RM, Byrne MF, Baillie J (2003) Pancreatitis. Lancet 361(9367):1447–1455

Moore EE, Cogbill TH, Jurkovich GJ et al (1990) Organ injury scaling, II: pancreas, duodenum, small bowel, colon, and rectum. J Trauma 30(11):1427–1429

Mortele KJ, Lemmerling M, de Hemptinne B et al (2000) Postoperative findings following the Whipple procedure: determination of prevalence and morphologic abdominal CT features. Eur Radiol 10(1):123–128

Mortele KJ, Wiesner W, Intriere L et al (2004) A modified CT severity index for evaluating acute pancreatitis: improved correlation with patient outcome. AJR Am J Roentgenol 183(5): 1261–1265

Rekhi S, Anderson SW, Rhea JT et al (2010) Imaging of blunt pancreatic trauma. Emerg Radiol 17(1):13–19

Scialpi M, Scaglione M, Volterani L et al (2005) Imaging evaluation of post pancreatic surgery. Eur J Radiol 53(3):417–424

Shanbhogue AK, Fasih N, Surabhi V et al (2009) A clinical and radiologic review of uncommon types and causes of pancreatitis. Radiographics 29(4):1003–1026

Smego DR, Richardson JD, Flint LM (1985) Determinants of outcome in pancreatic trauma. J Trauma 25(8):771–776

Soto JA, Alvarez O, Munera F et al (2001) Traumatic disruption of the pancreatic duct: diagnosis with MR pancreatography. AJR Am J Roentgenol 176(1):175–178

Steer ML, Waxman I, Freedman S (1995) Chronic pancreatitis. N Engl J Med 332(22):1482–1490

Tamura R, Ishibashi T, Takahashi S (2006) Chronic pancreatitis: MRCP versus ERCP for quantitative caliber measurement and qualitative evaluation. Radiology 238(3):920–928

Venkatesh SK, Wan JM (2008) CT of blunt pancreatic trauma: a pictorial essay. Eur J Radiol 67(2):311–320

Wallace MB, Hawes RH (2001) Endoscopic ultrasound in the evaluation and treatment of chronic pancreatitis. Pancreas 23(1):26–35

Whitcomb DC (2006) Clinical practice. Acute pancreatitis. N Engl J Med 354(20):2142–2150

White PH, Benfield JR (1972) Amylase in the management of pancreatic trauma. Arch Surg 105(2):158–163

Kidney, Ureter, Adrenal Gland

Michael K. Scherr and Ulrich Linsenmaier

Contents

Abstract

Today, multidetector computer tomography (MDCT), with its fast gantry rotation, enables large body volumes to be scanned with high temporal and spatial resolution. The fast rates of data acquisition and reconstruction result in multiphase protocols with short time intervals between consecutive scan series following the administration of a single bolus of intravenous contrast material (CM). Large scans obtained within a single breath-hold are possible and even the image data of non-cooperative or emergency patients are of acceptable quality. The acquired thin-slice raw data with isotropic sub-millimeter voxels can be visualized using different reconstruction algorithms and reformatted in all three spatial planes. The advantages of MDCT in the imaging of urologic emergencies are the excellent visualization of acute arterial and venous pathologies, detailed assessment of adrenal and renal parenchyma, and the precise depiction of the urinary tract (Foley 2002). Thus, in trauma and non-trauma settings a highly informative visualization of parenchymal patterns, bleeding, inflammatory disease is provided, allowing the differentiation of obstructive, post-traumatic, or post-therapeutic pathologies along the upper and lower urinary tract and including the adjacent retroperitoneal structures. Based on these MDCT findings, adequate decision-making in acute trauma, therapy planning, and interventional or surgical procedure planning can be carried out.

M. K. Scherr (✉) · U. Linsenmaier
Department of Clinical Radiology,
Ludwig-Maximilians-University,
80336 Munich, Germany
e-mail: michael.scherr@med.uni-muenchen.de

M. Scaglione et al. (eds.), *Emergency Radiology of the Abdomen*,
Medical Radiology. Diagnostic Imaging,
DOI: 10.1007/174_2011_470, © Springer-Verlag Berlin Heidelberg 2012

1   Kidney and Ureter

1.1   Anatomy and General Imaging Considerations

1.1.1   Kidney

The size of the kidney in its craniocaudal diameter ranges from 9 to 13 cm, with the left kidney being slightly larger than the right one. The upper aspects of the kidneys are partially protected by the 11 and 12th ribs. The kidneys and the adrenal glands are surrounded by two layers of perirenal and pararenal fat and by the renal fascia, which help to cushion these organs. The kidneys are located posteriorly high in the retroperitoneum, overlying the transverse aponeurosis, diaphragm, quadratus lumborum muscle laterally and psoas major muscle medially. Severe hemorrhage from these muscles can occur with blunt and, more likely, with penetrating injuries. The left kidney is crossed anteriorly by the pancreatic tail and is located behind the lower splenic pole; thus, concomitant injuries to the left colon, stomach, spleen, and pancreas are common. The right kidney is in immediate contact with the duodenum and liver; these organs, as well as the adrenal glands bilaterally, are likewise commonly identified as concomitant injuries.

The renal arteries arise from the aorta at the level of lumbar vertebra, 2 cm below the origin of the superior mesenteric artery. The renal arterial blood supply consists of four segments: superior, middle, lower, and posterior. The segmental arteries further divide into lobar arteries. Approximately 25% of all kidneys are perfused by accessory arterial vessels of different diameters that originate from the abdominal aorta and end in the renal sinus or the upper or lower poles.

The venous drainage of the renal cortex follows the arcuate and interlobar veins, further joining to a main renal vein. The renal veins are usually positioned anterior to the arteries. The left renal vein is much longer than the right renal vein and receives further venous branches-the left adrenal vein, the left gonadal vein inferiorly, and often a posterior lumbar vein-before joining the inferior vena cava (IVC).

1.1.2   Ureter

The ureter arises medially from the renal pelvis, descends to the bladder on the psoas muscle, and crosses the pelvi-ureteric junction near the bifurcation of the iliac arteries, which it traverses. After descending further postero-inferiorly on the lateral pelvic wall, the ureter turns anteromedially to enter the bladder from the backside, at the vesico-ureteric junction. The ureteral blood supply is particularly important in trauma surgery; branches originate from the adrenal and renal arteries in the upper third, from the aorta and gonadal arteries in the middle third, and from pelvic vessels in the lower third. These branches supply an anastomotic chain usually with a longitudinal vessel along the ureter.

1.1.3   Imaging Protocol

In emergency and trauma settings, there are no restrictions concerning sensitivity and specificity based on low-dose protocols. Modern MDCT scanners already provide dose reduction techniques, either as part of the latest-generation detectors or through the use of sophisticated reconstruction algorithms. However, in more subtle but important diagnoses, especially discrete parenchymatous and vascular lesions, low-dose protocols and single-shot strategies are not appropriate. In fact, the only remaining task for a single low-dose scan approach is the clinically uncomplicated suspicion of urinary calculi along the genito-urinary tract.

Renal Contrast Phases

Urogenital emergencies are quickly evaluated using MDCT in different contrast phases, including specific variations to facilitate the diagnosis (Table 1). Optimal timing of the scan following CM administration is mandatory to achieve highly distinct contrast phases and will depend on the patient's cardiac output as well as the flow rate and total volume of the CM. The main components of a scanning protocol are a non-enhanced phase (neP), a nephrographic (almost portal venous phase , (pvP) phase (ngP), and an excretory phase (exP). These three scanning phases can be accompanied or replaced by prior low-dose neP, arterial CT angiography (artP), and an angionephrographic corticomedullary phase (cmP) (Scherr 2009).

Non-Enhanced Phase

The neP provides good delineation of hyperdense concrements along the upper and lower urinary tract and depicts further previously unsuspected findings such as a dilated ureter or collecting system. Non-enhanced scans already provide excellent anatomic

Table 1 Summary of the renal contrast phases in MDCT

Contrast phases	Non-enhanced phase	Non-enhanced phase low-dose	Arterial phase (CT-angiography of the kidney)	Angionephrographic/corticomedullary phase	Nephrographic phase (almost portal-venous)	Excretory phase
Abbreviation	neP	neP ld	artP	cmP	ngP	exP
Scan parameters						
Tube voltage (kV)	120					
Rotation time (s)	0.5					
Tube current (mAs)	50–300 dose-modulated at noise index 29	30, non-modulated, up to 60 in obesity	50–300 dose-modulated, noise index 29			
Collimation (mm)	0.33–0.625					
Normalized pitch	1					
Scan Field	Diaphragm to lower margin of symphysis	Diaphragm to lower margin of symphysis	Diaphragm to crista iliaca		Complete abdomen	Diaphragm to lower margin of symphysis
Scan direction	Craniocaudal					
Scans	1					1, additional if applicable
Reconstruction parameters						
Increment (mm)	4	2	4	4		2
Slice thickness (mm), primarily axial	5	2.5	5	5	2.5	2.5
Kernel	Standard					
Archiving strategy						
Primary reconstruction axial (mm)	5	2.5 or 5	2.5	5	5	2.5
Secondary reconstructions (mm)	Cor 3–5, sag 3–5	Cor 3, sag 3	Cor 3, sag 3, MIP cor/sag 10 mm, optional VR/SSD	Cor 3, sag 3		Cor 3, sag 3, MIP cor 100 mm, optional cMPR along ureter, VR, SSD
Contrast administration						
Concentration (mg iodine/ml)	0		300			

(continued)

Table 1 (continued)

Contrast phases	Non-enhanced phase	Non-enhanced phase low-dose	Arterial phase (CT-angiography of the kidney)	Angionephrographic/corticomedullary phase	Nephrographic phase (almost portal-venous)	Excretory phase
Abbreviation	neP	neP ld	artP	cmP	ngP	exP
Volume (ml)	0	0	1.5/kg body weight			
Injection rate (ml/s)	0	0	4	3–4		4
Saline flush (ml NaCl; ml/s)	0	0	50; 4	50; 3–4		50; 4
Scan delay (s)	0	0	Bolus tracking aorta at height of renal pedicle +0, or at 15–20	Bolus tracking aorta at height of renal pedicle +20, or at 30–40	Bolus tracking aorta at height of renal pedicle +60, or at 75–100	Minimum 300; better after 450; optional additional scan after 1200
Oral or rectal contrast	0		Optional positive oral and/or rectal			0

cor Coronal, *sag* sagittal, *VR* volume-rendering, *SSD* shaded surface display, MIP maximum-intensity projection, *cMPR* curved multiplanar reconstruction

orientation in the retroperitoneum, allowing the detection of the increased density in hematoma and the lower densities characteristic of other fluid collections, in addition to providing baseline density measurements of renal masses (for instance, complex cystic lesions or verification of fatty tissue in angiomyolipoma or adenoma). When the exclusive diagnostic issue in a young patient is the detection of calculi, a low-dose protocol might be sufficient despite the reduced assessment of parenchymal structures due to increased image noise.

Arterial Phase

The arterial contrast phase occurs approximately 15–20 s post-injection of CM, when the aortic contrast peak reaches the epigastrium, and provides the highest degree of contrast in imaging the aorta and its branches. While artP provides the best delineation of arterial anatomy, opacification of the renal veins occurs almost simultaneously. To exclude intra-individual variants in circulation, a bolus trigger/tracking technique (starting at an aortic threshold >120 HU) is useful and recommended (Kocakoc et al. 2005). The test bolus technique is comparable, but a scan start with fixed scan delay often misses the appropriate starting time. When there is evidence of vascular pathologies (e.g., aneurysm, vascular disruption, dissection, or occlusion) in an emergency setting, artP is almost always covered by either a whole-body CT (WBCT) scan or abdominal CT angiography.

Angionephrographic/Corticomedullary Phase

A few seconds later (~30- to 40-s delay), angionephrographic contrast is achieved, with persistent arterial inflow, already vibrant venous drainage, and a homogeneous cortical enhancement due to CM transit in the medullary parenchyma (corticomedullary). The most sensitive depiction of pathologies in renal perfusion and of lesions in the renal cortex is obtained during cmP, which continues up to a delay of 60 s.

Nephrographic Phase

The ngP reflects the time during which the renal cortex and medulla are enhanced homogeneously and CM just reaches the renal collecting system. This phase begins 75–100 s after contrast injection and is therefore almost comparable to a standard pvP scan. Focal masses arising in the cortex or medulla (usually hypodense) and pathologic pooling of CM, as a sign of infection or other loss of function, are detected during ngP. In the emergency setting, this phase is replaced by the usually performed pvP CT scan of the abdomen and pelvis.

Excretory Phase

The exP or urographic phase is used to evaluate the renal collecting system and subsequently the ureters. It begins as early as 3 min after the start of CM injection but in some cases as late as 20 min, reflecting a wide range of intra-individual differences (Kemper et al. 2006; Akbar et al. 2004; Van Der Molen et al. 2008). Thus, while most authors recommend a delay of 7 or 10 min, an additional scan at 20 min might be necessary in individuals with delayed excretion. Although the intensity of the nephrogram has already declined at exP, CM excretion results in a very hyperdense opacification of the calyces, renal pelvis, ureter, and, in a final step, the urinary bladder. With exP, bilateral comparisons of functional excretion, the integrity of the renal collecting system and ureters (to rule out urine leakage), and the detection of an obstruction (blockage of the contrast column) are possible. To include the urinary bladder in this scan, prior occlusion of a Foley catheter or retrograde bladder filling for CT cystography are reasonable options (see "The Pelvis").

Image Processing and Postprocessing

The almost isotropic datasets can be reconstructed in multiplanar reformations (MPR) in fixed standard orientations (axial, sagittal, coronal) or as curved multiplanar reformations (cMPR) along a structure of interest such as the lumen of the ureter or the renal artery in center-line or lumen-view reconstructions. Further reconstruction methods are thick- or thin-slice maximum intensity projections (MIPs), e.g., the projection of a hyperdense arterial vessel or of excretion by the collection system of a predefined volume, resulting in CT-based angiograms or urograms. In complex alterations, surface shaded display (SSD) or volume rendering (VR) technique can serve as a roadmap for surgical planning or summarize a pathology in an anatomic surrounding.

1.2 Non-Traumatic Emergency

1.2.1 Non-Infectious Causes

Acute colicky flank pain, renal-angle tenderness, and macro- or microhematuria are often symptoms of obstructing or non-obstructing renal or ureteral stone formations. Intermittent or continuous urinary tract obstruction during passage evokes different patterns of pain. Stone size is the single most reliable indicator of possible stone passage. Whereas 80% of concrements <4 mm are passed spontaneously, with increasing size (especially >8 mm) the number of complications, such as total obstruction, secondary infection, abscess, rupture, and, finally, renal insufficiency, increases in parallel (Furlan et al. 2008). If the urologic examination is inconclusive, or the location, origin, and extent of the obstruction are of interest, or other abdominal differential diagnoses have to be ruled out, MDCT is indicated. The reported sensitivity and specificity of neP are as high as 97 and 96%, respectively, such that following the introduction of single-slice capability, in the 1990s, CT has widely replaced conventional abdominal X-ray and intravenous pyelogram (IVP). Nowadays, with MDCT and thin-collimation MDCT, almost all urinary tract calculi can be detected as radio-opaque structures on neP, without any prior patient preparation (Akbar et al. 2004). A considerable reduction in the radiation dose is possible using specific calculi detection protocols (l-d neP), which are especially recommended in younger individuals or in case of sonographic evidence of hydronephrosis caused by the concrement.

The ureters anteriorly cross the iliac arteries near the bifurcation at the pelvic entrance, a common site for the impaction of kidney calculi. Two other bottlenecks for kidney stones are the ureteropelvic junction (UPJ), where the renal pelvis meets the ureter and the ureter enters the bladder.

A typical finding is the "rim sign", seen as a 1–2 mm soft-tissue thickening around a calculus as a correlate of focal ureteral wall edema at the position of stone impaction (Heneghan et al. 1997). This sign has a specificity of 92% and helps to discriminate phleboliths or other confusing calcifications that are often found along the ureteral passage. Further CT findings of urolithiasis are dilatation of the ureter or collecting system, asymmetric enlargement and/or a decreased density of the kidney, and perinephric or periureteral stranding of surrounding fatty tissue.

If CT in (low-dose) neP does not display evidence of stones, a high-grade hydronephrosis with risk of fornix rupture is excluded, but subsequent imaging with IV contrast in ngP should be performed to rule out the seldom case of non-radio-opaque calculi. With the aid of MPRs or cMPRs, an exact localization of the stone(s) is usually possible. Together with a

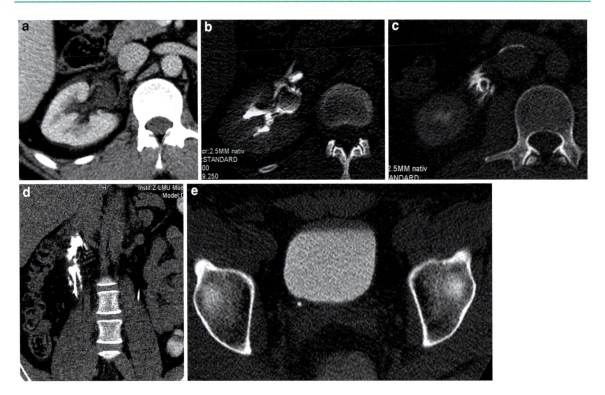

Fig. 1 Forniceal rupture in a patient presenting with acute abdomen, macrohematuria, and flank pain. **a** Perirenal fluid/stranding and a dilated renal pelvis in nephrographic phase (*ngP*). **b–d** Excretory phase (*exP*) depicts CM extravasation (urine) at the level of the renal pelvis (**b**), along the proximal ureter (**c**), and both in the coronal plane (**d**). **e** The rupture was due to the impaction of a calcified stone at the *right* ostium of the urinary bladder

precise measurement of stone size the likelihood of spontaneous passage can be determined. The advantage of CT in calculi detection is the ability to assess the entire abdomen and pelvis, allowing for a quick and easy exclusion of differential diagnoses such as appendicitis, diverticulitis, biliary colic, symptomatic ovarian cyst, or the seldom case of ruptured aortic aneurysm. Patients with these conditions may have similar findings (Foley 2003), sometimes even in neP.

If ngP is performed in a timely manner, the homogeneous distribution of renal CM provides functional information. An additional delayed phase after 7–10 min then enables the dedicated visualization of the renal collection system and the ureteral course, thus revealing possible filling defects or, with interruption of the contrast column, e.g., compression by extrauteral masses (Kemper et al. 2006; Silverman et al. 2009; Sheth and Fishman 2004).

Longer-lasting obstruction and hydronephrosis, especially in patients suffering from diabetes or who are immune-compromised, may lead to infection and thus pyelonephritis and pyonephrosis or result in forniceal rupture (Fig. 1).

1.2.2 Infections

For the vast majority of patients suffering from genitourinary infection, further imaging is neither necessary nor recommended due to history, clinical presentation, and typical laboratory findings. If these infections are recurrent, resistant to antibiotics, have a fulminant clinical course, or occur in association with immune deficiency, diabetes, or clinically inconclusive disease patterns, MDCT can be helpful and is indicated for diagnosis and further therapy planning. Based on differences in the perfusion patterns, MDCT performed in artP and ngP enables disease differentiation among chronic inflammatory changes, acute pyelonephritis (acute lobar nephronia), and the severe occurrence of xanthogranulomatous and emphysematous forms of pyelonephritis.

Pyelonephritis

The most common CT findings of acute pyelonephritis (PN) are ill-defined, wedge-shaped lesions of

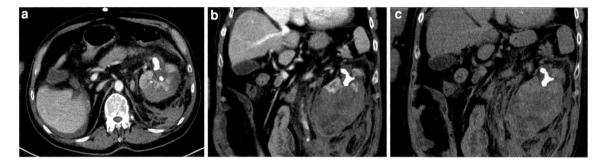

Fig. 2 Prolonged pyelonephritis. Due to obstruction by a complex-shaped forniceal staghorn-like calculus (hyperdense formation in renal pelvis in ngP; **a** axial and **b** coronal views), prolonged pyelonephritis resulted in renal rupture with severe retroperitoneal and intraperitoneal hemorrhage. **b** Only small areas of remaining CM enhancement of the renal parenchyma are seen. **c** Delayed scan in exP does not show any urine along the collection system nor extravasation from the already non-functioning *left* kidney

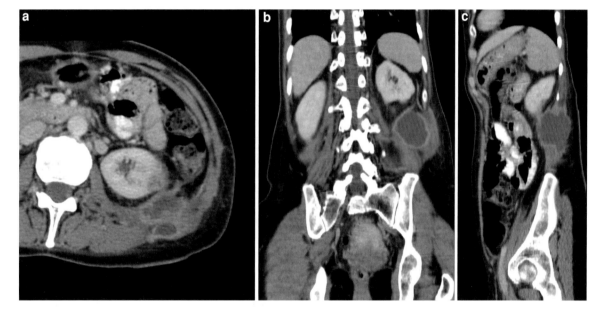

Fig. 3 Renal abscess in a patient with acute flank pain, fever, and high laboratory inflammation parameters. **a** MDCT in ngP depicts the hypodense and irregular parenchyma at the dorsal lower pole of the *left* kidney continuing in the *left* dorsal lumbar muscles. **b, c** Liquefied low-density abscess formation extends within the muscle (20–30 HU) and shows typical rim enhancement in the reformatted planes. The patient underwent surgery

decreased contrast enhancement radiating from the papilla to the cortex as a result of tubulo-interstitial inflammation (Akbar et al. 2004; Kawashima and LeRoy 2003). While the altered attenuation may be subtle in cmP, this perfusion abnormality often is better delineated in ngP (Browne et al. 2004; Demertzis and Menias 2007). Further characteristic changes in parenchymal enhancement are a striated nephrogram, consisting of linear bands of hypoattenuation and hyperattenuation oriented along the axes of the tubules and collecting ducts. Retained concentrated CM in the tubules, caused by, e.g., debris obstruction, local ischemia, and adjacent interstitial edema, accounts for this CT appearance (Craig et al. 2008). Acute PN at this stage is a non-liquefying infection typically due to gram-negative rods (*E. coli*). Clinically, these patients present with flank pain, fever, leukocytosis, and pyuria, often caused by urinary tract abnormalities or urine reflux. Associated thickening and enhancement of the

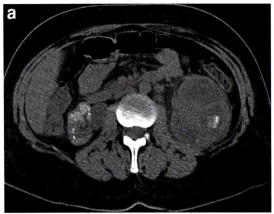 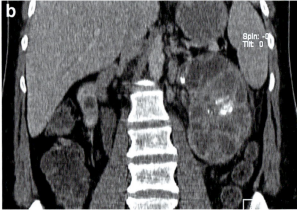

Fig. 4 Renal abscess in a patient with diabetes and recurrent renal and urinary tract infections who presented with sepsis. Non-enhanced MDCT image reveals a small *right* kidney with a hydronephrotic collection system, parenchymal loss, and calcifications. **a** Extreme swelling of the *left* kidney with parenchymal alterations and thickening of the fascia of Gerota. **b** Coronal MPR in ngP shows confluent hyodensities (renal abscesses) as a complete picture of an xanthogranulomatous pyelonephritis. The patient underwent bilateral nephrectomy

urothelium along the pelvicalyceal wall, focal or global swelling of the kidney, perirenal stranding of surrounding fatty tissue, and thickening of the fascia of Gerota are additional findings. The differential diagnoses consists of arterial/venous infarction and contrast-associated nephrotoxicity (striated nephrogram).

Pyonephrosis

In addition to the inflammatory presentation of the affected kidney seen in PN, in pyonephrosis there is further extensive infection of the dilated ureter. In some cases fluid–fluid levels, gas in the collection system, or urothelial thickening occurs. This condition is mostly the result of a prolonged hydronephrosis caused by concrements (Fig. 2), tumors, retroperitoneal fibrosis, or iatrogenic strictures with a secondary infection. It is known as "pus under pressure" and is a ticking time bomb since once the pus-filled system ruptures, there is a high probability for systemic septic spread and thus a life-threatening condition. A therapeutic approach is decompression by CT-guided nephrostomy.

Renal Abscess

Intra-, peri-, und pararenal abscesses present as acute or delayed complications in severe renal infections formed by colliquative necrosis or transforming the tissue into a liquefactive mass. Hematogenous spread or the extension of an extrarenal inflammatory process (e.g., diverticulitis) seldom is the origin. MDCT can delineate the extent and course

of the abscess and sometimes the origin of the infection. The typical appearance is a low-attenuation fluid or pus collection with a capsule showing rim contrast enhancement. Perinephric abscess may result from the rupture of an intrarenal abscess into the perirenal space or can develop directly from acute PN. It can extend through the fascia of Gerota to the pararenal space, may involve the psoas muscle, and extend retro- or intraperitoneally into the pelvis and groin (Fig. 3). Within the same session, CT-guided puncture to determine the pathogen for targeted antibiotics or therapeutic CT-guided drainage can be carried out.

Emphysematous Pyelonephritis

Emphysematous PN is a fulminant gas-forming infection of the kidney parenchyma that usually occurs in patients suffering from poorly or uncontrolled diabetes or from severe immunosuppression (Craig et al. 2008). Type I emphysematous PN is characterized by destruction of the parenchyma, with scattered or streaky regions of gas within the parenchyma and little or no fluid entrapment. In type II, there is a large renal or perirenal fluid accumulation with additional bubbly or confluent gas. Patients with the type II pattern have a better prognosis than those with type I, in which surgical nephrectomy is usually required.

Xanthogranulomatous Pyelonephritis

Subsequent to ureteral or pelvic obstructive calculus or external compression, a prolonged urinary

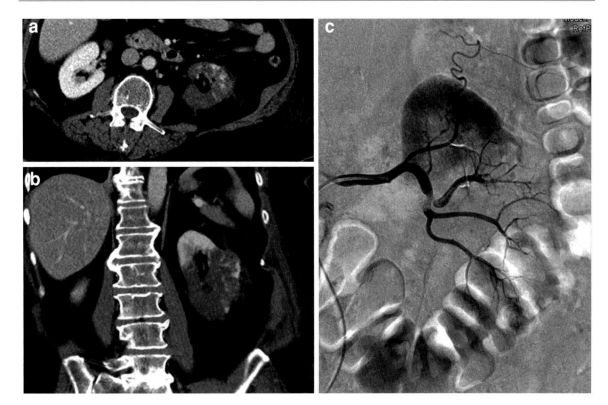

Fig. 5 Renal thrombembolism in a patient with acute *left*-sided flank pain, atrial fibrillation, and microhematuria. MDCT in ngP depicted homogeneous enhancement of the *right* kidney (**a**), whereas the *left* kidney lacks enhancement in the lower two thirds (**b**). DSA reveals persistent thrombembolic material at the hilar ramification of the *left* renal artery. **c** The upper pole branch is not affected, resulting in early upper pole opacification. The patient underwent intra-arterial lysis

tract infection can result in xanthogranulomatous pyelonephritis, a rare chronic infection (Craig et al. 2008). Typical causative germs are *E. coli* and *Proteus mirabilis*. The highest incidence is seen in middle-aged women with clinical presentation of flank pain, fever, and a history of recurrent low-grade urinary tract infections and a typical staghorn calculus.

MDCT in ngP usually demonstrates an enlarged non-functioning kidney, a staghorn calculus, and multiple, round, hypodense masses representing a hydronephrotic collecting system. Over time, extension of the inflammatory process to the perirenal and pararenal spaces and adjacent organs is not uncommon. Further complications are cutaneous and reno-enteral fistulas. Nephrectomy is often required for treatment (Fig. 4). The differential diagnose includes diffuse tumor infiltration (lymphoma/metastatic/renal cell carcinoma) and tuberculosis.

1.2.3 Vascular, Non-traumatic Renal Pathologies
Renal Artery Aneurysm/Renal Artery Infarct

Non-traumatic cases of emergency seldom involve the renal arteries. Pre-existing aneurysm of the renal artery (RAA) can rupture or become clinically apparent as flank pain. Embolic vascular occlusion and spontaneous isolated dissection of the renal artery are the result of atherosclerosis of the involved renal arterial segment. A further cause of (partial) vascular occlusion is dissection following minor trauma or the continuous extent of a type B aortic dissection membrane. These three conditions can be precisely evaluated by CT angiography/artP (Foley 2002; Fleischmann 2003). While RAA is predominantly a congenital condition, later accompanied by fibromuscular dysplasia, atherosclerotic and post-inflammatory or (delayed) post-traumatic (total incidence 0.01–1.0%) disorders, a dissection of the renal-artery wall may be an iatrogenic complication

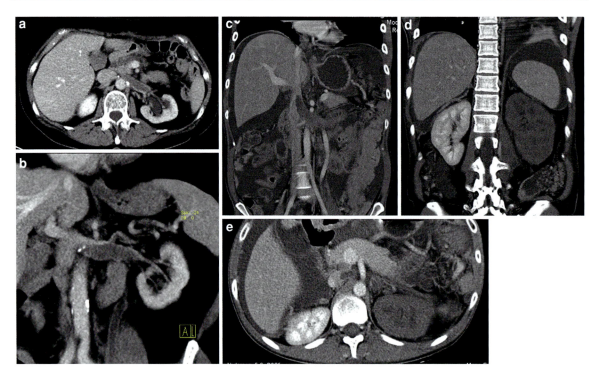

Fig. 6 Renal vein thrombosis. Two different cases of paraneoplastic *left*-sided renal vein thrombosis. **a, b** The first patient presented with a large thrombus in the *left* renal vein but still sufficient venous drainage, resulting in still normal bilateral perfusion of the renal parenchyma in ngP. The persistent thrombus in the second patient completely occludes the *left* renal vein and extends into the inferior vena cava (**c**), resulting in a complete *left*-sided venous renal infarction with limited parenchymal perfusion and edematous parenchymal swelling (**d, e**)

following stenting and angioplasty maneuvers. In patients with RAA rupture, MDCT during the early stage typically shows retroperitoneal hematoma in artP, often progressive and with active CM extravasation in ngP or exP. Patients with rupured RAA often are initially free of pain and simply present with hypertension. A (partial) reduced enhancement of the renal parenchyma as vital sign of malperfusion or a complete loss of renal perfusion as a correlate of ischemia can appear in all three vascular alterations and is best estimated in ngP (Fig. 5).

Thin-slice ($\leq$1 mm) acquisition in artP with additional reconstructions (MPR, cMPR, and MIP) often clearly depicts the site of the stenosis or occlusion and in case of active bleeding is useful in pre-interventional vascular-anatomic mapping of the true vessel lumen (Regine et al. 2007).

Renal Vein Thrombosis / Venous Renal Infarction

Acute or chronic renal vein thrombosis is predominately caused by a renal cell carcinoma or adrenal carcinoma with venous invasion or tumor/thrombus extension into the renal vein and/or IVC. By far more seldom is a progressive thrombosis in the underlying tissue, e.g., of the left ovarian/testicular vein, or a coagulopathy arising from a clotting disorder. A rapid extension of the thrombus or the formation of secondary arterial emboli may give rise to an acute loss of renal function, observed as delayed corticomedullary enhancement of the affected kidney. An additional, secondary imaging sign is global renal enlargement due to the venous blockage, together presenting the imaging features of venous renal infarction. On ngP, the typical hypodense thrombus in a distended and parathrombotic enhancing vein is seen. A false-positive diagnosis due to incomplete venous contrast in ngP can be avoided by a further scan with a scan delay of 90–120 s (Urban et al. 2001). An assessment of the different scan phases will confirm or rule out direct venous compression by a pathologic mass. Depending on the origin, decompression surgery, anticoagulation, or thrombus extirpation can be carried out (Fig. 6).

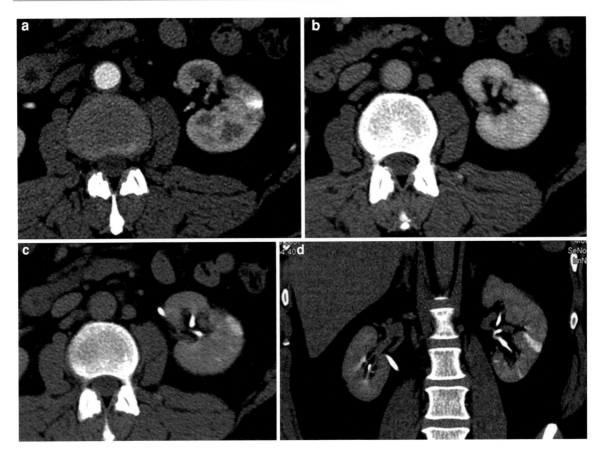

Fig. 7 Renal arterial infarction after stenting of the renal artery (*RA*) in a patient with acute flank pain and microhematuria following stenting of a *left* RA stenosis. MDCT in arterial/corticomedullary phase depicts blush of CM in *left* renal cortex (**a**), persistent in ngP (**b**) and with evidence of washout in exP (**c** axial, **d** coronal views), interpreted as slight peri-interventional parenchymal bleeding and diagnosed as a segmental infarction. There was no further complication and no need for further treatment

Non Traumatic Renal Bleeding

Besides renal bleeding following blunt or penetrating or iatrogenic trauma, there is the risk of spontaneous bleeding in benign and malignant renal masses. Larger angiomyolipomas (>4 cm, typically composed of blood vessels, smooth muscle and fatty tissue) (Zagoria 2000), rapidly expanding malignomas, and extensive renal cysts can be the origin of spontaneous life-threatening renal bleeding or occur following minor trauma involving the kidney. Complicating factors that predispose these patients to a fatal outcome are severe coagulopathy or anticoagulation. Clinical signs are progressive flank pain and sometimes hematuria. Large amounts of hemorrhage in the renal parenchyma and retroperitoneal space and an invasion in the peritoneal cavity can already be depicted in the neP (non-enhanced phase) (e.g. in the aberrant search for renal or ureteral concrements). To localize active bleeding and its vascular-anatomic origin, CT angiography (artP) is useful for intervention planning (access path and feasibility of embolization) and/or prior to a surgical procedure. It also allows estimation of the amount of parenchymal damage. A sign of active bleeding is an irregular or linear focus of high-density contrast extravasation that remains as such and may increase in size in a delayed scan (Fig. 7).

1.3 Traumatic Emergencies

1.3.1 General Clinical Considerations and Other Imaging Modalities

Renal injuries can lead to significant morbidity and mortality whereas renal trauma is uncommon,

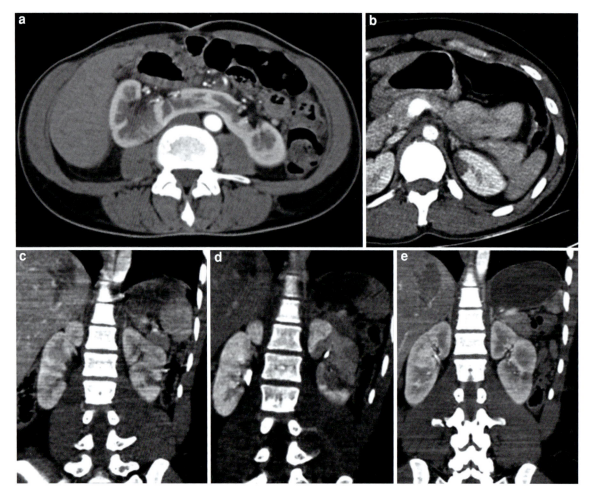

Fig. 8 Renal trauma (grade I, two cases). **a** Slight hypoperfusion due to contusion in the vertebra and adjacent dorsal lip in the *right* part of a horseshoe kidney. **b** More obvious hypoperfusion due to post-traumatic segmental infarction of the *left* kidney. Sequence at 1, 2.5, and 9 h after a suicidal jump resulting in liver laceration. Subtle (**c**), extensive (**d**), and complete recovery of a post-traumatic perfusion defect that was due to compression. The differential diagnosis included partial shock kidney (**e**)

accounting for only 1.4–3.25% of all traumatic injuries (Santucci et al. 2004; Miller and Shanmuganathan 2005). Most of the cases (70–80%) occur in patients <44 years, the mean age being 20–30 years, and are more common in males, supposedly attributable to their higher involvement in risk activities. A large percentage of renal trauma (75–85%) represents minor injuries that generally can be managed conservatively. These lesions include renal contusions, subcapsular hematomas, minor lacerations with limited perinephric hematoma, and small cortical infarcts. Serious renal injuries with persistent, life-threatening hemorrhage caused by renal parenchymal lesion or pedicle avulsion are rare and require surgical exploration. Penetrating renal trauma ranges from 4.6 to 18.4%, and blunt renal trauma from 81.6 to 95%, with coexisting further injuries in up to 90% (Alonso et al. 2009; Heyns 2004; Kawashima et al. 2001). Parameters such as incidence, severity of injury, and adequate treatment have not been clearly evaluated in prospective trials so far. A significant number of papers discuss treatment options of renal trauma, but geographic differences are obvious and outcome studies are not available. In 2004, a consensus conference was convened by the WHO, which published its results on "Evaluation and management of renal injuries" (Santucci et al. 2004).

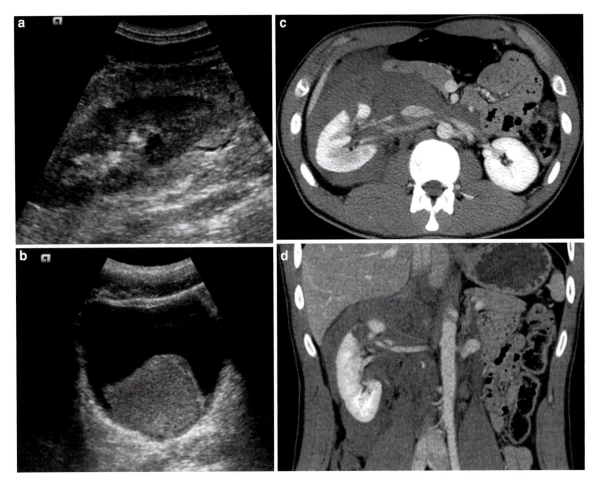

Fig. 9 Renal trauma (grade III). Lesion of the *right* kidney in a young man after a kick in the *right* flank, resulting in moderate pain but macrohematuria. Suspicion of *right* perirenal hematoma (**a**) and blood clots in the urinary bladder (**b**) based on the FAST examination. A deep 3 cm laceration of the *right* kidney accompanied by extensive perirenal, pararenal, and beginning intraperitoneal hematoma as seen on ngP MDCT (**c, d**). On exP, there was no evidence of collection system involvement. The patient was successfully treated conservatively

Blunt ureteral and ureteropelvic injuries are very rare and difficult to diagnose. Motor vehicle accidents and falls are obvious causes of renal injury; deceleration trauma leads to injuries of the renal pedicle and ureteropelvic junction (UPJ) (Ortega et al. 2008). Direct impact or secondary collision with the ribs and or the abdominal wall can result in organ acceleration and collision, inducing parenchymal lacerations and hematoma.

Many of these injuries can be missed on the initial CT trauma evaluation and delays in diagnosis occur in over 50% of the cases. Today, MDCT provides the safest and most comprehensive means of initial diagnostic and follow-up examinations of renal injuries in emergency radiology. MDCT can accurately identify parenchymal laceration, vascular injury and urinary extravasation, as well as perirenal hemorrhage (Alonso et al. 2009). Alternative imaging methods are ultrasonography (US), intravenous urography, renal arteriography, high-field magnetic resonance imaging (MRI), and retrograde pyelography. US is useful in detecting abdominal mass bleedings; however, its sensitivity for parenchymal renal injuries and retroperitoneal hemorrhage is limited. Intravenous urography in emergency situation is no longer in use and only an option if CT is not available. Selective angiography is used when, based on CT findings, interventional treatment is planned. Retrograde pyelography is valuable in assessing ureteral and renal pelvic integrity in suspected UPJ injury. Patients with

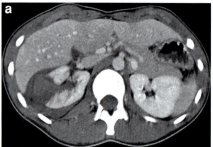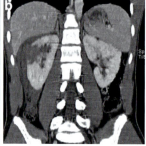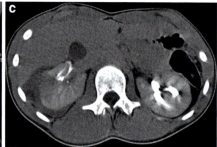

Fig. 10 Renal trauma (grade IV). Lesions of the *right* kidney. **a, b** Laceration extends through the renal cortex, medulla, and collecting system, with a devitalized and devascularized renal fragment and extensive perinephric hematoma, as seen on ngP CT. **c** Additional delayed exP CT reveals the typical sign of renal pelvis rupture, with the extravasation of hyperdense urine into the *right* perinephric space

pre-existing kidney abnormalities are at increased risk of complications. Extrarenal pelvis and/or hydrone-phrosis may result in higher rate of pelvic or UPJ disruption; renal cysts or tumor may predispose the patient to renal hemorrhage or rupture; and horseshoe kidneys (Fig. 8a) are more fragile. Albeit very seldom, iatrogenic renal bleeding may occur following, e.g., biopsy or lithotripsy.

Indications for CT are penetrating trauma with microscopic hematuria (>5 RBC/field), blunt trauma with gross hematuria, microscopic hematuria with hypotension (<90 mmHg at any time), significant accompanying injuries (flank contusion, lower rib fracture, thoracolumbar spinal fracture, or retroperi-toneal hematoma), blunt trauma and hematuria in children, and any positive US finding on emergency room FAST (focused assessment with sonography in trauma) studies. In these cases, MDCT detects, characterizes, and stages injury patterns and con-comitant injuries, enables priority-oriented therapy planning, illustrates renal function, and confirms a functioning contralateral kidney.

Urine analysis is the most important laboratory test. Hematuria is present in 80–94% of cases, although it does not correlate with the severity of injury. Gross hematuria, however, can predict major injuries; nonetheless, it can be transient or even absent and may be negative in penetrating trauma or pedicle injuries.

1.3.2 Renal Trauma
Grading of Renal Trauma

The grading of renal trauma is essential to properly diagnose lesions in terms of quantification, the extent of the traumatic damage, therapeutic decision-making, and outcome controls (Santucci et al. 2004; Kuan et al. 2006).

Grade I. Low-grade injuries comprise parenchyma contusions, focal areas of decreased enhancement in the renal parenchyma with sharply or poorly defined margins, and small subcapsular hematomas, not exp-anding in the pararenal space and without parenchymal lacerations. Clinically, these lesions can be associated with microscopic or gross hematuria (Fig. 8).

Grade II. With increasing severity, hematomas become larger, expand perirenally, but are confined to the renal retroperitoneum. Parenchymal lacerations are first seen, but with a depth of <1.0 cm and no urinary extravasation.

Grade III. Parenchyma lacerations reach a depth >1.0 cm but without rupture of the collecting system and no urinary extravasation (Fig. 9).

Grade IV. The main features are lacerations extending through cortex, medulla, and collecting system, resulting in urinary extravasation, best diag-nosed on exP. The most recent literature advocates a wait and see approach to treatment, but a surgical procedure is in fact indicated. Included in this grade are also vascular injuries of the main renal artery or vein resulting in active but contained hemorrhage (Fig. 10).

Grade V. Lacerations result in a completely shattered kidney while vascular injuries can lead to life-threatening avulsion of renal hilum structures, with active bleeding and or devascularized kidneys. These injuries usually require immediate surgery (Fig. 11).

In renal trauma, delayed renal opacification is due to the increased resistance to arterial perfusion.

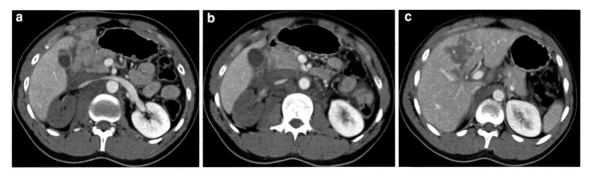

Fig. 11 Renal trauma (grade V). **a, b** *Right* renal artery occlusion due to dissection and thrombosis, with expanding retroperitoneal hematoma. Consecutively, no opacification of the *right* renal parenchyma is observed. Associated injuries are minor laceration of pancreatic head (grade 1), liver laceration, and severe grade III duodenal injury (**a–c**)

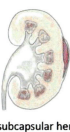
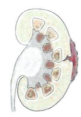
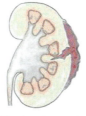
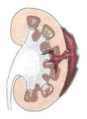

I: subcapsular hematoma parenchymal contusion, subsegmental infarction

II: superficial renal laceration <1cm, segmental infarction

III: >1cm laceration without urinary extravasation

IV: deep laceration involving the collection system with urinary extravasation

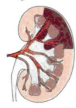
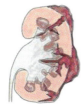
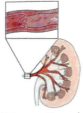
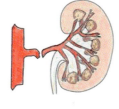

IV: segmental thrombosis of renal arterial branch and/or contained hemmorhage

V: multiple deep lacerations resulting in shattered kidney

V: traumatic occlusion of the main renal artery

V: renal arterial avulsion resulting in devascularization

Fig. 12 MDCT-based classification of renal trauma, including a modified organ injury scale and vascular injury patterns. (Adapted from the AAST)

If active bleeding is detected, angiographic embolization, if available, is the preferred treatment. Surgery may be required when there are multiple bleeding sites and high-grade injuries (>grade IV) in order to achieve bleeding control but nephrectomy is often inevitable. Delayed images are useful and mandatory to diagnose injury to the collection system (grade IV) as well as in renal vascular injury. A reduction of the radiation dose in a delayed scan is possible (Stuhlfaut et al. 2006). Clinical hypertension related to a renin-angiotensin-aldosterone mechanism can be caused by local ischemia after trauma.

Figure 12 The modified AAST organ injury severity scale in renal trauma

The original AAST organ injury scale (Santucci et al. 2004), devised by Federle et al., did not consider parenchymal contusions and vascular injuries. Federle recently revised the scheme to include a five-grade system similar to the one developed by the committee (Table 2) (Federle 2000). Most renal injuries are minor (grades I–III; 75–85%) and can be treated conservatively. Significant injuries (grade IV–V; 15–25%) are more frequent in penetrating than in blunt trauma (27–68% vs. 4–25%). Nephrectomy is

Table 2 The modified American association for the surgery of trauma (AAST) organ injury severity scale in renal trauma

Grade[a]	Injury type	Injury description
I	Contusion	Focal area of decreased enhancement in the renal parenchyma, sharply or poorly defined margins (microscopic or gross hematuria)
	Hematoma	Subcapsular, non-expanding, without parenchymal laceration
	Vascular	Small subsegmental cortical infarction
II	Hematoma	Non-expanding perirenal, confirmed to renal retroperitoneum
	Laceration	Parenchymal depth <1.0 cm, no urinary extravasation
	Vascular	Segmental parenchymal infarction
III	Laceration	Parenchymal depth >1.0 cm, without collecting system rupture or urinary extravasation
IV	Laceration	Parenchymal laceration extending through the cortex, medulla, and collecting system
	Vascular	Injury to main renal artery or vein but with contained hemorrhage
V	Laceration	Completely shattered kidney
	Vascular	Avulsion of the renal hilum devascularizes the kidney

[a] Advance one grade for bilateral up to grade III

deemed necessary in 0.8–7% while major injuries with gross hematuria and arterial hypotension (RRsys <90 mmHg) are seen in 0.2–2.0% of patients. Whether a shattered kidney (grade V), when associated with pedicle and hilar injuries, indeed implies irretrievable tissue loss and a worse clinical outcome remains to be established. The presence of multiple cortical lacerations should result in a higher grade (grade IV). Future changes based on further developments in MDCT imaging will allow the differentiation of pseudoaneurysm from segmental hemorrhage and the quantification of hematoma and tissue loss. This information will better identify patients best treated by a radiological intervention and those absolutely requiring surgical therapy.

Absolute indications for surgical renal exploration are persistent, life-threatening renal hemorrhage, renal pedicle avulsion (grade V), expanding, and pulsatile or uncontained retroperitoneal hematoma, also indicating renal pedicle avulsion. Relative indications for surgical exploration are large lacerations of the renal pelvis, avulsion of the UPJ, grade III and IV injuries with coexisting bowel or pancreatic injuries, persistent urinary leakage, post-injury urinoma, perinephric abscess, failed percutaneous or interventional treatment, and the development of renovascular hypertension. Post-traumatic complications include infected urinoma, perinephric abscesses, urinary leakage, and secondary hemorrhage.

Renal Vascular Trauma

Vascular injuries include arterial cut-off, arterial avulsion, perforation, and intimal tears or dissections as well as false aneurysm and, very rarely, arteriovenous fistulas (Regine et al. 2007). More common are traumatic sub- and segmental infarctions; these have been integrated in a modified organ injury scale. In 6–14% of renal traumas, there are concomitant renal vascular injuries; 30% involve veins or both arterial and venous vessels.

Segmental or subsegmental renal infarctions typically appear as wedge-shaped areas of parenchyma with reduced CM enhancement, best seen on cmP and ngP CT. Segmental infarcts may be solitary or multiple and are often associated with other renal injury patterns. The term "shattered" with respect to the kidney refers to extended multiple infarctions with multiple areas of decreased CM enhancement, sometimes with very irregular patterns. Active bleeding must be differentiated from traumatic pseudoaneurysm, which is seen on post-contrast CT as round areas of high density along renal arterial vessels. They are best detected on arterial images with an early washout and as a decrease in density on delayed images (Alonso et al. 2009). Pseudoaneurysm and arteriovenous fistulas are usually post-traumatic or iatrogenic; however, pseudoaneurysms also occur in inflammatory disease. They represent major renal injuries, may rupture, and result in hemodynamically significant hemorrhage (Fig. 13).

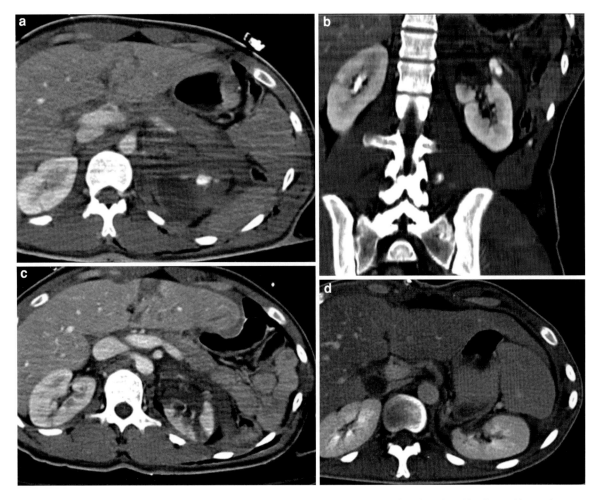

Fig. 13 Renal traumatic pseudoaneurysm in a patient with severe abdominal trauma due to a motor vehicle accident. **a, b** Besides liver laceration, peritoneal and retroperitoneal hemorrhages, ngP depicts a circumscribed nodular CM pooling in the projection of the renal upper pole laceration, typical for pseudoaneurysm with washout in a delayed phase or a differential diagnosis of active bleeding with persistent or expanding CM extravasation. **c** Control scan several days after conservative treatment shows the almost resolved enhancement of the pseudoaneurysm. **d** Over the next 2 months, there was further regression of the hematoma with renal scarring

Urgent radiological interventional treatment with endovascular embolization and occlusion of the affected arterial branch should be carried out whenever possible as this approach best preserves the renal parenchyma. If the renal artery is occluded or the kidney is devascularized due to an isolated vascular injury, parenchymal hemorrhage as well as clinical hematuria may be absent. CT imaging signs of renal infarction are occlusion of the renal arterial lumen, the presence of thrombus or a dissecting membrane in the lumen, and retrograde CM filling of the renal veins. CT imaging signs of a traumatic renal venous thrombosis include the presence of thrombus in the vein, a persistent opacification in ngP, and reduced enhancement in the renal vein. Traumatic occlusions of the renal artery should be rapidly diagnosed since after 120 min of warm ischemia there is progressive and permanent loss of renal tissue. Traumatic intimal dissection or occlusion of the main-stem renal artery requires immediate interventional recanalization and endovascular stenting. In these cases, technical success is reported even after several hours of warm ischemia, but interventional treatment should be concluded within 4 h of injury to effectively preserve renal function. After more than 4 h, the decision should be made based upon the presence of a

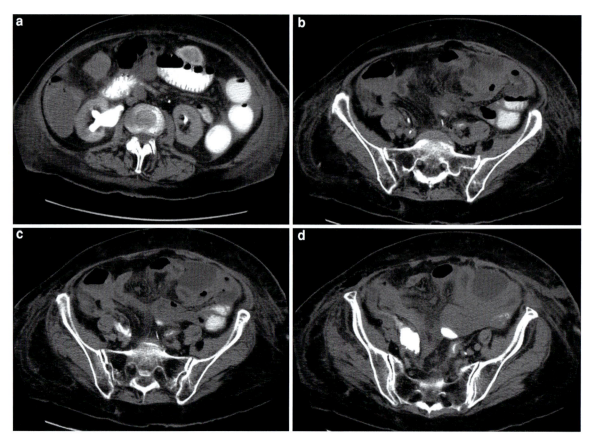

Fig. 14 Ureteral injury (grade IV) is typically located at the distal three-quarters of the *right* ureter. Secondary signs of injury are adilated collection system (**a**) and retroperitoneal hemorrhage (**b–d**) are seen on exP. Urinary extravasation starts at the uretero-iliac crossing, expanding along the distal ureter and intraperitoneally (**d**), requiring surgical therapy

contralateral normal uninjured kidney. If in very rare cases there is bilateral trauma or a single kidney before trauma, interventional treatment or, reconstructive surgery is strongly indicated.

Ureteral Trauma

Ureteral involvement in urogenital injury occurs in 1% of cases while the incidence in the setting of abdominal trauma is very low (0.25%). The majority (75%) of ureteral injuries are iatrogenic (incision, perforation, ligature, endoureteral procedures) but they also occur during blunt (18%) and penetrating (7%) trauma. In 75% of the cases, the UPJ or the distal third of the ureteral course is involved (Kawashima et al. 1997) (Fig. 14).

Further causes of ureteral leakage are prolonged obstruction or stone passage. Urine extravasation (urinoma) starts perirenally, contained by the fascia of Gerota, and penetrates intraperitoneally at a later stage (Titton et al. 2003) (Fig. 15).

Both conventional (intraoperative) IVP and exP MDCT are appropriate to depict the level and extent of damage and the extravasation. As a specific sign, often the distal ureter is non-opacified and the proximal portion may be dilated. Non-specific signs comprise perinephric stranding, low-density fluid around the kidney and ureters, blood or fluid in the pararenal spaces, and thickening of the renal fascia. More specific signs are contrast extravasation from the genito-urinary tract, which can only be diagnosed on exP images. Subtle leakage is predominantly missed on primary pvP/ngP CT, with non-specific signs of a dilated renal collection system, retroperitoneal hematoma, pararenal fluid collection, and perinephric stranding. Therapy for grade II and III injuries is operative closure or JJ-stenting, Grade IV and V injuries require sophisticated reconstruction techniques.

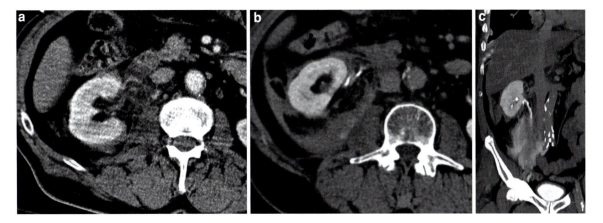

Fig. 15 Ureteral injury (grade V). **a** Extensive transection and devascularization of the ureter. Immediate whole-body CT after polytrauma with ngP of the abdomen reveals perinephic and retroperitonal fluid collections. **b** A follow-up scan with late CM excretion of the first examination in ngP shows urinary extravasation from the proximal *right* ureter and increasing retroperitoneal hematoma. **c** Additional exP obtained during the second examination demonstrates extensive hyperdense urinary (CM) extravasation from the proximal *right* ureter due to extensive transection in the coronal reformation

Table 3 The AAST organ injury severity scale in ureteral trauma

Grade[a]	Injury type	Injury description
I	Hematoma	Contusion or hematoma without devascularization
II	Laceration	Transection <50%
III	Laceration	Transection >50%
IV	Laceration	Complete transection with <2 cm devascularization
V	Laceration	Avulsion with >2 cm of devascularization

[a] Advance one grade for bilateral up to grade III

Grading of Ureteral Trauma

As for renal trauma, ureteral trauma is graded according to an AAST severity scale that recognizes five (I–V) grades of injury (Table 3).

2 Adrenal Gland

2.1 Anatomy and General Considerations

The adrenal glands are positioned in the perirenal space, usually cranial to the kidneys. The right adrenal gland lies cranial to the kidney, medial to the liver, lateral to the diaphragm crus, and posterior adjacent to the IVC. The left adrenal gland lies cranial and medial to the upper kidney pole, posterior to the pancreas and the splenic vein. Although variations of the blood supply to the adrenal glands are common, there are usually three arteries that supply each one, originating from the inferior phrenic artery, abdominal aorta, and the renal artery. The right adrenal vein drains directly into the IVC, while the left adrenal vein usually enters the left renal vein or the inferior phrenic vein. The destruction of >90% of functional adrenal tissue leads to the abrupt life-threatening onset of primary adrenal insufficiency.

The high spatial and temporal resolution of MDCT provides sufficient adrenal imaging to depict pathologies even in free-breathing or uncooperative patients and at the height of phrenic excursion.

2.2 Non-Traumatic Emergency

2.2.1 Non-Traumatic Hemorrhage

Non-traumatic adrenal hemorrhage is a rare and uncommon condition that is infrequently diagnosed

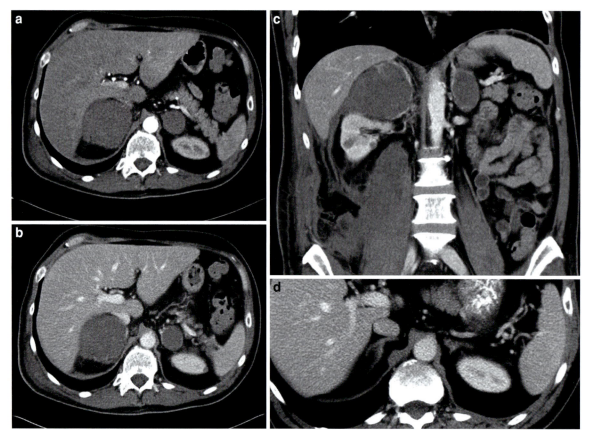

Fig. 16 Adrenal gland hemorrhage. Extensive bilateral bleeding following a hypertensive episode and simultaneous anticoagulation therapy. **a, b** Dual-phase MDCT (arterial, nephrographic phases) demonstrates bilateral adrenal masses with persistent 70-HU density in both scans. **c** Reformation in arterial phase illustrates the typical contained hemorrhage on the *left* and the more severe and expanding hematoma on the *right* side. **d** No obvious adrenal pathology was seen 6 weeks before

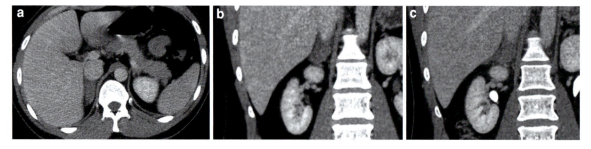

Fig. 17 Adrenal gland hemorrhage. **a, b** *Right* adrenal mass representing a subtle adrenal bleeding following minor (grade I) abdominal trauma. **c** The increase in size and stranding within 2 h rules out the differential diagnosis of adrenal adenoma

while the patient is alive but is an under-recognized cause of decompensation and multisystemic organ failure (Kawashima et al. 1999). Reported triggers are postoperative antiphospholipid-antibody syndrome, heparin-associated thrombocytopenia, hemorrhagic diathesis, sepsis, neoplastic infiltration, or in the setting of severe physical stress and multi-organ failure. Most of these conditions provoke either an increased blood inflow or/and a reduced blood output, resulting in hemorrhage. Another trigger is direct venous obstruction by thrombosis of the IVC or the renal veins. On non-enhanced CT, a hyperdense (50–90 HU) mass

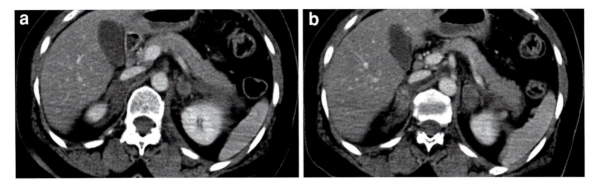

Fig. 18 Adrenal gland trauma. **a, b** MDCT shows a pancreatic tail injury, a grade I lesion of the *left* kidney (**b**) and bilateral adrenal hemorrhage with evidence of bilateral major parenchymal destruction, consistent with grade V adrenal trauma

Table 4 The AAST organ injury severity scale in adrenal trauma

Grade[a]	Injury description
I	Contusion or hematoma without devascularization
II	Laceration involving only the cortex (<2 cm)
III	Laceration extending to the medulla (≥2 cm)
IV	Parenchymal destruction >50%
V	Total parenchymal destruction (including massive intraparenchymal hemorrhage); avulsion from blood supply

[a] Advance one grade for bilateral up to grade V

within or originating from the adrenal gland may be depicted. MDCT in pvP shows a persistent hyperattenuation. The most important sign is periadrenal fat stranding, indicating acute hemorrhage or edema extending into the surrounding fat planes. This sign can help differentiate adrenal hematoma from adenoma or metastasis (Kawashima et al. 1999). In ambiguous cases, a short-term repeat scan may show the gland's persistent hyperdense appearance, an increase in the extent, and stranding in case of bleeding (Fig. 16).

2.3 Traumatic Emergency

2.3.1 Bleeding

Although relatively uncommon, adrenal injuries have been recognized as an important indicator of the severity of associated abdominal trauma. They have been associated with increased overall patient morbidity and mortality during high-energy-induced trauma. In blunt abdominal trauma, adrenal gland bleeding is unilateral in 80% of the cases (right > - left) and bilateral in 20%. Unilateral limited bleeding

tends to be clinically unapparent (Sinelnikov et al. 2007; Vella et al. 2001) (Fig. 17).

Life-threatening cases of acute adrenal insufficiency, with fatigue, nausea, and vomiting combined with abdominal, lumbar, or thoracic pain up to manifested shock occur predominantly in the seldom cases of bilateral hemorrhage, which has a mortality rate of 15%. This severe state necessitates steroid replacement therapy. The appearance of post-traumatic bleeding on MDCT does not differ from that of non-traumatic hemorrhage but is often associated with further severe abdominal-organ injury (Fig. 18).

One further abnormal presentation of the adrenal gland on CT is that due to hypovolemic shock. While many of the abdominal shock organs show reduced contrast enhancement (kidneys, liver, pancreas, and intestine with wall thickening), the adrenal glands continue to be normally perfused for a long time or become hyperperfused, which can be confusing in establishing a differential diagnosis of adrenal bleeding in a gland with preserved integrity. The differential diagnosis in this setting includes adenoma and metastasis.

2.3.2 Grading of Adrenal Trauma

Adrenal trauma is also graded on an AAST scale, again with five (I–V) grades (Table 4).

References

Akbar SA, Mortele KJ, Baeyens K, Kekelidze M, Silverman SG (2004) Multidetector CT urography: techniques, clinical applications, and pitfalls. Semin Ultrasound CT MR 25:41–54

Alonso RC, Nacenta SB, Martinez PD, Guerrero AS, Fuentes CG (2009) Kidney in danger: CT findings of blunt and penetrating renal trauma. Radiographics 29:2033–2053

Browne RF, Zwirewich C, Torreggiani WC (2004) Imaging of urinary tract infection in the adult. Eur Radiol 14 (Suppl3):168–183

Craig WD, Wagner BJ, Travis MD (2008) Pyelonephritis: radiologic-pathologic review. Radiographics 28:255–277 (quiz 327-8)

Demertzis J, Menias CO (2007) State of the art: imaging of renal infections. Emerg Radiol 14:13–22

Federle MP (2000) Renal trauma. In: Pollack HM, McClennan BL (eds) Clinical urography. WB Saunders, Philadelphia, pp 1772–1784 (P 13)

Fleischmann D (2003) Multiple detector-row CT angiography of the renal and mesenteric vessels. Eur J Radiol 45 (Suppl1):S79–S87

Foley WD (2002) Special focus session: multidetector CT: abdominal visceral imaging. Radiographics 22:701–719

Foley WD (2003) Renal MDCT. Eur J Radiol 45 (Suppl1):S73–S78

Furlan A, Federle MP, Yealy DM, Averch TD, Pealer K (2008) Nonobstructing renal stones on unenhanced CT: a real cause for renal colic? AJR Am J Roentgenol 190:W125–W127

Heneghan JP, Dalrymple NC, Verga M, Rosenfield AT, Smith RC (1997) Soft-tissue "rim" sign in the diagnosis of ureteral calculi with use of unenhanced helical CT. Radiology 202:709–711

Heyns CF (2004) Renal trauma: indications for imaging and surgical exploration. BJU Int 93:1165–1170

Kawashima A, LeRoy AJ (2003) Radiologic evaluation of patients with renal infections. Infect Dis Clin North Am 17:433–456

Kawashima A, Sandler CM, Corriere JN Jr, Rodgers BM, Goldman SM (1997) Ureteropelvic junction injuries secondary to blunt abdominal trauma. Radiology 205:487–492

Kawashima A, Sandler CM, Ernst RD et al (1999) Imaging of nontraumatic hemorrhage of the adrenal gland. Radiographics 19:949–963

Kawashima A, Sandler CM, Corl FM et al (2001) Imaging of renal trauma: a comprehensive review. Radiographics 21:557–574

Kemper J, Regier M, Stork A, Adam G, Nolte-Ernsting C (2006) Improved visualization of the urinary tract in multidetector CT urography (MDCTU): analysis of individual acquisition delay and opacification using furosemide and low-dose test images. J Comput Assist Tomogr 30:751–757

Kocakoc E, Bhatt S, Dogra VS (2005) Renal multidector row CT. Radiol Clin North Am 43:1021–1047 viii

Kuan JK, Wright JL, Nathens AB, Rivara FP, Wessells H (2006) American association for the surgery of trauma organ injury scale for kidney injuries predicts nephrectomy, dialysis, and death in patients with blunt injury and nephrectomy for penetrating injuries. J Trauma 60:351–356

Miller LA, Shanmuganathan K (2005) Multidetector CT evaluation of abdominal trauma. Radiol Clin North Am 43:1079–1095 (viii)

Ortega SJ, Netto FS, Hamilton P, Chu P, Tien HC (2008) CT scanning for diagnosing blunt ureteral and ureteropelvic junction injuries. BMC Urol 8:3

Regine G, Stasolla A, Miele V (2007) Multidetector computed tomography of the renal arteries in vascular emergencies. Eur J Radiol 64:83–91

Santucci RA, Wessells H, Bartsch G et al (2004) Evaluation and management of renal injuries: consensus statement of the renal trauma subcommittee. BJU Int 93:937–954

Scherr MK (2009) Multi-detector computed tomography in non-traumatic urologic emergencies. Radiologe 49:516–522

Sheth S, Fishman EK (2004) Multi-detector row CT of the kidneys and urinary tract: techniques and applications in the diagnosis of benign diseases. Radiographics 24:e20

Silverman SG, Leyendecker JR, Amis ES Jr (2009) What is the current role of CT urography and MR urography in the evaluation of the urinary tract? Radiology 250:309–323

Sinelnikov AO, Abujudeh HH, Chan D, Novelline RA (2007) CT manifestations of adrenal trauma: experience with 73 cases. Emerg Radiol 13:313–318

Stuhlfaut JW, Lucey BC, Varghese JC, Soto JA (2006) Blunt abdominal trauma: utility of 5-minute delayed CT with a reduced radiation dose. Radiology 238:473–479

Titton RL, Gervais DA, Hahn PF, Harisinghani MG, Arellano RS, Mueller PR (2003) Urine leaks and urinomas: diagnosis and imaging-guided intervention. Radiographics 23:1133–1147

Urban BA, Ratner LE, Fishman EK (2001) Three-dimensional volume-rendered CT angiography of the renal arteries and veins: normal anatomy, variants, and clinical applications. Radiographics 21:373–386 (questionnaire 549-55)

Van Der Molen AJ, Cowan NC, Mueller-Lisse UG, Nolte-Ernsting CC, Takahashi S, Cohan RH (2008) CT urography: definition, indications and techniques. A guideline for clinical practice. Eur Radiol 18:4–17

Vella A, Nippoldt TB, Morris JC (2001) 3rd. Adrenal hemorrhage: a 25-year experience at the Mayo Clinic. Mayo Clin Proc 76:161–168

Zagoria RJ (2000) Imaging of small renal masses: a medical success story. AJR Am J Roentgenol 175:945–955

Gastrointestinal Tract

Mariano Scaglione, Veronica Di Mizio, Antonio Pinto, Maria Antonietta Mazzei, Luigia Romano, and Roberto Grassi

Contents

M. Scaglione (✉)
Department of Radiology, Pineta Grande Medical Center,
Via Domiziana Km. 30, 81030 Castel Volturno, Italy
e-mail: mscaglione@tiscali.it

V. Di Mizio
Radiology Service,
Santa Maria della Misericordia Hospital,
Rovigo, Italy

A. Pinto · L. Romano
Department of Radiology, Cardarelli Hospital,
Naples, Italy

M. A. Mazzei
Department of Radiology, University of Siena,
Siena, Italy

R. Grassi
Department of Radiology, Second University,
Naples, Italy

Abstract

The term "acute abdomen" is very comprehensive and traditionally related to the surgical gastrointestinal (GI) emergencies; nevertheless, only one quarter of patients who are previously classified with an acute abdomen actually receive a surgical treatment. Depending on a wide range of etiologies, the clinical assessment of such conditions remains equivocal in 4/5 of the cases in experienced hands and this data drops to 1\2 in the hands of young surgeons. In some cases, the clinical dilemma is if the patient needs a surgical treatment or not and, furthermore, in which cases the surgical option needs to be adopted urgently. Today, integrated imaging has revolutioned the classical clinical approach and the radiologists are asked to express in terms of clinical management in the emergency room more often than the past. In this chapter, the most commonly encountered etiologies of the GI emergencies will be discussed.

1 Gastrointestinal Tract

The term "acute abdomen" is very comprehensive and traditionally related to surgical gastrointestinal (GI) emergencies; nevertheless, only one quarter of patients previously classified with an acute abdomen actually undergo surgical treatment. Depending on a wide range of etiologies, the clinical assessment of such conditions remains equivocal in four-fifths of the cases in experienced hands and one half of the case in less experienced ones (Brinton 2000). Sometimes, the

M. Scaglione et al. (eds.), *Emergency Radiology of the Abdomen*,
Medical Radiology. Diagnostic Imaging,
DOI: 10.1007/174_2011_471, © Springer-Verlag Berlin Heidelberg 2012

clinical question is whether or not the patient requires surgical treatment, and in which cases the surgical option needs to be urgently implemented. Today, integrated imaging has revolutionized the classical clinical approach such that radiologists are much more likely to be asked to contribute to patients' clinical management in the emergency room.

In this chapter, the most commonly encountered etiologies of GI emergencies are discussed.

1.1 Small-Bowel Obstruction

1.1.1 Terminology and Clinical Issues

Small-bowel obstruction (SBO) is responsible for about 15% of laparotomies of the acute abdomen. The most frequent causes include adhesions (60%), hernias (20%), and neoplasms (15%). SBO is characterized by an interruption of luminal integrity with acute changes of canalization. The obstructive fulcrum causes dilatation of the proximal loops and collapse of the distal loops. The intestinal stasis is always mixed, gaseous, and liquid. SBO has an intrinsic dynamism: in other words, it may evolve to hypotonic and/or paralytic ileus, for example.

In SBO, the crux of the clinical and radiologic problem is to differentiate obstruction in which the risk is purely occlusive from the obstruction in which there is additional vascular risk.

Pure obstruction allows a less hurried preparation to surgery and a more complete restoration of the patient's hydro-electrolytic equilibrium status. Naso-gastric intubation may avoid urgent surgical intervention. On the other hand, obstruction in which there is also vascular risk will not show significant clinical improvement after the naso-gastric probe placement and unnecessary delays in surgery must be avoided.

On the basis of surgical and imaging findings, SBO can be simple, decompensated, or complicated (Di Mizio and Scaglione 2007). These entities are discussed below.

1.1.1.1 Simple SBO

In SBO the underlying pathophysiology is the distension of the bowel loops proximal to the obstructive site. The increased intraluminal tension distends the loop and causes a reduction in tone, with a progressive increase in the diameter of the affected segment.

Intestinal stasis is always of the mixed variety, gaseous and fluid. The extreme intraluminal tension compresses and thins the wall.

Following the intravenous administration of contrast medium (CM), contrast-enhanced CT (CECT) shows the bowel's thin walls with preserved and homogeneous contrast enhancement. Valvulae conniventes with their elegant completely circular pattern, rapidly appear, indicating the extreme tone resulting from the bowel's kinetic attempt to exceed the mechanically occlusive obstacle.

In simple SBO, the vascular supply is preserved and there is no peritoneal fluid. Nevertheless, simple obstruction has an intrinsic evolutionary dynamism.

1.1.1.2 Decompensated SBO

Usually, the GI tract handles 8–9 l of fluid every day, most of which is reabsorbed by the small bowel (SB). If the occlusive status persists, simple SBO evolves into decompensated SBO. The increasing intraluminal tension causes a change in the parietal microcirculation, which hampers the reabsorption bowel capability. This happens only when the intraluminal pressure is greater than the pressure within the capillary vessels, causing an alteration of vascular permeability. The bowel loop progressively, becomes decompensated. There is a definite flow of fluids out of the intestinal wall into the lumen and peritoneal cavity. Nevertheless, the wall does not thicken because the tension of the lumen squeezes it like a sponge. The stretched and compressed wall becomes thin and tight.

CECT following intravenous CM administration shows the thin walls with preserved and homogeneous enhancement.

The wall exudes liquid into and then out of the loop and a transudate appears in the peritoneal cavity. As in all states of imbalance, the decompensated bowel may be acute or chronic, and it may resolve or deteriorate. Both in simple and decompensated SBO, mortality is about 3%. However, both may resolve after medical therapy and placement of a naso-gastric tube.

1.1.1.3 Complicated SBO

This refers to an occlusive state complicated by vascular changes of the bowel wall. The complications may present with as vascular changes due to fight and those due to strangling–strangulation.

Regardless of the type, in the initial phase the vascular change within the loop is reversible, with the recovery of the intestinal vitality and function. In the absence of a timely resolution, the final condition of the acute secondary venous ischemia is necrosis, gangrene, perforation, and peritonitis.

Vascular changes due to fight. In the evolution of SBO, vascular compromise due to fight may appear. The origin of this event is multifactorial and unpredictable but the main factors are: (a) the obstructive mechanism, duration of occlusion, onset of complex mechanisms, (b) the mesenteric and enteric circulation, already uncertain because of diffuse atherosclerotic disease, (c) the pathological consequence, which alter the abdominal habitat, and (d) the general status and age of patient.

CECT following intravenous CM administration shows high contrast enhancement in the wall, with normal or borderline thickness. The continuous vascular efflux causes repeated engorgement and a vascular dilatation with intramural congestion: the wall therefore thickens.

Usually, a loop due to fight is near the obstructive site. The venous congestion of the loop may cause the passage of blood in the peritoneal cavity. Mesenteric involvement is absent or minimal.

Vascular changes due to strangling–strangulation. The mechanism of strangling–strangulation involves the loop and its mesentery. In these cases, the perfusion deficit affects the venous circulation, which is more easily compressible and collapsible. Impairment of the arterial circulation is very late. The inhibition of blood outflow causes intramural venous congestion with pathological wall thickening of the loop. The hemorrhagic engorgement of the mesentery forces the swollen and edematous mesenteric loops anteriorly, spacing them out. The vasculature becomes prominent, with numerous and dilated vessels. In addition, there is the early appearance of peritoneal fluid, initially in the recesses between the loops, then in the peritoneal recesses of the mesentery, and finally free in the peritoneal cavity.

Bowel strangulation is observed in 10–15% of patients undergoing surgery for SBO. The mortality in such cases is about 8% if the surgical intervention is performed within 36 h following the appearance of symptoms (Frager and Baer 1995). If surgery performed after 36 h, mortality increases to about 25%.

1.1.1.4 Volvulus

The term "volvulus" derives from the Latin verb *volvere*, to coil, and defines loop torsion on its mesenteric axis; that is, the mesentery coils on itself. This mechanism causes the abnormal location of loops and vessels, threatening torsion. Loops assume a spiral configuration, while vessels are stretched and twisted until the positions of the artery and vein are inverted.

Volvulus may spontaneously resolve. The formation of a volvulus does not necessarily imply strangulation of the feeding vessel pedicle. This ultimate event occurs only in cases of a particularly serrated strangulation.

1.1.1.5 Closed-Loop

Closed-loop refers to a loop obstructed at two adjacent points along its course. The mechanism by which a closed-loop forms consists of a single obstructed focus, such as an adhesive band, entrapped-incarcerated hernia or laparocele, or volvulus, that interacts on two points of the same segment of the intestinal tract. Numerous formation mechanisms of SBO may generate closed-loop.

It is important to be aware that evidence of a closed-loop is not synonymous with strangling or strangulation.

1.1.1.6 Intussusception

This is an unusual cause of bowel obstruction in which a proximal segment of bowel (intussusceptum) invaginates into the lumen of a distal, adjacent bowel segment (intussuscipiens). Intussusception may involve only the SB (ileo-ileal intussusception, typically in adults), both the small and large bowel (ileo-colic intussusception, typically in children) or be restricted to the colon (colo-colic intussusception). In adults, intussusception must be considered as a complication of a neoplasm, until proven otherwise. Based on the consequences regarding bowel canalization, three different types of intussusception are identified: (1) cold intussusception (asymptomatic), (2) incomplete and reversible hot intussusception (with recurrent and transient episodes of intestinal obstruction), and (3) complete and irreversible hot intussusception (complicated obstruction due to simultaneous involvement of both the bowel and its vascular supply).

1.1.2 Imaging

The radiographic and US findings of simple SBO are;

- Dilated proximal SB loops
- Multiple air-fluid levels
- Collapsed distal loops
- Absence of peritoneal fluid (US)
  The CT findings of simple SBO are:
- Dilated loops proximally to the transition zone, defined as the site of the abrupt change in the caliber of the dilated vs. the collapsed loops
- Collapsed loops distal to the point of obstruction
- Mixed enteric stasis, gaseous and liquid. A fecaloid enteric stasis (small-bowel feces sign) is sometimes visible and is considered a non-specific finding of SBO; it is also detectable on plain film and using US
- Normal and thin walls with homogeneous and regular contrast-enhancement
- At the jejunum, the presence of multiple, crowded, thin valvulae conniventes, equal to one another
- Scantly detectable or collapsed colon structure; preserved and homogeneous colon contrast-enhancement
- Normal and transparent mesentery
- Normal and preserved mesenteric vascularity
- Absence of peritoneal fluid

The imaging findings of decompensated SBO consist of the bowel changes of simple SBO in addition to findings related to the peritoneal cavity.

Radiographic and US findings:

- Dilated loops, with normal and thin walls (seen on both X-ray and US)
- Mixed enteric stasis (US)
- Extraluminal fluid between (X-ray and US) the dilated loops (US)
- Fluid in the peritoneal recesses of mesentery (US)
- Free fluid in the peritoneal cavity (US)
  On CT, decompensated SBO will present as:
- Dilated loops with normal and thin walls of homogeneous contrast enhancement; CE density may progressively decrease with decreasing vascular supply
- Mixed enteric stasis, mainly liquid
- Normal and transparent mesentery
- Normal and preserved mesenteric vascularity
- Extraluminal fluid between the dilated loops
- Fluid in the peritoneal mesenteric recesses
- Free fluid in the peritoneal cavity

Strangling and strangulation of the small intestine are characterized by thickened bowel walls and vascular changes, with significant involvement of the mesentery and the peritoneal cavity. Usually, CT only documents this clinical situation, with the following features:

- Dilated loops proximal to the transition zone
- Transition zone
- Collapsed loops distal to the point of obstruction
- Mixed enteric stasis, with marked prevalence of liquid stasis
- A thin bowel wall where vascular supply is normal; circumferential wall thickening with vascular compromise
- Bowel-wall abnormality on CECT: vascular changes in the intestinal wall may present different patterns according to the severity of the vascular injury, ranging from a strongly enhancing thickened bowel wall to the total absence of CE
- The thickened loop becomes rigid and loses its morphology
- Wall pneumatosis, with lamellar shape or intramural gas bubbles
- Hemorrhage of the mesenteric fat tissue, with a hazy, opaque, misty appearance and a thick shape accompanied by a loss of transparency perimesenteric fat.
- Congestion and engorgement of the mesenteric vessels, with prominent vasculature
- Gas in the superior mesenteric vein
- Gas in the portal vein
- Free fluid in the peritoneal cavity; due to a significant hemorrhagic component; the presence of fluid in some areas will result in higher attenuation values

In volvulus of the SB, there is topographic variation in the position of the bowel loops in the peritoneal cavity, with an abnormal spatial configuration and radial shape converging toward the site of obstruction. Similarly, the mesenteric vessels show an atypical and abnormal course, until finally there is an inversion of the normal disposition between the superior mesenteric artery (SMA) and vein. The mesenteric vessels are stretched and converge at the obstruction site. The rotation of the bowel and its mesentery results in the whirl sign (Fig. 1).

In closed-loop obstruction, CT may identify the two adjacent loops proximal to the obstructed site and the collapsed loops distal to it. Adhesional bands are rarely visible (Fig. 2).

Fig. 1 Small-bowel volvulus due to an adhesional band. Three contiguous contrast enhanced MDCT axial scans (**a–c**) show SBO with twisted mesenteric vessels, producing the whirl sign. Note also the free fluid within the loops and the peritoneal cavity and normal bowel wall enhancement, indicating the absence of ischemic changes of the dilated loops. **d** Multiplanar reconstruction (MPR) image shows spiral disposition of the non-ischemic dilated small bowel loops. Laparotomy was performed immediately. No ischemic bowel changes were found at surgery; the volvulus was derotated

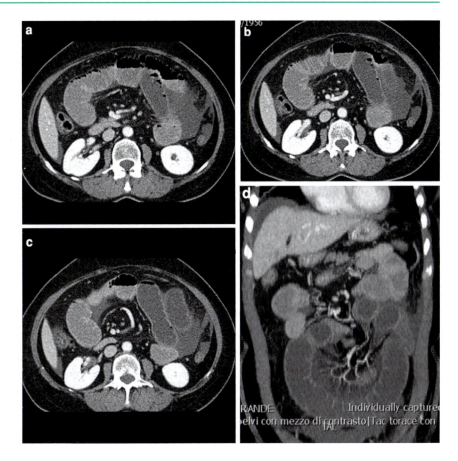

The CT findings of intussusception include the typical bowel within the bowel appearance (target sign), corresponding to alternating layers of low-attenuation mesenteric fat and high-attenuation bowel wall (Fig. 3). These findings can be also detectable on gray-scale, color Doppler US and on magnetic resonance imaging (MRI).

In SBO, post-processing CT techniques in any plane are a valid adjunct to the axial images and should always be performed to reach a more confident diagnosis (Frager and Baer 1995).

The essential imaging features of SBO are listed in Table 1.

1.1.3 Differentials

Acute intestinal behaviors:

- Reflex spastic ileus
- Reflex hypotonic ileus
- Paralytic ileus

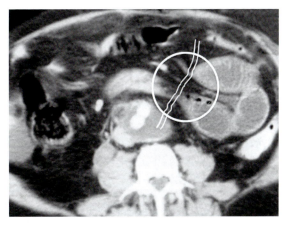

Fig. 2 Closed-loop obstruction. Blockage due to an adhesional band (*white lines*) at the transition zone acts on two adjacent points of jejunal loops (*circle*) forming a closed loop. Thin bowel walls and normal contrast enhancement are visible. There is free focal peritoneal fluid in the mesenteric recesses and a dilated, calcified, and thrombotic aorta

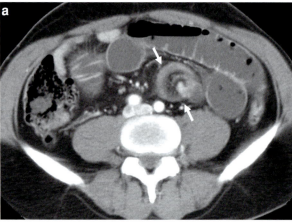 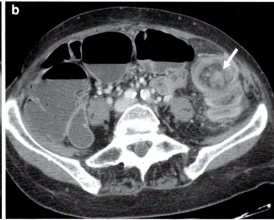

Fig. 3 Two cases of intussusception. **a** Hot ileo-ileal intussusception, with its typical target appearance (*arrows*), as a cause of SBO. **b** Hot colo-colic intussusception. At the left iliac fossa, there is a large, complex mass of invaginated left colonic segments; also note a polypoid lesion in the lumen of the colon, the leading point (*arrow*) responsible for the intussusception. A small amount of fluid and peri-visceral fat haziness are also detectable. The diagnosis was large-bowel obstruction. (Images courtesy of Dr. Vittorio Miele, Rome)

Table 1 Types of SBO and corresponding basic imaging features

SBO type	Bowel walls/ Valvulae conniventes	Fluid in the peritoneal cavity and/or within the loops	Mesenteric supply of the obstructed loops
Simple	Thin	Absent	Not involved
Decompensated	Thin	Present	Not involved
Complicated	Thick	Present	Hazy, misty, opaque

These three conditions can be readily distinguished on plain abdominal films (Di Mizio and Scaglione 2007). Other possibilities that must be considered are:

- Colonic obstruction
- Cystic fibrosis
- Functional obstruction of the SB due to thick, viscous bowel contents
- Fatty replacement of the pancreas, which on CT with also produce a SB feces sign.

1.2 Large-Bowel Obstruction

1.2.1 Terminology and Clinical Issues

In large-bowel occlusion, the colon is dilated due to mechanical or functional causes. In adults, the most common cause of large bowel obstruction (LBO) is malignancy, specifically adenocarcinoma (Fig. 4). Other causes include diverticulitis, volvulus, intussusception, ischemia, adhesions, fecal impaction, and strictures including radiation. A further possible cause of colonic occlusion is acute (toxic) or chronic megacolon. Given the risks of complications, such as sepsis, ischemia, and perforation, toxic megacolon is to be considered a real emergency. Patients with LBO typically present with abdominal distension, pain, nausea, and vomiting. Compared to SBO, the pain is more constant and often occurs over a distended cecum. The risk of perforation increases significantly when the diameter of the cecum exceeds 10 cm. The cecum always dilates to the largest extent regardless of the LBO site, according to Laplace's law. Another condition responsible for colonic occlusion is Ogilvie's syndrome (see Differentials), which is often encountered in hospitalized patients with significant underlying morbidity (Fig. 5).

When untreated, LBO has significant associated morbidity and mortality. Accordingly, timely diagnosis, which can be made on plain abdominal film images, can improve patient prognosis.

Fig. 4 Colonic obstruction due to a sigmoid colonic tumor. **a** Supine plain abdominal film shows colonic overdistension, with sudden caliber reduction of the sigmoid colon (*arrow*), and coprostasis in the ascending colon. **b, c** Two contiguous CT scans demonstrate a large, stenosing mass (*arrow*) obstructing the lumen of the sigmoid colon. Note the significant overdistension of the cecum

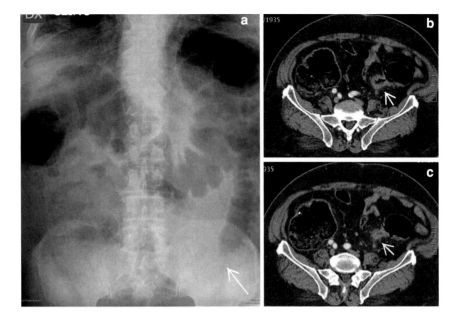

1.2.2 Imaging

Plain radiographs will show:

- Air- and fluid-filled loops of dilated colon
- Dilated proximal SB loops
- Multiple air-fluid levels

  In addition, CT identifies:

- Underlying cause of obstruction
- Initial signs of complication, such as perforation (small gas bubbles) and colonic ischemia.

1.2.3 Differentials

- Reflex hypotonic ileus
- Paralytic ileus
- Ogilvie's syndrome (colonic pseudo-obstruction).

In most cases, the plain film appearance is sufficiently characteristic: the haustra are smooth and regularly spaced, and the septa smooth, thin, and sharply marginated. The lumen is gas-filled and the wall contour is clearly demarcated (unlike obstruction, in which shaggy interfaces are often seen).

1.3 Acute Mesenteric Ischemia

1.3.1 Terminology and Clinical Issues

Acute mesenteric ischemia (AMI) is a life-threatening condition that accounts for approximately 2% of gastrointestinal illnesses, with a mortality of 50–90%, despite recent advances in surgery and intensive

therapy. Early diagnosis combined with timely treatment are essential to improving patient survival and quality of life (Brandt and Boley 2000; Yashura 2005). This goal, however, is still far from achieved, due to the non-specific clinical/laboratory findings and to the absence of specific and early radiologic findings typical of AMI.

The spectrum of diseases that encompass AMI may be classified as acute mesenteric arterial embolus and thrombus (60–70% of cases), primary or secondary mesenteric venous thrombosis (5–15%), and non-occlusive mesenteric ischemia (NOMI) (20%) (Table 2). These diseases have common clinical features. Another feature of AMI, typically observed in acute mesenteric arterial occlusion and in NOMI, is reperfusion injury, which may exacerbate the ischemic damage of the intestinal microcirculation. There is substantial evidence that the mortality associated with AMI varies according to the cause of the ischemia. NOMI is the most lethal form of (58–70%) because its poorly understood pathophysiology together with the mild and non-specific symptoms and signs at imaging often determine a delayed diagnosis. Mesenteric venous thrombosis is much less lethal (0–30%) than either acute thromboembolism of the SMA (17–90%) or NOMI. Thus, the etiology of AMI is an important prognostic factor and should thus be explored in imaging studies.

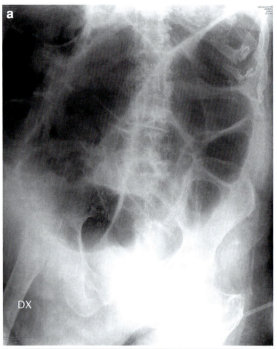

DX

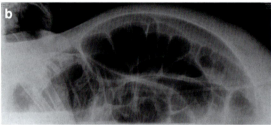

Fig. 5 Ogilvie's syndrome. **a, b** Anteroposterior and latero-lateral radiographs show abnormal distension of the colon in the absence of any mechanical obstruction

Table 2 Classification of acute mesenteric ischemia

Arterial occlusion: 60–70%	Venous thrombosis: 5–15%	NOMI: 20%
Emboli to the SMA	*Primary*	Systemic hypotension
Thrombotic occlusion	Deficiency of proteins C and S, antithrombin III, factor V Leiden, Antiphospholipid syndrome	Cardiac failure
Dissecting aortic aneurysm	*Secondary*	Septic shock
Vasculitis or arteritis	Paraneoplastic, pancreatitis, inflammatory bowel disease, cirrhosis and portal hypertension, splenomegaly or splenectomy, postoperative state, trauma, oral contraceptives	
Fibromuscular dysplasia		
Direct trauma		

1.3.2 Imaging

Diagnostic imaging of AMI has significantly improved with the advent of multidetector CT (MDCT) scanners (Moschetta et al. 2009; Wadman et al. 2010; Menke 2010; Furukawa et al. 2009). Many authors have demonstrated that MDCT is a valid diagnostic alternative to catheter angiography, based on its ability to identify the site, level, and cause of bowel ischemia and by showing abnormalities in the bowel wall, mesentery, and peritoneal cavity, and not only in the mesenteric vessels. It can also provide alternative diagnosis for patients in whom mesenteric ischemia is suspected. Today, catheter angiography should be limited to therapeutic purposes whereas MRI in some cases will allow detection of the early phase of ischemia.

The radiologic findings of AMI may vary widely according to the cause and underlying pathophysiology (Berritto et al. 2011; Tang et al. 2010). In addition, the CT appearance depends on the severity of the bowel ischemia (superficial mucosal or transmural bowel wall necrosis), location (only the SB vs. the small and large bowels), presence and degree of hemorrhage, and/or subsequent superinfections.

Acute mesenteric arterial occlusion. At CT, emboli and thrombi can be seen as defects in the SMA and its branches. Most emboli wedge at branching points around or distal to the middle colic artery, whereas thrombosis typically occurs at or near the origin of the mesenteric arteries. The bowel is contracted (reflex spastic ileus). Gas-filled appearance of the bowel may be seen in the intermediate phase of ischemia, reflecting a reflex hypotonic ileus, whereas in the final phase the bowel lumen may be filled with both gas and fluid or only fluid (paralytic ileus). Pneumatosis is typically observed in cases of transmural infarction, associated or not with portomesenteric venous gas. Coexisting embolism of other organs may also be see on CECT (Figs. 6, 7, 8, 9).

Acute mesenteric venous occlusion. Thrombosis of the mesenteric vein is primary or secondary to portal hypertension or infection or it can be associated with various hypercoagulopathy states. At CT, thrombi can be seen as defects in the SMV and its branches;

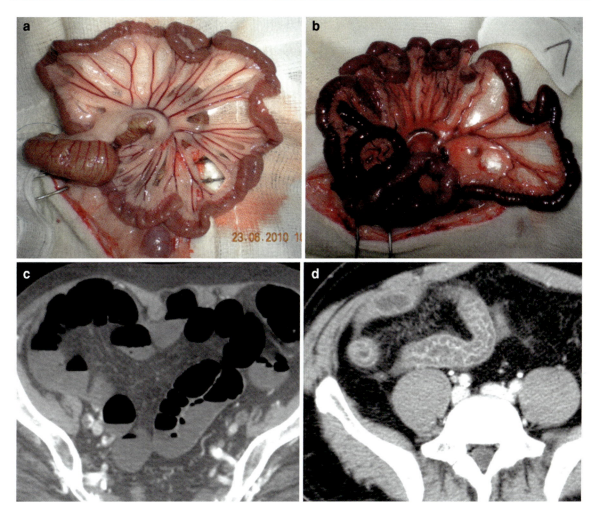

Fig. 6 Acute mesenteric ischemia. **a**, **b** Appearance of the mesentery. In experimental models, arterial occlusive ischemia results in a bloodless mesentery due to severe vasoconstriction (**a**), whereas the elevation of mesenteric venous pressure causes sudden mesenteric congestion (**b**). **c**, **d** Morphologic changes of the mesentery at CT. Depending on the specific etiology, the mesenteric vessels appear reduced in caliber in arterial occlusive ischemia (**c**) and increased in caliber in venoocclusive ischemia (**d**)

Fig. 7 Acute mesenteric ischemia: abdominal radiographs in the early phase.
a Reflex spastic ileus (gasless abdomen) in acute mesenteric arterial occlusion.
b Thickness of the small bowel wall (*arrowheads*) in venous mesenteric ischemia

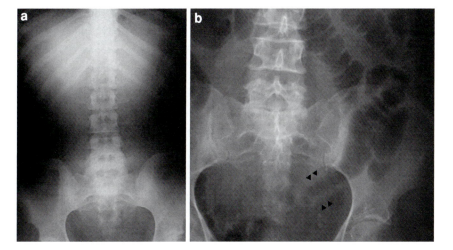

Fig. 8 Acute mesenteric ischemia of arterial etiology. Mesenteric vessels and bowel wall CT findings. **a** Coronal MPR image shows complete occlusion of the SMA. **b** Axial contrast-enhanced CT image demonstrates absent (*stars*) and diminished contrast enhancement of two adjacent ileal loops. **c** Reduction in the number and caliber of the mesenteric vessels and the contraction of small-bowel loops (reflex spastic ileus) in the early phase. **d** Dilated loops with gas (reflex hypotonic ileus) and gas and fluid in the intermediate phase of ischemia

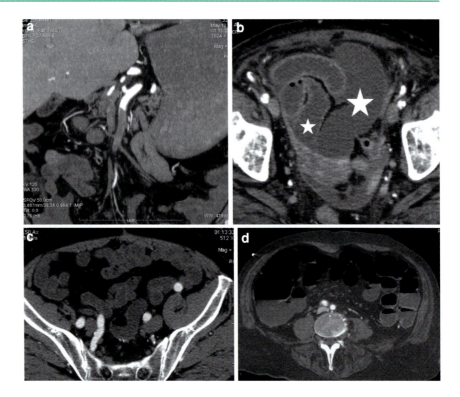

engorgement of the mesenteric veins is also observed. Fat stranding in the mesentery and ascites are common findings, also in the early phase of ischemia.

The bowel wall is thickened and shows different patterns after CM administration. Absent or diminished bowel wall enhancement usually indicates transmural infarction, particularly when it is associated with pneumatosis and portomesenteric venous gas. The degree of bowel wall thickening, mesenteric fat stranding, or ascites not always correlate with the severity of ischemic bowel damage (Fig. 10).

Non-occlusive mesenteric ischemia (NOMI). Ischemic injury may range from reversible superficial damage localized to the watershed areas to a more severe form involving the entire bowel. At CT, the early phase findings are identical to those observed in occlusive AMI: reduction of caliber of the SMA and poor evidence of its branches together with a bowel wall and contracted. Since there is no arterial flow, contrast enhancement of the involved bowel is absent or diminished. However, among the various types of AMI, the early phase of NOMI is the most difficult to diagnose on CT.

When reperfusion occurs, the CT features of NOMI change, resembling those of veno-occlusive ischemia. The bowel wall of the involved segments is thickened and the enhancement pattern may vary (absent, decreased, increased, halo or target type). Both fat stranding of the mesentery and ascites are visible (Fig. 11).

Finally, the approach to image interpretation in AMI should include the evaluation of the vessels bowel loops, mesentery.

1.3.3 Differentials

Crohn's disease. Fat mesenteric stranding, thickened bowel wall, mucosal hyper-enhancement, halo and target patterns do not have a vascular distribution, as in AMI; only ileal loops are involved in Crohn's disease; furthermore, enlarged lymph nodes can be also present, close to the loops involved or in the mesentery.

Shock bowel. This condition is usually seen following trauma or hypotension. There is mucosal hyper-enhancement or sub-mucosal edema, reflex spastic ileus. It is reversible with resuscitation.

Fibrosing mesenteritis. Idiopatic inflammation is accompanied by a fibrotic, misty mesentery and bowel wall thickening.

Lupus enteritis. The bowel wall is focally thickened and there is submucosal edema, and ascites.

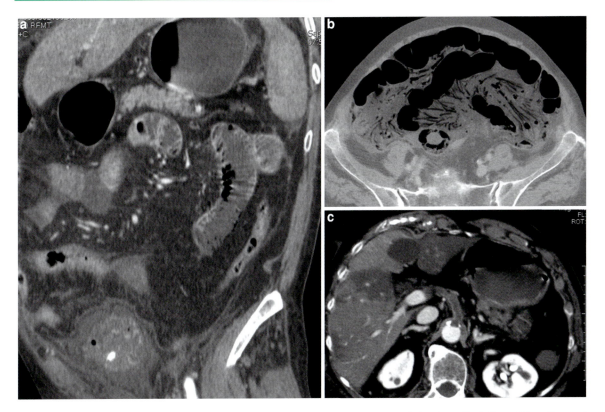

Fig. 9 **a** Coronal MPR image shows multiple foci of pneumatosis intestinalis mostly evident in the dependent aspect of the walls of small-bowel loops and **b** mesenteric pneumatosis in cases with transmural infarction. **c** Embolism of the celiac trunk associated with hypoperfusion of the liver parenchyma

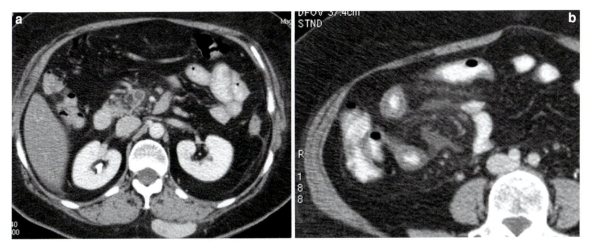

Fig. 10 Acute mesenteric ischemia of veno-occlusive origin. CT demonstrates mesenteric vessels and small bowel findings: **a** complete occlusion of the superior mesenteric vein; **b** increased number and caliber of mesenteric vessels and small-bowel wall thickening. Small quantity of fluid and fat stranding are also seen

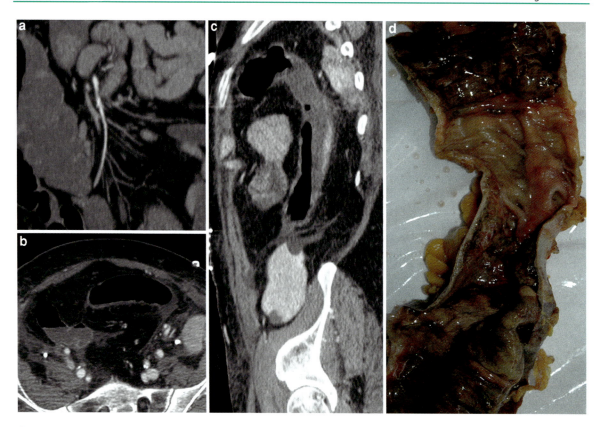

Fig. 11 Non-occlusive mesenteric ischemia with reperfusion. Mesenteric vessels and bowel CT findings: **a** reduction of caliber of the SMA and its branches, **b** dilated loops and peritoneal fluid in the intermediate phase of ischaemia, and **c** thickening of the wall of the colon due to reperfusion. **d** The surgical specimen shows multiple foci of necrosis in the colonic wall, confirming the diagnosis of non-occlusive mesenteric ischemia with reperfusion

1.4 Ischemic Colitis

1.4.1 Terminology and Clinical Issues

As the most frequent form of intestinal ischemia and the second-most frequent cause of lower gastrointestinal bleeding, ischemic colitis (IC) is a relatively common disease (Stamatakos et al. 2009; Cubiella Fernández et al. 2010; Koutroubakis 2008). It is generally a disease of the elderly, with the prevalence increasing with age. A plethora of conditions may favor the development of IC: mesenteric artery emboli, thrombosis; trauma, hypoperfusion states; mechanical colonic obstruction (tumors, adhesions, volvuli, hernias, diverticulitis); drugs (antibiotics, appetite suppressants, chemotherapeutic agents, cardiac glucosides, diuretics, illicit drugs); and iatrogenic causes (abdominal vascular surgery, colonic surgery, endoscopy). Generally, IC is the consequence of an acute interruption or it is part of a chronic decrease of the colonic blood supply, either occlusive or non-occlusive in origin (Gore et al. 2008). This results in ischemic necrosis of a variable severity, ranging from superficial mucosal involvement to full-thickness transmural necrosis. From a clinical viewpoint, IC presents in either a gangrenous (acute fulminant) or non-gangrenous (acute, transient or chronic) form, with a mortality rate ranging from 10 (non-occlusive disease) to 90% (occlusive mesenteric infarction due to embolus or thrombosis). The left colon is involved in 75% of the cases, and the right in the remaining 25%; the splenic flexure and the sigmoid colon are the areas most frequently affected. The incidence of IC is difficult to determine, as many mild cases are transient and are either not reported or misdiagnosed. CT is considered the best diagnostic modality in acute settings, revealing non-specific and late findings. Furthermore, a recent experimental study demonstrated that MRI can identify the pathological findings of acute IC, with optimal histopathological correlations (Iacobellis et al. 2012).

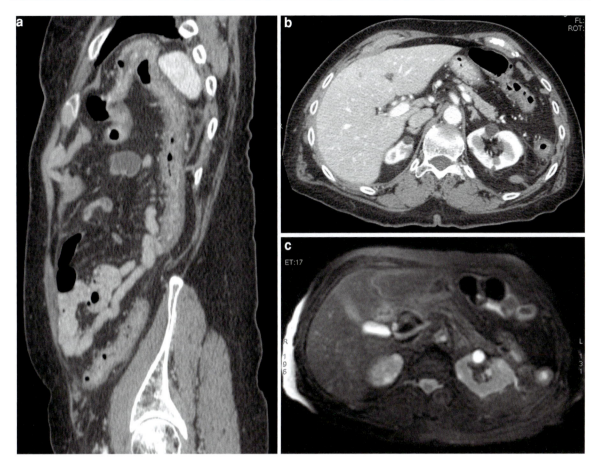

Fig. 12 Ischemic colitis of the left colon. Sagittal reconstruction image (**a**) and contrast-enhanced axial CT scan (**b**) show diffuse thickening of the colonic wall with submucosal hypodensity due to edema, pericolonic fat stranding, and small amount of peritoneal fluid. **c** On axial fat suppressed T2 weighted MRI, there is diffuse thickening of the colon wall with mild hyperintensity due to submucosal edema

1.4.2 Imaging

Endoscopy is generally considered as the method of choice in establishing the diagnosis of IC, even if this procedure is dangerous in the acute stages of the disease. However, endoscopic biopsy often cannot reveal the real extent of the ischemic injury throughout the wall of the colon. Instead, US and barium enema can detect the early colonic signs of ischemia as well as several abnormalities; but CECT is the best diagnostic modality in acute settings, providing suggestive findings related to the evolutionary stages of the disease and its complications or excluding other acute conditions (Romano et al. 2006; Taourel et al. 2008).

The CT findings (Figs. 12, 13) differ in the early, intermediate, and late stages of the disease:

Early phase. Arterial occlusion shows thin wall loops. In cases of reperfusion, extensive submucosal edema causes mural thickening and peri-colonic stranding with or without peritoneal fluid. Venous compromise results in thickening and mucosal hyperdensity due to hemorrhagic phenomena, moderate peritoneal in the peritoneal cavity, and the occlusion of mesenteric vessels.

Intermediate phase. Ischemic changes will cause symmetric/concentric colonic mural thickening if there is no arterial reperfusion. In the presence of reperfusion, colonic sub-mucosal edema may be strongly evident, with wall thickening and heterogeneous enhancement, loss of colonic haustra, and varying degrees of pericolic streakiness. In venous occlusion, mural stratification with concentric rings (double halo or target sign) is related to the submucosal hypodensity, due to mural edema. The involved colon has a shaggy contour, associated with pericolic

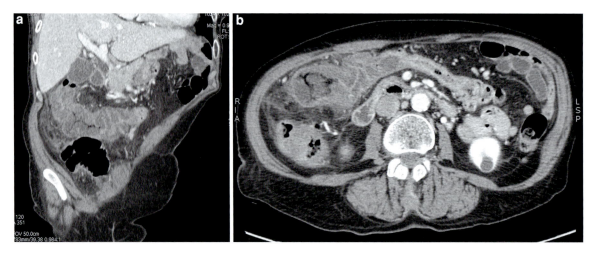

Fig. 13 Ischemic colitis of the ascending colon, right colic flexure, and transverse colon. Oblique coronal reconstruction (**a**) and axial CT (**b**) images show a diffuse thickening of the colonic wall with submucosal hypodensity due to submucosal edema, pericolonic fat stranding, and peritoneal fluid

stranding. Variable amounts of peritoneal free fluid and mesenteric vascular occlusion are also seen.

Late phase. The colonic wall is thin and unenhanced in cases of total vascular occlusion without reperfusion. The lumen is dilated. Intramural/mesenteric or portal venous gas, with intraperitoneal fluid and pneumoperitoneum, may also be present. In venous infarction, the colon is thickened, with decreased enhancement. Pneumatosis and portal and mesenteric venous gas may be present: the occlusion of mesenteric vessels can be identified.

1.4.3 Differentials
- Diverticulitis
- Ulcerative colitis
- Crohn's disease
- Pseudomembranous colitis
- Antibiotic or *C. difficile* colitis
- Pancolitis: colonic wall thickening, accordion sign, ascites
- Colon carcinoma.

1.5 Ulcerative Colitis

1.5.1 Terminology and Clinical Issues
Ulcerative colitis (UC) is a chronic, idiopatic, diffuse inflammatory disease primarily involving the colorectal mucosa. Only the rectum is involved in about 30% of patients, both the rectum and colon in 40%, and a

pancolitis in 30%. The inflammatory process is generally limited to the mucosa and submucosa. Toxic megacolon, which is related to an abnormal gaseous distention of the colon (dilatation of the transverse colon >6 cm determined on plain abdominal film) is a complication of UC (Fig. 14). Expansion of the colon is not a sudden event; rather, it tends to develop over more than one day and is often anticipated by an increased gas content of the small bowel.

1.5.2 Imaging
The best diagnostic clue of UC is toxic megacolon. On abdominal plain film, about half of the patients with severe UC show jejunal-ileal gaseous stasis (pre-megacolon). In an interesting study (Caprilli et al. 1987), among 31 patients with severe UC including gaseous stasis in the SB, 7 developed toxic megacolon. On the other hand, it was never observed in a control group of 38 patients with severe UC but without abnormally large a mounts of gas in the small bowel.

To address radiation-dose-related issues, plain film follow-up studies are performed in patients with toxic megacolon. In the event of clinical regression, a reduction of the hydro-gaseous stasis and changes in loop caliber are noted, with the recovery of intestinal tone and motility. In case of disease worsening, both the amount of stasis fluid and the caliber of the involved bowel loops will increase, with a progressive decline in tone and motility that may end in paralysis. A possible event is a free perforation of the colon,

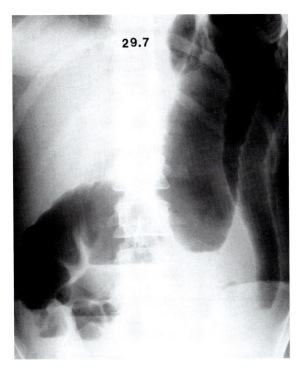

29.7

Fig. 14 Toxic megacolon in ulcerative colitis. Plain abdominal film in orthostasis. Relevant colonic distension and air-fluid levels with a prevalent gaseous component are seen. Functional repercussion of the SB due to metabolic toxicosis

resulting in communication with the peritoneal cavity. CT features include an enhancing inner ring (mucosa), non-enhancing middle ring (submucosa), enhancing outer ring (muscularis propria), and the target or halo sign

1.5.3 Differentials
- Paralytic ileus
- Ogilvie's syndrome
- Crohn's disease.

1.6 Crohn's Disease

1.6.1 Terminology and Clinical Issues

Crohn's disease (CD) is a recurrent, segmental, granulomatous inflammatory bowel disease that may appear acutely as an acute abdomen. The full-blown ulcerative form, particularly terminal ileitis, can mimic an acute appendicitis or an acute inflammatory disease of the female genital system. Fibrostenosing forms induce bowel movement changes until a mechanical occlusion results. Phlegmons and abscesses require a

correct and timely diagnosis. Toxic megacolon is a possible but infrequent complication of Crohn's colitis, with similar features to UC. Free perforations in the peritoneal cavity are rare.

1.6.2 Imaging

Although typically located in the terminal ileum (95%), CD may occur anywhere along the gut, from the mouth to the anus. Best imaging clues include segmental areas of ileo-colonic ulceration and wall thickening. At CT, wall thickness $\geq$a 3 mm is considered pathologic. A thickened wall that lacks stratification shows two patterns (Wittenberg et al. 2002), white attenuation and gray attenuation, while the fat halo sign and edema halo sign are seen in cases of wall thickening with stratification. Among the non-stratified forms of thickening, white attenuation represents a thickened loop, without stratification, with intense and homogeneous contrast enhancement involving the entire wall depth. It is an expression of both the parietal hyperemia of the acute inflammation and of mucosal and submucosal active ulcers. Gray attenuation evidences the modest homogeneous enhancement of the thickened wall, with attenuation values similar to those of the muscle. It is a typical pattern of fibrotic, inveterate, and inactive parietal disease.

In the stratified form of wall thickening, the fat halo sign consists of three concentric rings. The intermediate halo has a fatty attenuation with negative tomodensitometric values. It indicates fat deposition in the submucosal layer, in turn an expression of a reparative inveterate processes. It is typical pattern of an inactive and extinguished disease. The edema halo sign likewise shows three rings of stratification. The intermediate halo has positive tomodensitometric values higher than those of water, indicative of submucosal edema and a multicellular infiltrate and thus of the acute and ulcerative nature of the inflammation. It should be remembered that CD is a systemic disease and that these patterns are an exclusive expression of the activity state at the level of the bowel wall. Correct evaluation of the nature of the stenosis is essential in the management of a CD patient (Di Mizio 2002). Wall thickness is related to the degree of damage to the lumen, which loses its distensibility. Peri-ulcerative edema, responsible for parietal thickening, is a functional and reversible condition that is responsive to medical therapy (Fig. 15). The repair-scarring phenomena seen in

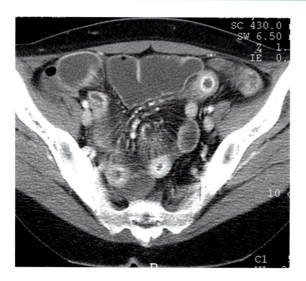

Fig. 15 Crohn's disease. CECT, axial view, shows multiple inflamed loops with reduced lumen. Thickened walls demonstrate white attenuation and the edema halo sign. The vascular network is thickened. This picture is indicative of functional, reversible disease responsive to medical therapy

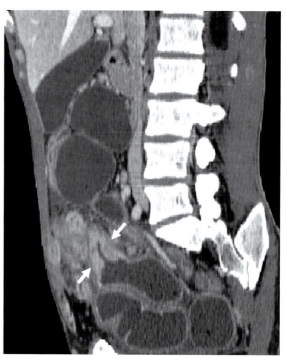

Fig. 16 Crohn's disease in a patient with small-bowel obstruction. Sagittal MPR image shows marked stenosis of the distal ileum with gray attenuation and a thickened wall (*arrows*) causing small bowel obstruction. Retroperitonal lymph nodes are visible. This ileal stenosis is fibrotic, organic, and irreversible. In this case, surgery is the treatment of choice

patients with inveterate disease entails formation of parietal fibrosis, with the increasingly hypo-distensible lumen ending in an organic irreversible stenosis requiring surgical therapy (Fig. 16).

1.6.3 Differentials
Ulcerative colitis
Ischemic colitis
Radiation enteritis
Therapeutic/excessive abdominal radiation at the terminal ileum with strictures, sinuses, fistulas
Metastases and lymphoma
Small-bowel metastases, melanoma, bronchogenic and breast carcinomas.
Non-Hodgkin lymphoma in the stomach and small bowel
Mesenteric adenitis
Enlarged lymph nodes and ileal wall thickening causing right lower quadrant pain in children.

1.7 Perforation

1.7.1 Terminology and Clinical Issues
Perforation of the GI tract is an emergent condition that requires prompt surgery. It can be due to peptic ulcer disease, inflammatory disease, blunt or penetrating trauma, iatrogenic factors, a foreign body or a neoplasm.

The clinical picture varies according to the site of perforation, its etiology, and any underlying diseases that may be present. There are various clinical manifestations of perforation: abdominal pain, nausea, vomiting, fever, peritonitis, localized abscess formation, inflammatory mass, fistulas, mechanical bowel obstruction, and gastrointestinal hemorrhage. Rare complications secondary to the perforation are septicemia, portal pyemia or pyogenic abscess, enterovascular fistulas, and even endocarditis. In many of the potential causative disorders, pain is initially localized to a relatively focal and suggestive site but may move to a different site by the time the patient is examined. An example is acute appendicitis, which typically starts with periumbilical or epigastric pain. Later, the patient develops visceral pain localized to the right lower quadrant. When rupture occurs, with the development of diffuse peritonitis, the clinical picture changes, culminating in diffuse, poorly localized abdominal pain. The clinical difficulty in evaluating the patient with acute abdominal pain increases when the patient is elderly, as he or she may have minimal findings at physical examination yet may harbor a significant pathology, perhaps requiring urgent intervention.

Correct diagnosis of the presence, level, and cause of the perforation is essential for appropriate management and surgical planning. Peptic ulcers are the main cause of gastroduodenal perforation, followed by necrotic or ulcerated malignancies. Penetrating ulcers of the anterior wall of the stomach or duodenum may perforate directly into the peritoneal cavity, whereas posterior stomach or duodenal ulcers often cause a walled-off or confined perforation. Duodenal ulcers are often located on the anterior bulb of the duodenum and are, therefore, a common cause of peritonitis. SB perforation is an emergency medical situation that presents as an acute abdomen, but it is only rarely diagnosed clinically. SB perforation can be caused by inflammatory, ischemic, traumatic, and neoplastic etiologies. Colonic perforation is a life-threatening condition requiring early recognition and treatment. Malignant neoplasms, diverticulitis, and spontaneous perforation are major causes of large-bowel perforation, followed by trauma, ischemia, different inflammatory lesions and iatrogenic causes (Furukawa et al. 2005).

1.7.2 Imaging

The radiologic hallmark of a perforated hollow viscus is the presence of air and/or fluid in the peritoneal cavity, in the retroperitoneum, or within abdominal organs. The extraluminal air may be in the peritoneal cavity, retroperitoneal spaces, mesentery, or ligaments of organs. Plain radiography remains the first imaging study: in addition to upright and supine abdominal radiographic images, upright chest films and/or left lateral decubitus abdominal films should be included for the assessment of GI tract perforation (Grassi et al. 2004). However, extraluminal air may not be demonstrable if the perforation is very small, self-sealed, or well-contained by adjacent organs. The reported sensitivity of plain radiography in the detection of extraluminal air is 50–70%. Other modalities include US, which may be particularly useful in patient groups in whom radiation burden should be limited, notably children and pregnant women. However, US should not be considered definitive in excluding a pneumoperitoneum. CT is very useful in

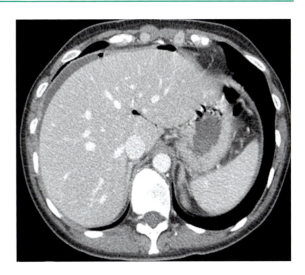

Fig. 17 Contrast-enhanced abdominal MDCT scan (wide window) of a patient with a perforated gastric ulcer. Evidence of peritoneal fluid and free air anterior to the liver surface. A small amount of air in the intrahepatic fissure for the ligamentum teres can also be seen

detecting extraluminal gas. MDCT is superior to single helical or conventional CT as it is able to provide rapid, high-volume coverage and diagnostic images even in patients unable to perform prolonged breath-holds. Moreover the thinner collimation of MDCT may improve the visualization of CT findings suggestive of colonic perforation (Ghekiere et al. 2007; Hainaux et al. 2006; Pinto et al. 2004).

Features that suggest perforated peptic ulcer (Fig. 17) on MDCT include extraluminal gas, extraluminal fluid, focal or diffuse gastroduodenal wall thickening >8 mm or abnormal enhancement, interruption of wall and inflammatory changes in the surrounding soft tissue or organs. Extraluminal free air is the most common and consistent finding of GD perforation, although it may be absent, especially at symptom onset. Free air or an air-fluid level crossing the midline and an accentuating falciform ligament (falciform ligament sign) and free air confined in the intrahepatic fissure of the ligamentum teres (ligamentum teres sign) are considered to be useful findings in patients with perforation of the duodenal bulb or stomach. Moreover, as a result of the anatomical relationship between the portal tract and the gastric antrum or duodenal bulb, in perforations of the upper GI tract free gas accumulates more frequently around the portal tract. This results in the peri-portal free gas

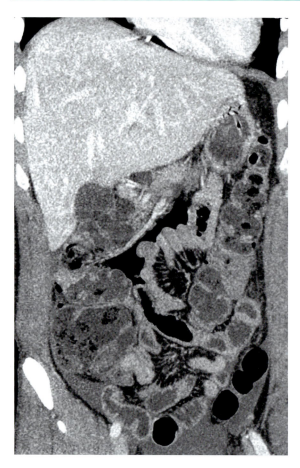

Fig. 18 Coronal MPR image (wide window) obtained in a 35-year-old man with a perforation of the jejunum after a motor vehicle accident. There is a large pneumoperitoneum in the middle abdominal quadrants close to some jejunal loops

sign, which is considered the most significant finding in distinguishing upper from lower GI tract perforation. On CT, direct visualization of the discontinuity of the bowel wall can specify the presence and site of GI tract perforation, which is marked by a low-attenuating cleft that usually runs perpendicular to the bowel wall. However, this cleft has been reported to be observed less frequently than free air on CT. Another specific finding of GI tract perforation is the extraluminal leakage of oral CM: thus, it is important to opacify the entire alimentary tract with a sufficient quantity of contrast agent. However, patients may not be able to cooperate because of pain, nausea, or vomiting and several authors have raised doubts about the added benefit of oral CM.

In SB perforations, the absence of pneumoperitoneum does not exclude perforation of a dilated fluid-filled SB loop. Even a small amount of peritoneal fluid may be the only sign indicating intestinal perforation. The usual ileal-perforating complications of CD are often sealed off because of inter-loop adhesions, leading to inflammation and abscess formation with localized peritonitis. Free perforation, although rare, is a life-threatening complication reported in up to 3% of cases. Jejunal diverticulitis is a rare cause of perforation: at CT, it manifests as a focal area of asymmetric thickening of the SB wall, most prominent on the mesenteric side of the bowel. The two most common etiologies that cause vascular impairment of the SB wall leading to perforation are direct vascular occlusion and strangulated SBO. Blunt abdominal trauma may result in SB perforation (Fig. 18). Shearing due to rapid deceleration injury may occur, for example, at the duodenojejunal flexure. CT findings include bowel wall thickening, pneumatosis, free gas, or a focal fluid collection adjacent to an injured SB loop. Ingested foreign bodies rarely cause GI perforation, as most pass uneventfully in the stool. Long, hard, or sharp objects, such as fish bones, chicken bones, and toothpicks may, however, cause perforation. Common sites of perforation include less fixed intestinal segments or segments with acute angulations, such as the ileum and the ileocecal and rectosigmoid segments.

Patients with colonic perforation, such as GD perforation, can present with a massive pneumoperitoneum, with free gas throughout the abdomen and pelvis. When free gas is present only in the pelvis, the colon, and not the SB, is the usual site of perforation. The reverse is true for supramesocolic free gas. However, exceptions occur, as sigmoid perforations may have free gas only in the supramesocolic compartment, in which case focal signs such as wall thickening and pericolonic stranding may be the only indications of the perforation site. Other CT findings observed in colonic perforation are: dirty mass (focal collection of extraluminal fecal matter containing small air bubbles), dirty fat sign (diffuse increase in attenuation of mesenteric fat), an extraluminal fluid collection, and interruption of the colonic wall (direct visualization of bowel wall discontinuity). Free retroperitoneal gas, often in the anterior pararenal space, may also be caused by colonoscopic perforations of the posterior walls of the sigmoid, ascending, and descending colon. Colonic carcinoma results in diffuse or focal bowel wall thickening and pericolonic stranding: once tumor invades the serosal fat, there is an increased possibility of perforation with abscess formation and gas leak. CT precisely determines the presence of free intra-abdominal gas, although the CT signs of perforation may be subtle and only indirectly related to the source. Findings such as a focal defect in the bowel wall, segmental bowel wall thickening, and concentrated bubbles of extraluminal gas in close proximity to the bowel wall have a high predictive value for the site of perforation. Stercoral perforation of the colon is a distinct clinical and pathologic entity. It occurs due to pressure necrosis of the colonic wall from a rock-hard fecaloma. In such cases, performing an immediate, optimal surgical procedure is mandatory to reduce the mortality rate from stercoral perforation; thus, it is important to be familiar with the CT findings of stercoral perforation.

1.7.3   Differentials

Acute pancreatitis
Acute cholecystitis
Acute non-perforated appendicitis
Gastro-enterocolitis
Small bowel obstruction
Ischemic bowel disease
Urolithiasis
Abdominal and pelvic hemorrhage.

1.8   Acute Gastrointestinal Bleeding

1.8.1   Terminology and Clinical Issues

Acute gastrointestinal bleeding (GIB) is an emergency situation requiring a fast and timely diagnosis. The annual incidence of GIB is 20–150 cases per 100,000 individuals, with a higher incidence in the upper GI tract (Manning-Dimmitt et al. 2005). The most frequent symptoms are: melena, hematemesis, decreasing hemoglobin, and even hemodynamic instability requiring stabilization of blood pressure and reinstatement of intravascular volume. Mortality ranges from 3.6 to 18% (Frager and Baer 1995) and increases to 21–40% in cases of massive bleeding (Van Leeerdam et al. 2003).

GIB is determined by upper and lower causes based on its originating proximal or distal to the ligament of Treitz. Upper GIB is approximately five times more common than lower GIB; lower GIB originates in the colon in 80% of the cases.

Localization of the bleeding site is essential to determine management. Nasogastric aspiration and lavage is an effective measure to determine whether there is an upper GIB. Endoscopy confirms the diagnosis in 95% of these cases in addition to offering therapeutic options (sclerotherapy, clipping, cauterizaton, or banding). In lower GIB, identification of the bleeding site is more difficult, with an overall reported success rate of 70%. Fortunately, up to 85% of the cases of lower GIB resolve spontaneously.

Several techniques have been established to discover the origin of acute GIB, including endoscopy, angiography, tagged red-blood cells nuclear scan, and CT. The choice of the most appropriate technique depends on local availability, examiner's experience, the nature and intensity of the hemorrhage, the origin of the bleeding, and the patient's condition. Endoscopy has a variable diagnostic yield of 48–90%; it often fails to localize the exact site of continued and massive bleeding (>1 ml/min); furthermore, the detection rate of bleeding lesions of the colon is low in the setting of incomplete intestinal preparation. Tagged red-blood cells scintigraphy is both very sensitive and non-invasive; it can help detect low rates (0.1 mL/min) of venous and arterial bleeding as well as intermittent bleeding. While it does not require patient preparation, it is a time-consuming procedure, does not exactly localize the site of bleeding, and it is not available 24/7 in many hospitals. Angiography is an expensive, time-consuming and invasive procedure that is not available in many institutions.

1.8.2   Imaging

MDCT-angiography is, potentially, the best diagnostic tool for detecting acute GIB. It is fast, available, and enables the acquisition of accurate arterial phase images, thus allowing mapping of the arterial vasculature and of CM extravasation into the intestinal lumen; the latter is indicative of GIB. Furthermore, isotropic spatial resolution and post-processing MDCT techniques have greatly expanded the diagnostic role of CT angiography, allowing the detection in multiple orthogonal planes of even very small vascular lesions responsible for bleeding (Yoon et al. 2006). MDCT-angiography may be superior to conventional angiography for detecting GIB, even at a bleeding intensity of 0.5 ml/min (Amarteifio et al. 2008).

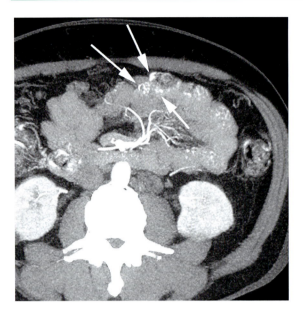

Fig. 19 Contrast-enhanced CT scan obtained in the arterial phase shows irregular enlargement of a jejunal loop vascular plexus due to angiodysplasia (*arrows*)

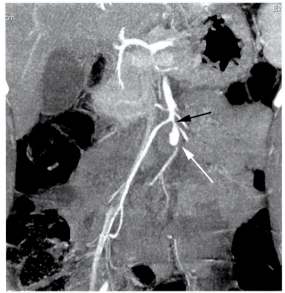

Fig. 20 Coronal MIP reformatted image acquired in the arterial phase shows a pseudo-aneurysm of a jejunal branch of the superior mesenteric artery, with a typical round morphology (*white arrow*) and narrow neck (*black arrow*)

Initial experience indicates that MDCT-angiography is a promising first-line modality for the detection and localization of acute GIB (sensitivity 91%, specificity 99%, accuracy 97.6%, positive predictive value 95%, and negative predictive value 98%).

Because of the intermittent nature of GIB, it is crucial to perform MDCT-angiography examination during an episode of active bleeding to maximize detection capabilities. Careful attention to MDCT technique is mandatory. A total CM volume of 100–120 ml with high concentrations of iodine at high injection rates (at least 4 ml/s) is recommended. Preliminary non-enhanced CT acquisition followed by an arterial-phase and at least one additional delayed acquisition may be necessary to detect GIB.

An unenhanced abdominal CT scan should be obtained to detect pre-existing hyper-attenuating material in the bowel lumen (see Differentials). The arterial phase is mandatory to identify arterial anomalies, early draining veins and vascular tufts, and initial extravasation of CM into the bowel lumen (Figs. 19, 20). Portal phase acquisition is useful to detect tumors causing GIB (Fig. 21). The late capillary phase allows ample time for the injected CM to pass through the GI wall vasculature, reaching the bleeding lesion and pooling in the bowel lumen. This phase is useful to detect the prolonged opacification

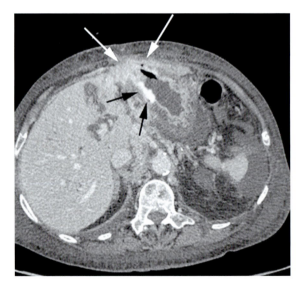

Fig. 21 Axial CT scan acquired in the portal phase shows a gastric fundus tumor that invades the peritoneal surface of the anterior abdominal wall (*white arrows*). The tumor is responsible for active hemorrhage with active bleeding in the gastric lumen (*black arrows*)

of intramural veins and the luminal extravasation of CM due to active bleeding. It also allows detection of slower bleeding sites that may not be evident at arterial phase scanning. Coronal maximum-intensity

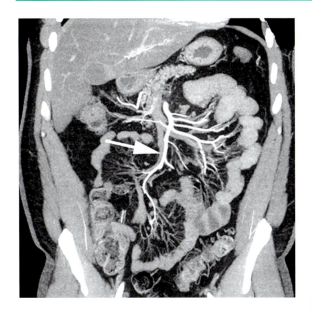

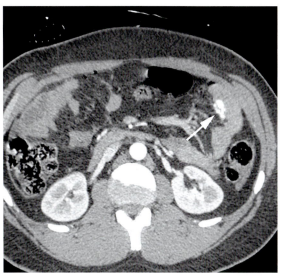

Fig. 22 Coronal MIP reformatted image shows the map of the superior mesenteric artery and its peripheral branches (*white arrow*)

Fig. 23 Axial CT scan depicts the extravasation of contrast material within the small bowel lumen due to active bleeding. The extravasated contrast material has a typical pooling morphology (*white arrow*)

projection (MIP) reformatted images are useful for localizing the bleeding bowel segment within the abdomen and to map the mesenteric arteries and their peripheral branches (Fig. 22).

The best CT image clue is hyper-attenuating extravasated CM within the GI lumen. Active bleeding is a focal area of high attenuation (>90 HU) that is detectable within the GI lumen (Fig. 23). Its shape may be linear and jet-like, swirled, ellipsoidal, spot or pooled; alternatively, it may fill the entire bowel lumen, resulting in a hyper-attenuating loop. Active arterial extravasation of CM can be differentiated from clotted blood by measuring CT attenuation. The attenuation of arterial active extravasation on MDCT scan ranges from 90 to 274 HU (mean 155), whereas that of clotted blood ranges from 28 to 82 HU (mean 54 HU). Minor CT findings include: high-attenuated peri-bowel fat, intestinal wall thickening, polyp, tumor, and vascular dilatation.

The site of CM extravasation on MDCT images corresponds exactly to the angiographically detected site of bleeding (Yoon et al. 2006). Compared to angiography, MDCT has a sensitivity of 90.9% and a specificity of 99% in the detection of acute GIB. In addition MDCT has an accuracy rate of 100% in localizing the site of acute GIB.

A negative CT-angiography excludes the necessity to perform angiography.

1.8.3 Differentials

- Pre-existing hyper-attenuating material in the bowel lumen (metallic clips, suture materials, foreign bodies, drugs, or retained contrast material)
- Hypervascular GI tumors (stromal tumors, carcinoid, and adenocarcinoma)
- Intraluminal hypervascular metastasis (melanoma, breast, and renal cell carcinoma)
- Solid density mass that does not show morphological changes during the arterial/portal acquisition phases
- Intestinal trauma
- Intestinal ischemia
- Gastric, duodenal ulcers
- Colonic angiodysplasia

An additional consideration in the differential diagnosis is a true diverticulum, which is the most frequent congenital malformation of the GI tract. It is located in the distal ileum, usually within about 60–100 cm of the ileocecal valve. The majority of people with Meckel's diverticulum are asymptomatic (Yashura 2005). However, the most common presenting symptom is painless rectal bleeding such as melaena-like black offensive stools, followed by intestinal obstruction, volvulus, and intussusception. Occasionally, Meckel's diverticulitis may present with all the features of acute appendicitis.

1.9   Acute Appendicitis

1.9.1   Terminology and Clinical Issues

Acute appendicitis is a common clinical problem in patients presenting to the emergency department with abdominal pain. In 80% of the cases, the clinical signs and symptoms are straightforward and imaging may not be necessary to make the diagnosis. However, in the remaining 20%, the clinical picture is atypical and the diagnosis is uncertain, especially in pediatric patients, thin young adults, and pregnant patients. In these patients radiation dose is an important consideration such that US is the first approach imaging modality. CT is used only in cases with inconclusive US findings, in obese/elderly patients, or in difficult/challenging cases.

Luminal obstruction due to appendicolith or hypertrophied Peyer patches and superimposed infection is the most common mechanism of appendiceal inflammation, causing a cascade mechanism in which there may be luminal distension, a pus-filled lumen, thickened appendiceal walls with infiltration by inflammatory cells, and even luminal perforation. Perforation of the appendix can lead to a peri-appendiceal abscess or diffuse peritonitis. The major reason for appendiceal perforation is a delay in diagnosis and treatment. In general, the longer the delay between diagnosis and surgery, the greater the likelihood of perforation. The risk of perforation 36 h after the onset of symptoms is at least 15%. Therefore, early diagnosis is essential; once appendicitis is diagnosed, surgery should be done without unnecessary delay.

1.9.2   Imaging

Abdominal radiography is of little clinical utility. In some cases, a calcified fecalith may be identified while signs of reflex ileus are frequently associated with appendiceal inflammation or perforation/peritonitis.

On US, the typical gray-scale signs include a non-compressible appendix ≥7 mm, sonographic McBurney's sign, shadowing, echogenic appendicolith, right lower quadrant fluid, inflammation, and abscess. Common color Doppler signs are flow within the appendiceal wall, which has 85% sensitivity and 90% specificity.

In most cases, non-enhanced CT is sufficient. CT signs include a dilated appendix ≥7 mm, peri-appendiceal fat stranding, and appendicolith (Nikolaidis et al. 2004). CECT is reserved for challenging cases (95% sensibility and specificity). A dilated appendix ≥7 mm, abnormal enhancement of the appendiceal wall, peri-appendiceal fat stranding are signs of acute appendicitis.

1.9.3   Differentials

A wide spectrum of diseases, not only loco-regional but also in the abdominal/retroperitoneal or thoracic compartments, make up the differential diagnosis. In these cases, CT evaluation should be widened and not limited to the right lower quadrant.

The most commonly signs include:

- Mesenteric adenitis: enlarged lymph nodes in the mesentery and right lower quadrant, normal appendix
- Crohn's disease
- Pelvic inflammatory disease: adnexal mass, dilated fallopian tube with fluid levels (pyosalpinx)
- Cecal diverticulitis: mural thickening with pericecal inflammatory changes
- Epiploic appendagitis: small oval-shaped pericolonic fatty nodule with a hyperdense ring
- Appendiceal tumor: soft-tissue density mass infiltrating the appendix with slight perivisceral infiltration
- Cecal carcinoma: a cecal mass with lymphadenopathy may obstruct the appendix; minimal surrounding changes (Fig. 24).

1.10   Acute Colonic Diverticulitis

1.10.1   Terminology and Clinical Issues

Acute colonic diverticulitis is the second most common cause of acute abdominal pain and leads to 130,000 hospitalizations in the USA annually. The prevalence, and thus the incidence, of diverticulosis increases with age (Jacobs 2007; Stollman and Raskin 2004). Among the general population, 10% of those younger than 40 years and >60% of people older than 80 years have diverticulosis. In 10–20% of this group, diverticulitis will develop, localized on the left side of

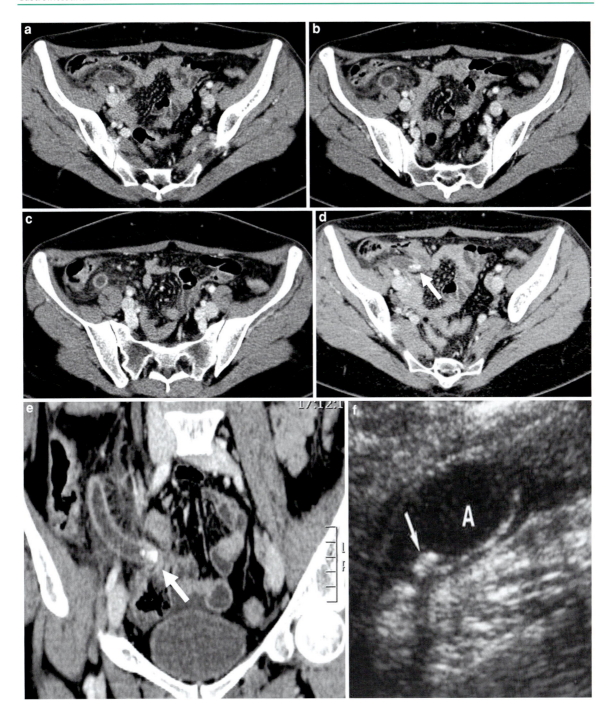

Fig. 24 Four contiguous axial CT scans show a long, fluid-filled, dilated, retrocecal appendicitis (**a–c**) in the right iliac fossa with an intraluminal appendicolith (**d**, *arrow*); haziness of the perivisceral fat is also visible. **e** Coronal MPR image shows a dilated appendicitis in its entire length and the appendicolith obstructing the visceral lumen. **f** US image shows the overdistended appendicitis (*A*) with a thickened bowel wall and intraluminal appendicolith (*arrow*)

the colon in 90% of cases. The process by which diverticulitis arises is similar to that of appendicitis: the neck of a diverticulum becomes obstructed by a fecolith, causing inflammation and localized ischemia, ultimately leading to perforation. Small perforations are contained by pericolic fat and cause

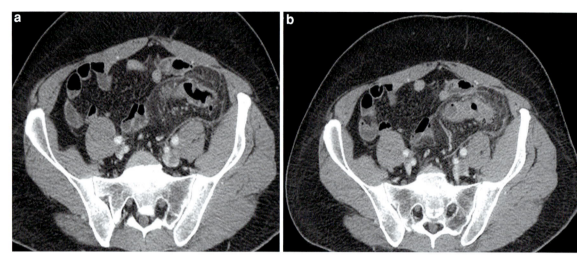

Fig. 25 A 45-year-old man with perforated sigmoid colon diverticulitis. Transverse MDCT scan shows segmental bowel-wall thickening, pericolic fat stranding and a diverticular outpouching (**a**); a diverticular abscess and a few extraluminal bubbles of air adjacent to the sigmoid wall are also seen (**b**)

pericolic inflammatory changes. Large perforations result in an abscess, which can be extensive and extend to other organs. Free perforation into the peritoneum causes feculent peritonitis but is rare.

Most patients with diverticulitis present with signs and symptoms sufficient to justify clinical diagnosis. Patients with acute colonic diverticulitis typically complain of generalized malaise, left lower abdominal quadrant pain, fever, nausea, vomiting, anorexia, and change in bowel habits, particularly constipation. On physical examination, left lower abdominal quadrant tenderness to palpation, rebound and involuntary guarding may be determined. Abdominal tenderness may be more midline or even in the right lower abdominal quadrant, when the sigmoid colon is redundant. Laboratory analysis may show an elevated white blood cell count. The severity of the clinical findings depends in large degree on the extent of paracolic inflammation that has spread from the point of the inflamed diverticulum.

1.10.2 Imaging

Until the 1980s, when it was replaced by CT, barium enema was the primary imaging modality for colonic diverticulitis (DeStigter and Keating 2009; Kaiser et al. 2005; Goh et al. 2007). Today, barium enema is not performed in the acute setting due to the risk of perforation and peritonitis. The advent of CT has revolutionized the diagnosis and

management of patients with diverticulitis. The following four criteria are considered diagnostic (Fig. 25): presence of diverticula, thickening of the bowel wall >4 mm, inflammatory pericolic fat, and pericolic abscess. The CT findings in complicated diverticulitis (Fig. 26) may include the presence of an abscess (defined as a fluid-containing mass with or without air and an enhancing wall) and contained or free extraluminal air bubbles or pockets. Other complications, such as bowel obstruction, hepatic abscess, fistula, and inferior mesenteric vein thrombosis, can often be demonstrated with CT. Fistulas frequently communicate with an abscess or other hollow viscus, and colovesicular fistulas are the most common.

In a recent meta-analysis, the accuracies of US and CT in the assessment and diagnosis of diverticulitis were not significantly different. Overall sensitivities were 92% for US and 94% for CT ($P = 0.65$), and overall specificities were 90% for US and 99% for CT ($P = 0.07$) (Lameris et al. 2008). The sensitivity of CT for the diagnosis of alternative diseases was higher (50–100%). Two frequently present CT findings that have high sensitivity for the diagnosis of diverticulitis are wall thickening (95% sensitivity) and fat stranding (91% sensitivity). CT is used not only to diagnose but also to stage disease. It assists in therapeutic decisions and in the detection of alternative diseases, according to the guidelines of the

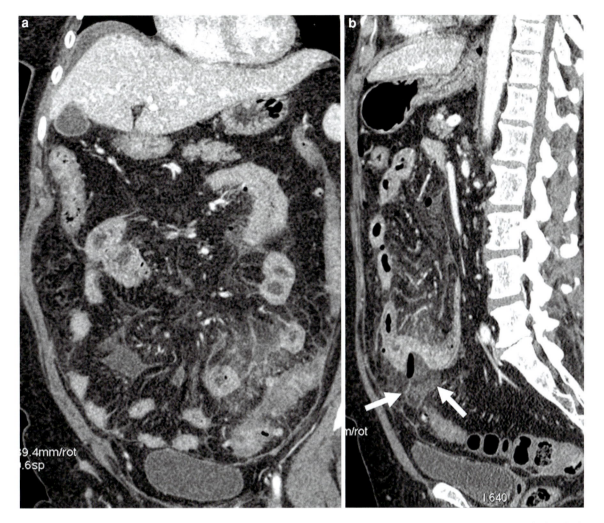

Fig. 26 A 56-year-old man with complicated sigmoid colon diverticulitis. **a** The MPR coronal image shows segmental bowel-wall thickening, pericolic fat stranding, and peritoneal fluid. **b** The MPR sagittal image shows a peri-diverticular abscess (*arrows*) and extraluminal air bubbles

American Society of Colorectal Surgeons: CT is helpful in identifying and/or excluding other causes of abdominal pain when diverticulitis is not the etiology. The disease stage in patients with diverticulitis is often determined by using the modified Hinchey classification system (Table 3).

Most patients with uncomplicated diverticulitis will respond to a conservative treatment regimen of antibiotics and diet modification. In mildly ill patients with a presentation clearly suggestive of uncomplicated diverticulitis (Hinchey stage 0 or 1a), the treatment decision is not based on the imaging results but rather on the patient's clinical status. In patients

Table 3 Modified Hinchey classification of disease stage in patients with diverticulitis

Stage	Characteristic
0	Mild clinical diverticulitis
1a	Confined pericolic inflammation, no abscess
1b	Confined pericolic inflammation with local abscess
2	Pelvic, retroperitoneal, or distant intraperitoneal abscess
3	Generalized purulent peritonitis, no communication with bowel lumen
4	Feculent peritonitis, open communication with bowel lumen

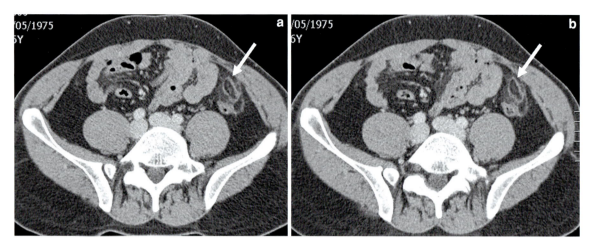

Fig. 27 A 35-year-old man with suspected colon diverticulitis. **a, b** Two contiguous axial CT scans show a small oval-shaped fatty nodule with a hyperdense ring (*arrow*), consistent with epiploic appendagitis located anterior to the distal discending colon. Note, peri-appendagitis soft-tissue haziness and a thickened lateroconal fascia

with Hinchey stage 1b diverticulitis in which there is a small (<2 cm) abscess, treatment can be conservative as well. Patients with larger abscesses are treated with percutaneous drainage. Diverticulitis-associated abscesses are found at CT in approximately 15% of patients. The majority of these collections (~36–59%) are mesocolic abscesses, which can be treated with percutaneous drainage. Percutaneous abscess drainage can obviate surgery or allow an elective one-step procedure in most cases. If patients do not respond to or deteriorate while undergoing conservative treatment, they will need to undergo surgery. However, correct imaging staging and therapy have today limited the surgical approach to a very few cases.

1.10.3 Differentials
- Acute cholecystitis
- Appendicitis
- Epiploic appendagitis
- Ischemic colitis
- Ovarian cystic disease
- Ureteral stone disease
- Inflammatory bowel disease
- Perforated colonic carcinoma

Primary colon carcinoma is the main concern in the differential for findings of diverticulitis on CT because it may present with eccentric or circumferential wall thickening, varying degrees of inflammation, and signs of obstruction (Fig. 27).

1.11 Bowel and Mesenteric Trauma

1.11.1 Terminology and Clinical Issues
Bowel and mesenteric trauma (BMT) is relatively uncommon, occurring in approximately 3–5% of patients undergoing laparotomy for blunt abdominal trauma. SB injuries typically occur in the proximal jejunum near the ligament of Trietz or at the distal ileum near the ileo-cecal junction, where mobile and fixed segments of the intestine are joined and can move during a blunt deceleration trauma. The mechanisms of blunt trauma that can cause intestinal and mesenteric injuries include crushing injury of the bowel between the vertebral bodies or steering wheels/handlebars; deceleration shearing of the SB at fixed points such as the Trietz ligament, the ileo-cecal valve, and around the mesenteric artery; closed-loop rupture caused by a sudden increase in intra-abdominal-pressure. The use of a seat-belt should raise suspicion for enteric and mesenteric injuries.

The clinical diagnosis of intestinal and mesenteric trauma and differentiation of the injuries requiring surgery from those that can be treated conservatively may be very difficult from a clinical viewpoint; signs and symptoms often require hours before they clinically appear. As a result, a delay in the diagnosis—and thus in the surgical repair of BMT—increases the incidence of fatal complications, such as acute bleeding, peritonitis, and abdominal abscesses. Mortality varies widely, from 5 to 65%. Mesenteric injuries are about three times more frequent than bowel injuries, with associated extra-GI injuries in at least half of all cases.

Blunt trauma accounts only for 5% of colonic traumatic injuries.

Injuries involving the colon are more frequently the result of a penetration trauma. The colon is the second most frequently injured organ after gunshot wounds and the third after stab wounds to the abdomen.

According to recent studies, morbidity after colonic injuries is in the range of 20–35% and mortality in the range of 3–15%. The incidence of infectious complications after a colonic injury is related to inadequate treatment or a delay in diagnosis. Several reports have confirmed that repair of a colonic injury within 3 h dramatically reduces the incidence of infectious complications.

1.11.2 Imaging

In many institutions, MDCT is the primary modality used in the emergency evaluation of patients with blunt abdominal trauma. Previous investigators have demonstrated the utility of CT for detecting solid-organ, vessel, and spine injuries. Numerous studies have evaluated the efficacy of CT for the diagnosis of BMT (Killeen et al. 2001; Malhotra et al. 2000; Scaglione et al. 2002; Brody et al. 2000).

Evaluation of the small intestinal tract with MDCT is not easy because the SB is several meters long, with a tortuous, variable course and a very thin wall. The large mesenteric fan and its arterial and venous supply are difficult to evaluate. In addition, BMTs have a low incidence, their characteristic appearance is less well known than that of solid-organ trauma lesions, and early signs may be subtle and easily overlooked at MDCT scan.

Preliminary NECT acquisition followed by CECT arterial and venous phases may be necessary to detect BMT. Contrast agents with higher concentrations of iodine (400 mg/ml) and high injection rates (at least 4 ml/s) are preferred and are followed by a 30–50 ml saline chaser, also injected at a rate of 4 ml/s. A volume of 100–120 ml of CM is generally sufficient for the post-contrast CT evaluation.

Preliminary NECT scan is performed to detect pre-existing hyper-attenuating material in the bowel lumen, such as metallic clips used for endoscopic hemostasis, suture materials, foreign bodies, drugs, or CM retained in the intestinal lumen.

The arterial phase is mandatory to identify arterial mesenteric bleeding, traumatic pseudo-aneurysm or thrombotic occlusion, and the early extravasation of CM within the bowel lumen. Portal phase acquisition results in maximum bowel wall enhancement and is useful to depict traumatic findings. A delayed phase may facilitate the detection of the mesenteric and endoluminal extravasation of CM due to late active bleeding. Evidence of active bleeding depends on multiple factors, including the patient's hemodynamic status and body mass index as well as the iodine concentration of the CM (Tang et al. 2010).

The use oral CM has been questioned by several authors (Stamatakos et al. 2009) based on literature reports of its lack of substantial added benefits for depicting bowel and mesenteric injuries. Moreover, intraluminal high-density oral CM can hide the wall of the injured intestinal loops, thereby delaying the diagnosis (Cubiella Fernández et al. 2010). Potential risks for unconscious patients include the aspiration of oral CM, with subsequent respiratory complications. At our institution, all initial CT scans for trauma patients are obtained without oral. The use of CM is reserved for follow-up/second look CT evaluations, in the restricted number of patients in whom bowel injuries have been previously suspected, or to confirm specific findings such as extravasation of oral CM.

CT findings of blunt BMT may be very subtle, difficult to detect, and easily overlooked at initial CT scans. These injuries are rarely isolated; rather, they are more often associated with other organ injuries, correlating with the type, site, and extent of the damage (Koutroubakis 2008).

The most important CT findings of BMT include:

- Free intra/retroperitoneal/mesenteric air or fluid
- Thickened bowel wall and or abnormal wall enhancement
- Bowel wall defect
- Active CM extravasation from a mesenteric vessel
- Focal mesenteric hematoma
- Vessel beading
- Abrupt vessel termination
- Mesenteric stranding or fluid between loops
- Extraluminal oral CM.

1.11.2.1 Bowel Loop Injury

Free intra- or retroperitoneal air or mesenteric air may indicate a bowel wall perforation (Fig. 28). Free air peritoneal bubbles can be distributed near the

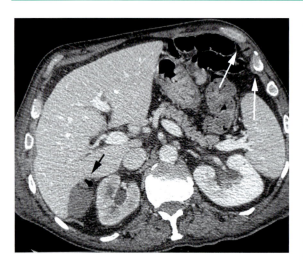

Fig. 28 Multiple intraperitoneal free air bubbles are localized near the left diaphragmatic rib attachment (*white arrows*) and within the subhepatic posterior space or Morison's recess (*black arrow*)

abdominal wall or can surround the liver and spleen. They can also accumulate in the hepatic hilum, in the mesenteric folds, and, rarely, in the portal lumen. Retroperitoneal gas bubbles indicate a rupture of the duodenum or the ascending or descending colon. A perforation of the right or left colon into the retroperitoneal spaces may be clinically silent for a long time. However, it should be emphasized that intraperitoneal free air is not a pathognomonic sign of bowel perforation but is also associated with traumatic bladder injury or the result of pneumothorax, pneumomediastinum, mechanical ventilation, iatrogenic, diagnostic peritoneal lavage or penetrating injury without organ damage.

Direct interruption of the bowel wall is rare; nevertheless, the use of thin axial slices might increase its recognition. Direct evidence of oral CM extravasation into the peritoneal spaces is also a rare observation and is indicative of a full discontinuity of the injured bowel wall.

The thickness of the normally distended bowel wall is 1–2 mm, whereas that of the collapsed wall is 3–4 mm. Segmental bowel wall thickening on CT is generally due to an intramural hematoma or edema, especially if associated with a mesenteric hematoma.

When the admission CT study demonstrates an isolated focal bowel wall thickening and non-operative management is initially accepted, a repeat CT should be performed after 6–8 h. If this new CT scan demonstrates imaging stability, conservative management is generally adopted.

Bowel enhancement is classified as abnormal when it is increased or decreased compared with the enhancement of adjacent bowel loops. An alteration in bowel wall enhancement can be related to intramural edema (hypodense) or hemorrhage (hyperdense). Sometimes there is a non-homogeneous patchy enhancement of the injured bowel loop that may be related to a slow blood perfusion. In this case, the damage to the submucosal vascular plexus can lead to ischemia and an intramural leakage of CM. In the bowel, vascular damage can also depend on an interruption of the blood supply by mesenteric injury, with thrombosis or leakage of the arterial vessels. In cases of arterial leak, MDCT can localize areas of active bleeding for angiographic embolization or surgery.

Mesenteric injury with active bleeding that secondarily causes a devascularized bowel will result in an ischemic bowel loop, a situation that requires surgical treatment.

The spectrum of injuries to the large intestine in blunt trauma, such as contusion, tears, intramural hematoma, and devascularization with ischemia, are similar to that of small intestinal loops. Bowel injuries requiring surgery include a full-thickness perforation or seromuscular tear or devascularized bowel loops.

Free fluid in the peritoneal spaces is a relatively frequent finding in abdominal trauma, associated or not with injuries to solid or hollow organs. Careful evaluation of the quantity, density, and location of the fluid is important for optimal management: large amounts of free (especially high-attenuation) fluid in more than one space or focal mesenteric fluid is suggestive of an underlying bowel/mesenteric injury and may warrant surgery, clinical observation, or CT follow-up, whereas a small amount of low-attenuation fluid (especially in females) should be initially considered as a benign finding, not necessarily associated with bowel or mesenteric injury. Thus, follow-up CT and close clinical/laboratory observations are critical measures in those situations.

1.11.2.2 Mesenteric Injury

Mesenteric injuries can appear as hazy infiltration, hematomas (Fig. 29), or active CM extravasation in the mesenterial folds. Hazy infiltration is generally associated with a mesenteric contusion without vascular leakage.

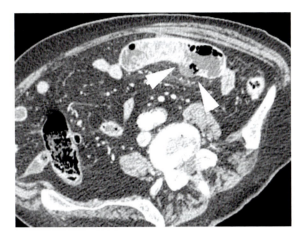

Fig. 29 Post-contrast CT axial scan demonstrates a discontinuity of a small bowel wall contour (*white arrows*) due to a traumatic injury

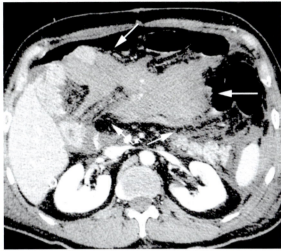

Fig. 31 Contrast-enhanced axial CT scan demonstrates a large homogeneously hyperdense transverse mesocolon hematoma (*white arrows*), without the extravasation of contrast medium

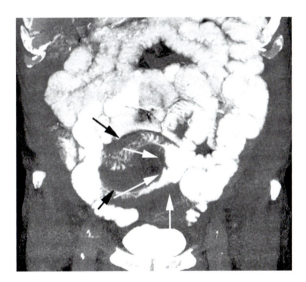

Fig. 30 Coronal MPR image demonstrates a large traumatic hematoma of the ileal loops (*black arrows*) and a large pooling of extravasated oral contrast medium outside the ileal lumen, due to a complete traumatic tear of the intestinal wall (*white arrows*)

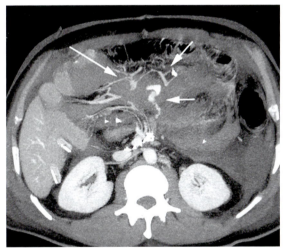

Fig. 32 Axial CT scan demonstrates a large mesenterial hematoma. The arterial mesenteric vessels have a beaded appearance, with irregular contours and abrupt termination (*white arrows*)

Irregularity of the mesenteric vessels includes a beaded appearance, with irregular contour and abrupt termination (Fig. 30) evidenced by the lack of continuity of the artery or vein.

CT attenuation values of mesenterial clotted blood are between 40 and 70 HU, whereas those of active hemorrhage vary from 70 to 370 HU. Active bleeding frequently occurs within a large mesenteric hematoma associated or not with a bowel injury.

Isolated mesenteric contusion or hematoma without active extravasation (Fig. 31) requires a follow-up CT evaluation after 6–8 h. If this scan demonstrates imaging stability, conservative management is generally adopted, whereas if a mesenteric vascular injury or bowel loop ischemia develops, the patient should undergo surgery and/or angiographic embolization (Fig. 32).

1.11.3 Differentials

In addition to bowel ischemia, the following should be considered:

Shock bowel. Mild to moderate diffuse small-bowel thickening and marked hyper-enhancement of the mucosa related to a reversible ischemic change

Coagulopathy. Segmental, extensive, localized bowel wall changes; spontaneous resolution, otherwise anticoagulant therapy

Vasculitis. Bowel wall and vascular changes related to polyarteritis nodosa, systemic lupus erythematosus, Henoch-Schonlein purpura

Ischemic enteritis. Segmental bowel wall thickening (>3 mm), focal or diffuse pneumatosis (later phase).

References

Amarteifio E, Sohns C, Heuser M et al (2008) Detection of gastrointestinal bleeding by using multislice computer tomography-acute and chronic hemorrhages. Clin Imaging 32(1):1–5

Berritto D, Somma F, Landi N, Cavaliere C, Corona M, Russo S, Fulciniti F, Cappabianca S, Rotondo A, Grassi R (2011) Seven-Tesla micro-MRI in early detection of acute arterial ischaemia: evolution of findings in an in vivo rat model. Radiol Med 116:829–841

Brandt LJ, Boley SJ (2000) AGA technical review on intestinal ischemia. Gastroenterology 118:954–968

Brinton J (2000) Acute abdomen. Oxford textbook of surgery. Oxford University Press, Oxford

Brody JM, Leighton DB, Murphy BL et al (2000) CT of blunt trauma bowel and mesenteric injury: typical findings and pitfalls in diagnosis. Radiographics 20:1525–1537

Caprilli R, Vernia P, Latella G, Torsoli A (1987) Early recognition of toxic megacolon. J Clin Gastroenterol 9:160–164

Cubiella Fernández J, Núñez Calvo L, González Vázquez E, García García MJ, Alves Pérez MT, Martínez Silva I, Fernández Seara J (2010) Risk factors associated with the development of ischemic colitis. World J Gastroenterol 16(36): 4564–4569

DeStigter KK, Keating DP (2009) Imaging update: acute colonic diverticulitis. Clin Colon Rectal Surg 22:147–155

Di Mizio R (2002) Morbo di Crohn del tenue. Atlante di Radiologia. Verduci Editore, Roma

Di Mizio R, Scaglione M (2007) Small bowel Obstruction. CT features with plain film and US correlations. Springer, Milano

Frager DH, Baer JW (1995) Role of CT in evaluating patients with small bowel obstruction. Semin Ultrasound CT MR 13:127–140

Furukawa A, Sakoda M, Yamasaki M et al (2005) Gastrointestinal tract perforation: CT diagnosis of presence, site, and cause. Abdom Imaging 30:524–534

Furukawa A, Kanasaki S, Kono N, Wakamiya M, Tanaka T, Takahashi M, Murata K (2009) CT diagnosis of acute mesenteric ischemia from various causes. AJR 192:408–416

Ghekiere O, Lesnik A, Hoa D et al (2007) Value of Computed Tomography in the diagnosis of the cause of nontraumatic gastrointestinal tract perforation. J Comput Assist Tomogr 31:169–176

Goh V, Halligan S, Taylor SA et al (2007) Differentiation between diverticulitis and colorectal cancer: quantitative CT perfusion measurements versus morphologic criteria–initial experience. Radiology 242:456–462

Gore RM, Yaghmai V, Thakrar KH, Berlin JW, Mehta UK, Newmark GM, Miller FH (2008) Imaging in intestinal ischemic disorders. Radiol Clin North Am 46(5):845–875

Grassi R, Romano S, Pinto A et al (2004) Gastro-duodenal perforations: conventional plain film, US and CT findings in 166 consecutive patients. Eur J Radiol 50:30–36

Hainaux B, Agneessens E, Bertinotti R et al (2006) Accuracy of MDCT in predicting site of gastrointestinal tract perforation. AJR Am J Roentgenol 187:1179–1183

Iacobellis F, Berritto D, Somma F, Cavaliere C, Corona M, Cozzolino S, Fulciniti F, Cappabianca S, Rotondo A, Grassi R (2012) MRI: could it be a new tool for the diagnostic management of acute ischemic colitis? An experimental study. World J Gastroenterol (in press)

Jacobs DO (2007) Clinical practice: diverticulitis. N Engl J Med 357:2057–2066

Kaiser AM, Jiang JK, Lake JP et al (2005) The management of complicated diverticulitis and the role of computed tomography. Am J Gastroenterol 100:910–917

Killeen KL, Shaunmuganathan K, Poletti PA et al (2001) Helical computed tomography of bowel and mesenteric injury. J Trauma) 1:26–36

Koutroubakis IE (2008) Ischemic colitis: clinical practice in diagnosis and treatment. World J Gastroenterol 14: 7302–7308

Lameris W, van Randen A, Bipat S et al (2008) Graded compression ultrasonography and computed tomography in acute colonic diverticulitis: meta-analysis of test accuracy. Eur Radiol 18:2498–2511

Malhotra AK, Fabian TC, Katsis SB et al (2000) Blunt bowel and mesenteric injuries: the role of screening computed tomography. J Trauma 48:91–100

Manning-Dimmitt LL, Dimmitt SG, Wilson GR (2005) Diagnosis of gastrointestinal bleeding in adults. Am Fam Phys 71:1339–1346

Menke J (2010) Diagnostic accuracy of multidetector CT in acute mesenteric ischemia: systematic review and metanalysis. Radiology 256(1):93–101

Moschetta M, Stabile Ianora AA, Pedote P et al (2009) Prognostic value of multidetector computer tomography in bowel infarction. Radiol Med 114:780–791

Nikolaidis P, Hwang CM, Miller FH, Papanicolaou N (2004) The nonvisualized appendix: incidence of acute appendicitis when secondary inflammatory changes are absent. AJR Am J Roentgenol 183(4):889–892

Pinto A, Scaglione M, Giovine S et al (2004) Comparison between the site of multislice CT signs of gastrointestinal perforation and the site of perforation detected at surgery in forty perforated patients. Radiol Med 108:208–217

Romano S, Lassandro F, Scaglione M, Romano L, Rotondo A, Grassi R (2006) Ischemia and infarction of the small bowel and colon: spectrum of imaging findings. Abdom Imaging 31(3):277–292

Scaglione M, Lassandro F, Romano L et al (2002) Value of contrast enhanced CT for managing mesenteric injuries after blunt trauma: review of five year experience. Emerg Radiol 9:26–31

Stamatakos M, Douzinas E, Stefanaki C et al (2009) Ischemic colitis: surging waves of update. Tohoku J Exp Med 218(2):83–92

Stollman N, Raskin JB (2004) Diverticular disease of the colon. Lancet 363:631–639

Tang ZH, Qiang JW, Feng XY, Li RK, Sun RX, Ye XG (2010) Acute mesenteric ischemia induced by ligation of porcine superior mesenteric vein: multidetector CT evaluations. Acad Radiol 17(9):1146–1152

Taourel P, Aufort S, Merigeaud S, Curros Doyon F, Devaux Hoquet M, Delabrousse E (2008) Imaging of ischemic colitis. Radiol Clin N Am 46:909–924

Van Leeerdam ME, Vreeburg EM, Rauws EA et al (2003) Acute upper GI bleeding: did anything change? Time trend analysis of incidents and outcome of acute upper GI bleeding between 1993/1994 and 2000. Am J Gastroenterol 98:1494–1499

Wadman M, Block T, Ekberg o, Sky I, Elmstahl S, Acosta S (2010) Impact of MDCT with intravenous contrast on the surival in patients with acute superior mesenteric artery occlusion. Emerg Radiol 17(3):171–178-13

Wittenberg J, Harisinghani MG, Jhaveri K et al (2002) Algorithmic approach to CT diagnosis of the abnormal bowel wall. RadioGraphics 22:1093–1107

Yashura H (2005) Acute mesenteric ischemia: the challenge of gastroenterology. Surg Today 35:185–195

Yoon W, Jeong YY, Shin SS et al (2006) Acute massive gastrointestinal bleeding: detection and localization with arterial phase multi-detector row helical CT. Radiology 228:743–750

The Pelvis

Lorenzo Mannelli, Claudia T. Sadro, Bruce E. Lehnert,
Manjiri K. Dighe, and Joel A. Gross

Contents

L. Mannelli · C. T. Sadro · B. E. Lehnert · J. A. Gross (✉)
Department of Radiology, Harborview Medical Center,
University of Washington, 325 Ninth Ave,
Box 359728 Seattle, WA 98104-2499, USA
e-mail: jagross@uw.edu

M. K. Dighe
Department of Radiology, University of Washington,
1959 NE Pacific Street, Box 357115
Seattle, WA 98195, USA

Abstract

This chapter reviews emergency imaging of the pelvis, and is divided into sections for the male and female patient, and for common imaging of both genders. The non-pregnant female pelvis is initially discussed, with a review of abnormal uterine bleeding in the pre- and post-menopausal patient, fibroids, cervical cancer, endometritis, functional ovarian cysts, polycystic ovarian syndrome, endometriosis, teratomas, pelvic inflammatory disease, tubo-ovarian abscess, ovarian torsion, and ovarian masses and cysts. This is followed by a review of the pregnant patient, including evaluation of the pregnancy itself, and of the acute abdomen in pregnancy. Emergency imaging of the male pelvis is then discussed, with a review of epididymo-orchitis,

M. Scaglione et al. (eds.), *Emergency Radiology of the Abdomen*,
Medical Radiology. Diagnostic Imaging,
DOI: 10.1007/174_2011_475, © Springer-Verlag Berlin Heidelberg 2012

testicular abscess, torsion of the testis and appendix testis, Fournier's gangrene, scrotal trauma, palpable scrotal lesions, varicoceles, hydroceles, the undescended testis, prostatic infection and abscess, and benign prostatic hypertrophy, Non-gender specific emergencies are next reviewed starting with trauma, and include pelvic osseous trauma, traumatic pelvic hemorrhage and bladder trauma. We finish up with a discussion of additional bladder emergencies including bladder fistulae and cancer.

1   Introduction

This chapter is divided into sections addressing the male and female patient, and common imaging in the two genders. Imaging of the non-pregnant female is initially presented, including evaluation of the uterus and ovaries for pain, abnormal uterine bleeding, infection, and neoplasms. This is followed by a brief review of complications during and after pregnancy. Imaging of the male pelvis is then presented, including traumatic and non-traumatic emergencies of the testes, scrotum, and prostate. The chapter concludes with a brief review of pelvic osseous trauma and hemorrhage, and imaging of traumatic and non-traumatic bladder emergencies.

2   Female Pelvis

2.1   Abnormal Uterine Bleeding in Premenopausal Patients

2.1.1   Terminology and Clinical Issues
In non-pregnant pre-menopausal patients, systemic factors (such as hormonal therapy or abnormalities, coagulopathy, etc.) are the most common cause of dysfunctional uterine bleeding, which may not present with abnormalities visible on imaging studies. This section will focus on those causes that can be imaged.

2.1.2   Imaging
An intrauterine device (IUD) can cause bleeding due to malposition, migration, or uterine perforation (Williams et al. 2003). Ultrasound (US) is the study of choice for suspected IUD related complications. Occasionally, radiographs or computed tomography (CT) may be helpful for further evaluation. Adenomyosis can present

with dysfunctional uterine bleeding due to functional endometrial tissue in an ectopic location within the myometrium. The US appearance includes myometrial cysts and ill-defined areas of heterogeneous and distorted myometrial echotexture in a globular or enlarged uterus. Asymmetric thickening of the myometrium may be seen in the setting of focal adenomyosis. The magnetic resonance imaging (MRI) criteria for the diagnosis of adenomyosis are a non-uniform, thickened junctional zone measuring >12 mm, with T1w hyperintense areas in the myometrium corresponding to the myometrial cysts. A specific sign of adenomyosis is foci of T1w high intensity in the myometrium, which represent cysts containing pooled blood. A focus of poorly defined myometrial heterogeneity could represent focal adenomyoma (Williams et al. 2003). Cervical carcinoma can cause bleeding in premenopausal patients, especially those who are sexually active; however, this is better evaluated with clinical examination as early cervical carcinoma may not be apparent on US (Williams et al. 2003). Endometriosis, fibroids, and pelvic inflammatory disease can also cause abnormal uterine bleeding in premenopausal patients and is discussed separately.

2.2   Abnormal Uterine Bleeding in Postmenopausal Patients

2.2.1   Terminology and Clinical Issues
In postmenopausal patients, the endometrial thickness is normally <5–7 mm (Williams et al. 2003). In the setting of hormone replacement therapy, it may be non-pathologically increased to 8–10 mm. The most common cause of posmenopausal uterine bleeding is atrophy of the endometrium. An endometrial thickness of ≤4 mm in a patient with postmenopausal bleeding is typical for endometrial atrophy and is associated with a very low (<1%) risk of malignancy Endometrial hyperplasia is most commonly encountered in perimenopausal women and can result in irregular bleeding.

2.2.2   Imaging
On US, echogenic endometrial thickening is noted, sometimes containing tiny cystic spaces (Williams et al. 2003). Blood clots, endometrial hyperplasia, endometrial polyps, endometrial carcinoma, and submucosal fibroids can have a similar US appearance. Sonohysterography may help to differentiate between these entities (Williams et al. 2003), as endometrial

hyperplasia demonstrates a uniform endometrial thickening, unlike polyps and carcinoma, which appears as focal masses. Polyps are usually seen as smooth pedunculated or sessile masses with a central vascular stalk. Endometrial carcinomas are hypoechoic or hyperechoic with an irregular shape and may extend into the myometrium. Submucosal fibroids are usually hypoechoic and heterogeneous in appearance and have a broad base with the endometrium; however, some submucosal fibroids are completely contained within the endometrium and have a stalk (Williams et al. 2003). Because of cost, limited availability, and low spatial resolution, the role of MRI in the workup of abnormal vaginal bleeding is limited.

2.3   Fibroid (Leiomyoma)

2.3.1   Terminology and Clinical Issues

Fibroids are common, occurring in 30% of women older than 30 years of age. They are responsible for many symptoms including menorrhagia, dysmenorrhea, urinary frequency, pelvic pain and pressure, and infertility. Acute fibroid-related pain is usually due to acute fibroid degeneration (Vandermeer and Wong-You-Cheong 2009; Kamaya et al. 2008) Fibroids are classified by location as submucosal, intramural, or subserosal.

2.3.2   Imaging

Although US is usually diagnostic for fibroids, large fibroids may not be completely or adequately evaluated on US. MRI may be used for further characterization of large fibroids or in patients undergoing fibroid embolization or surgical resection (Williams et al. 2003; Bennett et al. 2002) CT is not recommended for the diagnosis or characterization of fibroids, although due to their high prevalence in women, fibroids are often incidentally noted on CT performed for other reasons.

The typical US appearance is a well-defined, hypoechoic mass; however, fibroids can be heterogeneous, hyperechoic, or calcified with acoustic shadowing (Vandermeer and Wong-You-Cheong 2009; Cano Alonso et al. 2009) Hypoechoic areas within a fibroid may represent cystic degeneration, while anechoic, irregular spaces can be present in necrotic fibroids (Vandermeer and Wong-You-Cheong 2009). On US, submucosal fibroids may be difficult to differentiate from endometrial pathologies,

and pedunculated fibroids can simulate adnexal pathologies. In these cases MRI can be useful in further evaluation (Cano Alonso et al. 2009).

The CT appearance depends on the presence of intravenous contrast and the degree of degeneration. The fibroid uterus is enlarged with lobulated contours and has heterogeneous attenuation. Post-contrast images demonstrate heterogeneous enhancement, with the degenerated portions demonstrating less enhancement and lower attenuation (Bennett et al. 2002; Cano Alonso et al. 2009) Coarse dystrophic calcification within a uterine mass is a very specific CT sign for a leiomyoma.

MRI is the most accurate imaging technique for the detection and characterization of uterine fibroids. Non-degenerated fibroids appear as well-circumscribed intrauterine masses with a homogeneously decreased signal on T2w images, and enhancement on post-gadolinium T1w images. Degenerated fibroids have a variable appearance on unenhanced and enhanced MRI depending on the type of degeneration. The multiplanar and volumetric capabilities of MRI enable better anatomic localization of fibroids protruding into the adnexal region, allowing differentiation of a fibroid from an ovarian mass. Recognition of separate normal ovaries and/or the continuity of the adnexal mass with the myometrium assists in the diagnosis of a pedunculated fibroid (Williams et al. 2003; Vandermeer and Wong-You-Cheong 2009).

2.4   Cervical Cancer

Cervical cancer is usually staged clinically; however it is often detected incidentally on CT or during an evaluation for vaginal bleeding or pelvic pain. Findings of distorted pelvic anatomy, infiltrating masses, or enlarged pelvic lymph nodes at CT must be further evaluated with physical exam and/or biopsy (Sahdev 2010). The clinical and imaging features and staging of cervical cancer are beyond the scope of this chapter.

2.5   Endometritis

In non-obstetric patients, endometritis can occur in patients with cervical stenosis or recent pelvic instrumentation. CT may be helpful for excluding associated complications such as septic pelvic thrombophlebitis, ovarian vein thrombosis, and phlegmon (Bennett et al. 2002). US may be normal, but suggestive findings include an enlarged uterus with fluid and debris within a distended endometrial cavity, and an irregular heterogeneous intrauterine mass-like appearance. These findings overlap with those of retained products of conception and intrauterine hematoma (Vandermeer and Wong-You-Cheong 2009). Air and fluid may be seen within the endometrium in patients with endometritis, however these imaging findings are non-specific following recent procedural intervention.

2.6 Functional Ovarian Cysts

Functional ovarian cysts are a common finding on US, CT, and MRI. Asymptomatic cysts do not require follow-up in premenopausal patients if <5 cm, but symptomatic cysts causing pain, discomfort or menstrual irregularities can be followed with US. Subtypes of functional cysts include follicular, corpus luteal, and theca-lutein cysts (Stany and Hamilton 2008). Follicular cysts are thin-walled, unilocular, simple cysts. They are hypoechoic on US and demonstrate homogeneous signal intensity on MRI (low T1w, high T2w). Hemorrhagic corpus luteum cysts have a variable appearance at US and demonstrate high signal intensity on T1w MR images (Funt and Hann 2002). Potential complications of both follicular and corpus luteal cysts are intraperitoneal rupture with hemoperitoneum. At US, acute intracystic hemorrhage may be isoechoic or echogenic in appearance. In chronic hemorrhage, a clot within the cyst will appear as an echogenic mass with absence of vascularity on color Doppler imaging (Fig. 1). On CT, a hemorrhagic ovarian cyst appears as a mixed-attenuation adnexal mass with a hyperdense component (45–100 HU). On MRI, hemorrhagic cysts will demonstrate relatively high-signal intensity on T1w images and intermediate to high-signal intensity on T2w MR images. Ruptured cysts will produce free intrapelvic fluid (Fig. 2).

2.7 Polycystic Ovarian Syndrome

2.7.1 Terminology and Clinical Issues

Symptoms of polycystic ovarian syndrome (PCOS) vary greatly among women and include menstrual irregularity and pelvic pain, infertility, and obesity.

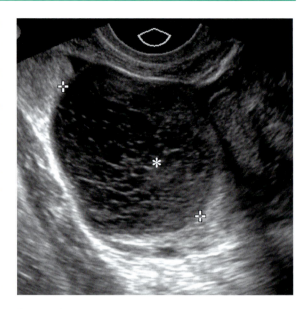

Fig. 1 US demonstrates an ovarian hemorrhagic cyst (*asterisk*) with a lace-like reticular pattern of internal echoes without internal color flow

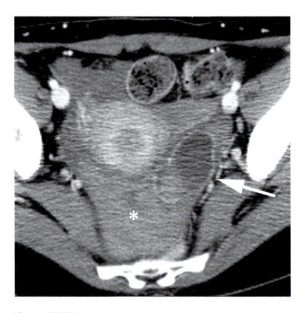

Fig. 2 CECT demonstrates ruptured ovarian hemorrhagic cyst (*arrow*) resulting in hemoperitoneum with a sentinel clot in the pelvis (*asterisk*)

The European Society for Human Reproduction and Embryology/American Society for Reproductive Medicine consensus criteria for the US diagnosis of PCOS are the presence of ≥12 follicles in each ovary measuring 2–9 mm in diameter or an increased ovarian volume (>10 cm^3) (Balen et al. 2003).

2.7.2 Imaging

The MRI-specific criteria have not yet been defined; however, MRI is very helpful when the ovaries are not visualized by US, for example in obese patients. The typical MRI features of PCOS are slightly enlarged ovaries with multiple small, peripherally located follicles around the normal central stroma. On T2w images, the follicles appear as multiple tiny, hyperintense, peripheral cysts while the central stroma is hypointense.

2.8 Endometriosis

2.8.1 Terminology and Clinical Issues

Endometriosis is defined by the presence of ectopic endometrial tissue outside the uterus. Symptoms include pelvic pain, dysmenorrhea, and dyspareunia (Brosens et al. 2004). Pelvic locations commonly involved are the ovaries, broad and round ligaments, fallopian tubes, cervix, vagina, and pouch of Douglas (Brosens et al. 2004).

2.8.2 Imaging

While US has low sensitivity in the detection of small endometrial implants, it is excellent in detecting endometriomas; these typically demonstrate diffuse, low-level internal echoes and hyperechoic foci in the wall. On CT, the imaging findings of endometrioma overlap those of an abscess, ovarian cyst, and malignant lesions, as endometriomas may appear solid, cystic, or mixed solid and cystic. On MRI, endometriomas are hyperintense on T1w images and hypointense on T2w images (referred to as "T2 shading").

2.9 Teratoma

2.9.1 Terminology and Clinical Issues

Mature cystic teratomas, also referred to as dermoid cysts, are well-differentiated neoplasms composed of at least two of the three germ cell layers (ectoderm, mesoderm, and endoderm). Mature cystic teratomas are usually asymptomatic, but can cause pain or other non-specific symptoms.

2.9.2 Imaging

On US, these tumors may have a variety of appearances:
- Cystic lesion with a densely echogenic tubercle projecting into the cyst lumen.
- Diffusely or partially echogenic mass with the echogenic area usually demonstrating posterior

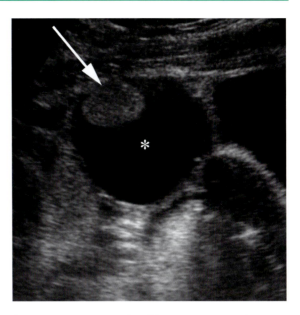

Fig. 3 US demonstrates the different components of a mature ovarian teratoma. The cyst contains an echogenic mural nodule (*arrow*), the "dermoid plug" that represents hair, teeth or fat. The cystic component (*asterisk*) is sebum, which is liquid at body temperature

attenuation owing to sebaceous material and hair within the cyst cavity.
- Multiple thin, echogenic bands caused by hair in the cyst cavity.

Hypoechoic or anechoic areas usually represent sebum (Fig. 3). Sebum floating above aqueous fluid may present as a fluid–fluid level. Echogenic foci with shadowing may be due to adipose-tissue calcifications or hair. The diagnosis is easier to make on CT and MRI due to their higher sensitivity in identifying fat within the cyst, which is diagnostic for teratoma (Fig. 4) (Buy et al. 1989).

Immature teratomas are rarer and usually larger than mature teratomas and may demonstrate malignant behavior. Large non-specific soft-tissue component masses, and discontinuity of the capsule are findings suggestive of immature teratomas, but on imaging they often cannot be differentiated from mature teratomas.

2.10 Pelvic Inflammatory Disease

Pelvic inflammatory disease (PID) should be suspected in patients presenting with pelvic pain, fever, and leukocytosis. The imaging findings depend on the

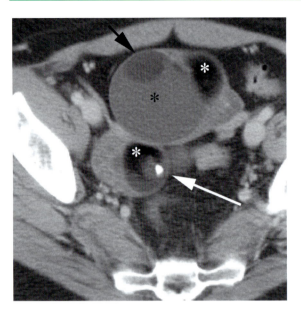

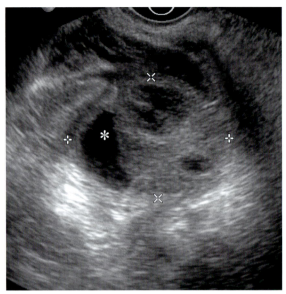

Fig. 4 CECT demonstrates bilateral ovarian dermoid cysts containing solid (black *arrow*) and fluid (*black asterisk*) components, fat (*white asterisks*), and calcifications (*white arrow*)

Fig. 5 US demonstrates complex cystic mass in the left adnexa representing a tubo-ovarian abscess, with solid and fluid (*asterisk*) components

disease severity (Vandermeer and Wong-You-Cheong 2009). In uncomplicated cases, US findings are frequently normal (Vandermeer and Wong-You-Cheong 2009). More severe cases may demonstrate uterine enlargement, endometrial thickening, endometrial fluid, enlarged ovaries, and complex free fluid with internal echoes. A very specific finding is visualization of a thick-walled, tubular adnexal mass, representing a distended or thickened Fallopian tube, with or without intrapelvic free fluid. CT is more sensitive than US for mild inflammatory changes. Typical CT findings include: pelvic fat stranding, obscuration of the pelvic fascial planes, thickening of the uterosacral ligaments, abnormal endometrial enhancement with fluid in the endometrial cavity, enhancement and thickening of the fallopian tubes, and abnormal enhancement and enlargement of the ovaries. At MRI, inflammation appears hyperintense on fat-suppressed T2w images and demonstrates intense enhancement on contrast-enhanced fat-suppressed T1w images.

2.11 Tubo-Ovarian Abscess

Tubo-ovarian abscesses (TOA) may result as a complication of PID, diverticulitis, appendicitis, inflammatory bowel disease, and gynecologic or obstetric surgery. Risk factors for TOA include: history of PID,

multiple sexual partners, IUD use, and immunosuppression. On US, TOAs are seen as complex cystic adnexal or cul-de-sac masses with thick irregular walls, septations, and internal echoes (Fig. 5). On CT and MRI, typical findings are thick-walled cystic adnexal masses with internal septations and surrounding inflammatory changes (Fig. 6). Hydroureter and hydronephrosis may also be present secondary to mass effect or inflammation (Kalish et al. 2007). On MRI, TOA appears as a mass of low signal intensity on T1w images and heterogeneous high signal intensity on T2w images. Hydrosalpinx, pyosalpinx, and hematosalpinx may accompany TOA and PID.

2.12 Ovarian Torsion

Ovarian torsion can occur at any age, but is most common in women of reproductive age (Varras et al. 2004). Ovarian enlargement, often due to cysts or neoplasms, predisposes the ovary to torsion. US with Doppler imaging is the study of choice, typically demonstrating an enlarged hypoechoic ovary (which becomes more heterogeneous over time) and an absence of venous and arterial flow (Fig. 7). Nevertheless, intraovarian arterial flow may occasionally be present in torsion, due to the dual blood supply from the ovarian artery and the ovarian branch of the uterine

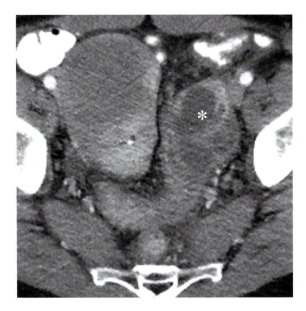

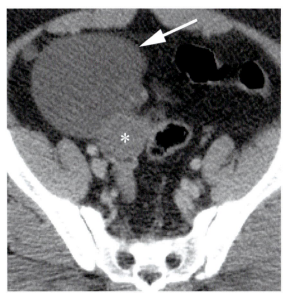

Fig. 6 CECT demonstrates the complex appearance of a tubo-ovarian abscess, with solid and fluid (*asterisk*) components

Fig. 8 CECT demonstrates displacement of the left ovary (*asterisk*) to the right. The large left ovarian cyst (*arrow*) predisposes the ovary to torsion

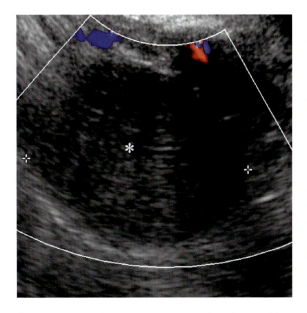

identifiable with torsion and US is usually required for a definitive diagnosis.

2.13 Ovarian Masses and Cysts

Ovarian masses should undergo clinical, laboratory, and imaging evaluation to exclude malignancy. Imaging findings raising concern for malignancy include: solid component, thick septations (>2–3 mm), Doppler flow to the solid component of the mass, and presence of ascites. These findings should prompt a gynecological consult and possibly further imaging and/or surgery. Most other ovarian lesions are addressed in the 2009 SRU Consensus Conference Statement (Levine et al. 2010), which focuses on asymptomatic ovarian and adnexal cysts but may also be applicable in symptomatic patients.

Fig. 7 Color Doppler US demonstrates an enlarged ovary without internal vascularity (*asterisk*), diagnostic for ovarian torsion

artery. Free pelvic fluid may be present. On CT and MRI, findings may include: an enlarged ovary displaced from its normal location with deviation of the uterus to the twisted side, obliteration of fat planes, thickening of the fallopian tube, ascites, non-enhancement of the ovary, and twisted vascular pedicle (Fig. 8). However these findings are not always

3 The Pregnant Patient

When a female patient presents to the emergency department with abdominal pain and/or bleeding, it is important to determine whether or not she is pregnant, with a serum pregnancy test. This influences clinical decision making.

3.1   Ectopic Pregnancy

3.1.1   Terminology and Clinical Issues

In the first trimester of pregnancy, the most common causes of pelvic pain and vaginal bleeding are an ectopic pregnancy or threatened or spontaneous abortion. When the serum beta-HCG concentration is >1000 mIU/mL (First International Reference Preparation or FIRP), in a normal pregnancy one should always be able to identify an intrauterine gestational sac with endovaginal US (EVUS) (Bree et al. 1989). If the beta-HCG concentration is is >1000 mIU/mL (FIRP) and an intrauterine gestational sac is not visualized, the differential diagnosis is a spontaneous abortion or an ectopic pregnancy. If the beta HCG is positive but <1000 mIU/mL, the differential diagnosis also includes a normal early pregnancy. It is important to remember that an ectopic pregnancy may be present even when the beta HCG is <1000 mIU/mL.

If an intrauterine pregnancy is identified, an ectopic pregnancy is effectively ruled out except in very high risk populations. A heterotopic pregnancy is an ectopic pregnancy that occurs in conjunction with an intrauterine pregnancy, and occurs in approximately 1 in 40,000 natural pregnancies; however, its incidence may be as high as 1 in 7,000 pregnancies in patients who have undergone assisted reproductive techniques (Hann et al. 1984).

3.1.2   Imaging

A normal intrauterine gestational sac is eccentrically situated within the endometrium. It has a thick decidual reaction which appears echogenic on US. Early on, the double decidual sac sign may be seen when the decidua capsularis is separated from the decidua parietalis by a small amount of fluid in the endometrial canal. A pseudogestational sac of an ectopic pregnancy occurs in 10–20% of ectopic pregnancies (Fig. 9) (Nyberg et al. 1983). It represents fluid or blood within the endometrial canal and should not be confused with a true intrauterine gestational sac. In order to definitively diagnose an intrauterine pregnancy and rule out an ectopic pregnancy, one must at least identify a yolk sac within the gestational sac (Fig. 10).

In a normal pregnancy, a yolk sac should always be visible on EVUS when the gestational sac measures >8 mm. When the gestational sac measures >16 mm, a yolk sac and embryo should be visible on EVUS. When

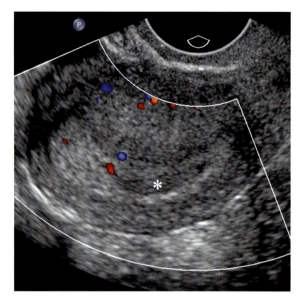

Fig. 9 EVUS shows no intrauterine pregnancy. There is a small amount of fluid in the endometrial cavity without color flow, representing a pseudogestational sac of an ectopic pregnancy (*asterisk*). It is oblong and centrally situated in the endometrial canal

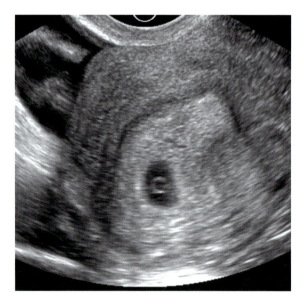

Fig. 10 EVUS demonstrates an intrauterine pregnancy with an intrauterine gestational sac and yolk sac

the embryo measures >5 mm, embryonic cardiac activity should be detectable in normal pregnancies.

The most specific sonographic finding in ectopic pregnancy is the identification of a gestational sac in the adnexa containing a yolk sac and/or fetal pole. Other, non-specific findings include an empty uterus,

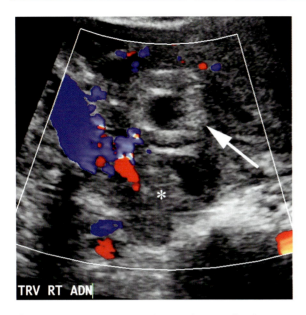

Fig. 11 On US, there was no intrauterine gestational sac (*not shown*). The ectopic pregnancy demonstrates an echogenic ring (*arrow*) separate from the right ovary (*asterisk*)

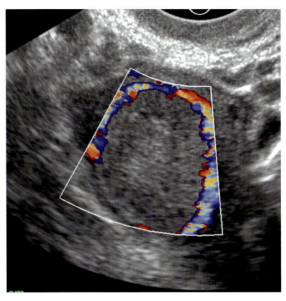

Fig. 12 Echogenic cyst in the right ovary with peripheral hyperemia is consistent with a hemorrhagic corpus luteum

pseudogestational sac, hemoperitoneum, or adnexal mass (Fig. 11). One should always evaluate the upper abdomen for free fluid in addition to evaluating the pelvis. Most ectopic pregnancies are located in the fallopian tube, although less commonly one may encounter a cornual or cervical ectopic pregnancy. An ectopic pregnancy should not be confused with a hemorrhagic corpus luteum. A corpus luteum is situated within the ovary, whereas the ectopic pregnancy is most often situated outside of the ovary. The wall of a corpus luteum is usually less echogenic than the wall of an ectopic pregnancy. Both demonstrate peripheral hyperemia on color Doppler (Fig. 12). A ruptured hemorrhagic corpus luteum may also cause pelvic pain and hemoperitoneum.

3.2   Placental Abruption

3.2.1   Terminology and Clinical Issues

Pregnant patients with subchorionic hemorrhage or placental abruption may also present with vaginal bleeding and/or pelvic pain. In the first trimester of pregnancy, a subchorionic hemorrhage demonstrates hypoechoic fluid between the chorion and endometrium. (Fig. 13)

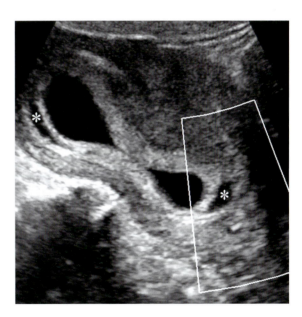

Fig. 13 US demonstrates a small subchorionic hemorrhage that is hypoechoic without internal color flow (*asterisk*)

Placental abruption occurs in second and third trimester pregnancies when the placenta separates from the uterine wall. Risk factors include trauma, drug and tobacco use, hypertension, multiparity, and fibroids. Patients present with uterine pain and irritability.

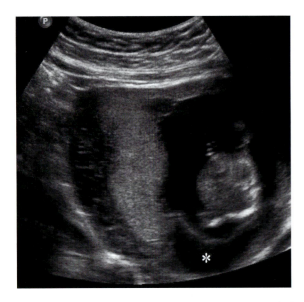

Fig. 14 Placental abruption. US demonstrates a marginal retroplacental hemorrhage that is hypoechoic without internal color flow (*asterisk*). It is located at the inferior margin of the posterior placenta and extends over the internal os of the cervix

3.2.2 Imaging

'Placental abruption is often diagnosed with US but it is an insensitive test (24% sensitive and 96% specific), producing false-negative results in most cases (Glantz and Purnell 2002). When the placenta separates from the uterine wall, there is retroplacental bleeding, which changes in appearance over time. Acutely, the retroplacental clot is heterogeneously hyperechoic. Over time, it becomes hypoechoic (Fig. 14). When isoechoic, it may be indistinguishable from normal placenta, simulating a thickened placenta on gray-scale US (Nyberg et al. 1987). Absence of internal flow on color Doppler assessment helps to differentiate a clot from placenta. The most sensitive test to diagnose placental abruption is external fetal monitoring with devices that measure uterine tone and contractility and fetal heart rate.

3.3 Retained Products of Conception

Retained products of conception (RPOC) may cause vaginal bleeding post-partum and following spontaneous or therapeutic abortion. It is due to retained trophoblastic tissue in the endometrial cavity. There is

an increased risk of RPOC in patients with placenta accreta. On US, there may be a mixed echogenicity mass in the endometrium or complex endometrial fluid. The leading differential diagnosis is a retained blood clot. RPOC may demonstrate vascularity within the mass, although this is not always present, and the absence of vascularity does not rule out the diagnosis (Fig. 15). An endometrial thickness measuring <10 mm makes RPOC very unlikely (Durfee et al. 2005).

3.4 Pregnancy and Trauma

Trauma is the leading cause of non-obstetric maternal mortality. The most common causes of trauma in pregnancy are motor vehicle crashes, domestic violence, and falls. Both major and minor traumas are associated with an increased risk of fetal loss. Maternal death almost always results in fetal death. With high-energy trauma such as motor vehicle crashes, all efforts are initially made to save the mother. The pregnant trauma patient is imaged the same way as a non-pregnant trauma patient, utilizing radiography, CT, and angiography as needed. Intravenous iodinated contrast is an FDA category B agent with no known adverse effects to the pregnancy and should be administered if indicated. In major trauma, the risks of ionizing radiation to the pregnancy are less than the risks of delayed diagnosis of maternal trauma, and imaging should be performed without delay. MRI is not a viable option in the acute trauma setting. US is performed to determine fetal viability, to date the pregnancy, and to evaluate for placental abruption, which is the most common cause of fetal death in surviving mothers (Fig. 14).

3.5 Pregnancy and the Acute Abdomen

3.5.1 Terminology and Clinical Issues

Acute appendicitis is the most common non-obstetrical condition requiring surgery in pregnancy, affecting 1 in 776 pregnancies (Patel et al. 2007). Clinical exam is difficult in the pregnant patient and the WBC count may be elevated in a normal pregnancy.

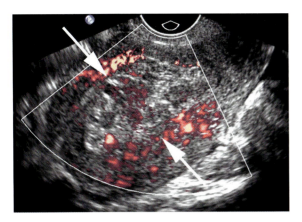

Fig. 15 Retained products of conception. EVUS demonstrates vascular hyperechoic heterogeneous material (*arrows*) within the endometrial canal

3.5.2   Imaging

The most sensitive and specific imaging test to diagnose appendicitis in pregnancy is contrast-enhanced CT (92% sensitive, 99% specific, 99% negative predictive value for diagnosing appendicitis in pregnancy).

The risk of perforation in appendicitis in pregnancy is higher than in non-pregnant patients due to delayed diagnosis, resulting in a fetal loss rate of 10.9% (Cohen-Kerem et al. 2005). The first-line imaging test to diagnose appendicitis in pregnancy is US. It is most effective in the first trimester of pregnancy, but becomes less diagnostic as the pregnancy advances. A positive US for appendicitis is very specific (Fig. 16), although many US examinations for appendicitis in pregnant patients are non-diagnostic due to non-visualization of the appendix.

MRI without gadolinium (which is an FDA category C agent) may be performed in pregnancy (Patel et al. 2007). MRI is most useful in the first trimester of pregnancy. Visualization of a normal appendix without edema in the surrounding fat results in a very high negative predictive value (Pedrosa et al. 2006). A positive diagnosis of appendicitis may be made upon visualization of a fluid-filled appendix measuring >7 mm with T2 hyperintensity in the appendiceal wall and edema in the periappendiceal fat. Unfortunately, MRI in the second and third trimesters of pregnancy may be non-diagnostic due to non-visualization of the appendix or equivocal radiologic findings. In the second and third trimesters and in patients in whom the index of suspicion is high and there may be a delay in performing MRI, CT is obtained with oral and

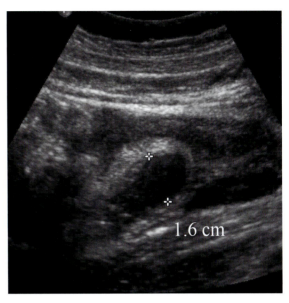

Fig. 16 Appendicitis in pregnancy. Right lower quadrant US demonstrates a dilated non-compressible appendix measuring 1.6 cm, diagnostic of acute appendicitis

intravenous contrast (Long et al. 2011). Informed consent should be obtained. A single CT scan of the pelvis in pregnancy results in a fetal dose of approximately 13–25 mGy, depending on the region covered and technique used (McCollough et al. 2007). At this dose, there is no risk of pregnancy loss, growth disturbance, mental retardation or organ malformation. The only risk to the fetus is a very minimal increased risk of childhood cancer. In 1977, the National Council of Radiation Protection and Measurements issued the following policy statement: "The risk (of abnormality) is considered to be negligible at 50 mGy or less when compared to other risks of pregnancy, and the risk of malformations is significantly increased above control levels only at doses above 150 mGy."

4   The Male Pelvis

4.1   Epididymo-orchitis

4.1.1   Terminology and Clinical Issues

Acute epididymitis and epididymo-orchitis are the most common causes of acute scrotal pain in adults. Acute epididymitis most commonly involves the epididymal head; however, the body may also be involved in up to 50% of cases.

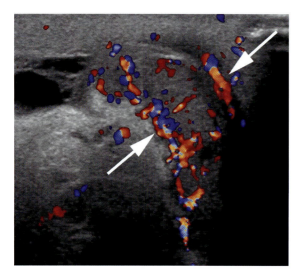

Fig. 17 US demonstrates typical findings of acute epididymitis: abnormally increased blood flow in an enlarged and hypoechoic epididymis (*arrows*)

4.1.2 Imaging

The modality of choice for initial evaluation of the scrotum is US, particularly in the emergency department (ED), as it permits detailed anatomic evaluation and provides physiologic information in the form of blood flow analysis with color and spectral Doppler. The examination is typically performed with a high frequency (7.5–12 MHz) linear-array transducer with a short focal zone while the patient is in the supine position. CT and MRI are rarely used to emergently image the prostate or scrotum, but testicular, scrotal, or prostatic abnormalities may be incidentally detected by these modalities when the patient is being imaged for other indications.

The epididymis may appear enlarged and heterogeneous on US, with relative hyperemia on color Doppler (Fig. 17). Visualization of an enlarged and heterogeneous epididymis with increased blood flow compared to the contralateral, asymptomatic side is usually sufficient for making the diagnosis of acute epididymitis. Although not routinely evaluated, a peak systolic velocity (PSV) of ≥ 15 cm/s or a PSV ratio ≥ 1.7 (symptomatic:asymptomatic side) have been shown to improve diagnostic accuracy, and may be helpful in equivocal cases (Brown et al. 1995). Secondary US findings of acute epididymitis may include a reactive hydrocele and/or scrotal skin thickening.

Isolated orchitis is relatively rare and is typically due to viral infection (particularly mumps) or as a result of trauma (Luker and Siegel 1994). Epididymo-orchitis develops in 20–40% of acute epididymitis cases as a result of the direct spread of infection. The testis in epididymo-orchitis may appear enlarged, hypoechoic, and heterogeneous in echotexture although it may also appear normal in echotexture. The process may be diffuse or multifocal. Asymmetric hyperemia of the painful testis as demonstrated on color Doppler is characteristic and may be the only finding, as the testicular parenchyma can also appear normal on gray-scale US. As with acute epididymitis, a PSV of ≥ 15 cm/s in the testis improves the diagnostic accuracy for orchitis, as does a PSV ratio ≥ 1.9 (Brown et al. 1995). Epididymo-orchitis may be complicated by infarction, abscess, or pyocele, as well as more long-term sequelae, including decreased fertility and chronic pain.

4.2 Abscess

Intratesticular abscess is usually due to epididymo-orchitis, however, other etiologies, such as trauma and infarction, should be considered. Findings on US include a heterogeneous hypoechoic intratesticular lesion with low level internal echoes, shaggy irregular walls, and occasional surrounding hyperemia (Fig. 18). The absence of vascularity and the clinical features of an infection, including fever and elevated white cell count, may allow differentiation from a complex cystic testicular neoplasm. Follow-up US after appropriate antibiotic treatment may be helpful in equivocal cases.

4.3 Torsion of the Appendix Testis

The appendix testis is located near the superior pole of the testis in a groove made with the epididymis. The structure is isoechoic to the epididymis and is not typically visible in the absence of a hydrocele. Torsion of the appendix testis is a common cause of acute scrotal pain in prepubertal boys. The torsed appendix testis may appear as an echogenic heterogeneous extratesticular mass measuring up to 17 mm with no blood flow at Doppler imaging (Baldisserotto et al. 2005). Associated findings include enlargement of the epididymal head, reactive hydrocele, and scrotal skin thickening. Significant overlap exists between the sonographic

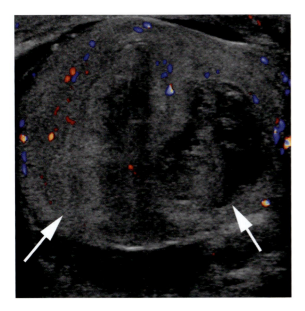

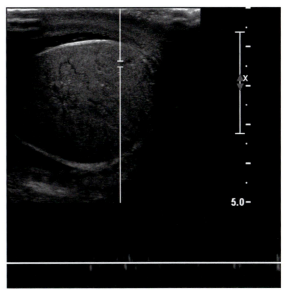

Fig. 18 US appearance of this testicular abscess is non-specific. There are ill-defined regions of heterogeneously increased and decreased echogenicity representing complex fluid, debris, and edema (*arrows*), indistinguishable from those seen in a malignant neoplasm, particularly a non-seminomatous germ cell tumor. Clinical correlation with signs and symptoms of infection is critical. Follow-up US after appropriate antibiotic treatment is often obtained in equivocal cases

Fig. 19 Spectral Doppler US in the setting of complete (≥360°) torsion demonstrates no blood flow within the testis

appearance of appendix testis torsion and that of acute epididymitis or torsion of the appendix epididymis, therefore reliable differentiation of these entities may not be possible in the absence of a visualized avascular, enlarged appendix testis (Yang et al. 2011).

4.4   Torsion of the Testis

4.4.1   Terminology and Clinical Issues

In addition to acute epididymo-orchitis and torsion of the appendix testis, testicular torsion should be included in the differential diagnosis for an acute scrotum as these entities can be difficult to differentiate clinically. While torsion of the testis can occur at any age, it is most common in adolescents. Extravaginal and intravaginal types of torsion exist. The extravaginal form is found exclusively in newborns and is not reviewed here. The intravaginal form occurs within the tunica vaginalis and the most common predisposing factor is the "bell clapper" deformity, in which the

tunica vaginalis completely encircles the testis, epididymis, and distal spermatic cord rather than attaching the posterolateral testis to the scrotal wall. This configuration allows the testis to rotate freely in the hemiscrotum, increasing the probability of torsion.

As the spermatic cord twists, venous outflow is compromised first, resulting in increased arterial vascular resistance and decreased or reversed diastolic flow compared to the unaffected side, as seen with spectral Doppler (Dogra et al. 2003). As the twisting becomes more severe (>360°), arterial flow becomes compromised, resulting in no visible blood flow with Doppler in the affected testis (Fig. 19).

4.4.2   Imaging

Ultrasound is an effective tool for diagnosing testicular torsion and for differentiating this condition from the more common epididymo-orchitis. The appearance of the torsed testis on gray-scale imaging is nonspecific and may be nearly normal, particularly in the hyperacute setting. Within 4–6 h of torsion, the testis may appear enlarged and hypoechoic which evolves into a heterogeneous pattern as the testis infarcts and begins to necrose (Fig. 20) (Dogra et al. 2003). Occasionally, twisting of the spermatic cord may be visible at the external inguinal ring.

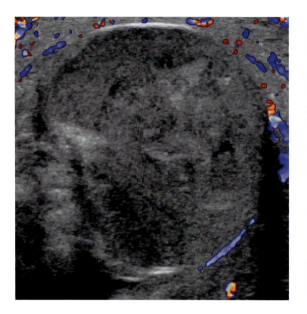

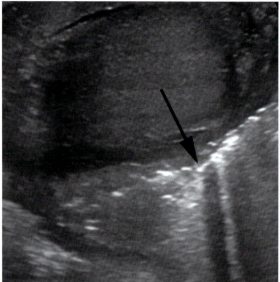

Fig. 20 Within 4–6 h, the torsed testis enlarges and becomes hypoechoic on US. The testicular parenchyma begins to appear heterogeneous and irregular, consistent with infarcts and hemorrhage

Fig. 21 US demonstrates gas within the scrotal wall or perineum, suggestive of necrotizing fasciitis (Fournier's gangrene). Soft-tissue emphysema appears as scattered and confluent foci of markedly increased echogenicity with somewhat hazy or "dirty" posterior acoustic shadowing (*arrow*)

4.5 Scrotal Cellulitis and Fournier's Gangrene

Scrotal wall thickening is a non-specific finding at US and may result from a myriad of conditions, including heart failure, liver failure, venous or lymphatic obstruction, infection or trauma. Cellulitis of the scrotum may demonstrate relative hyperemia with color Doppler, but this finding is non-specific and clinical correlation is critical for accurate diagnosis. A thickened scrotal wall with multiple discrete foci of increased echogenicity and "dirty" shadowing representing soft-tissue emphysema is an ominous finding, indicating necrotizing fasciitis of the scrotum, also known as Fournier's gangrene (Fig. 21).

4.6 Scrotal Trauma

Trauma to the scrotum may result from blunt, penetrating, or degloving mechanisms or from thermal injury. Scrotal US is the first-line imaging modality to evaluate scrotal trauma and is highly accurate in identifying injuries requiring surgical intervention, such as testicular rupture (Buckley and McAninch 2006a).

Blunt trauma is the most common cause of scrotal injury and may result in hematoma, fracture of the testis, or frank testicular rupture. A hematoma may appear as a focal region of decreased echogenicity and heterogeneous echotexture without demonstrable blood flow. Hematomas may be difficult to distinguish from a testicular neoplasm and a follow-up US is indicated for equivocal cases.

A fracture of the testis manifests sonographically as a linear band of decreased echogenicity that traverses the testicular parenchyma without distorting the contour of the testis or disrupting the tunica albuginea. Doppler is critical to demonstrate flow to the affected testis, as increased intratesticular pressure due to hemorrhage and edema contained by the tunica can result in ischemia and infarction.

A ruptured testis occurs when there is disruption of both the testicular parenchyma and its surrounding tunica albuginea, often with extrusion of testicular contents into the scrotum. US features include disruption of the tunica, testicular contour deformity, and heterogeneous areas of increased and decreased echogenicity in the testicular parenchyma, representing infarction and hemorrhage (Fig. 22). Scrotal wall thickening and hematocele frequently coexist.

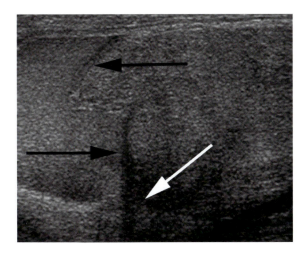

Fig. 22 US demonstrates an irregular hypoechoic line through the mid testis, representing parenchymal fracture (*black arrows*). The posterior tunica albuginea is irregular and not well seen (*white arrow*), suggesting testicular rupture in a blunt scrotal trauma victim

The US diagnosis of testicular rupture can be difficult if frank disruption of the tunica and extrusion of testicular contents are not present; however, the findings of heterogeneous parenchymal echogenicity and loss of contour definition have been reported to be highly sensitive and specific. Rupture is managed with prompt surgical reconstruction, resulting in salvage rates as high as 83% (Buckley and McAninch 2006a, b).

4.7 Palpable Scrotal Lesions

4.7.1 Terminology and Clinical Issues

Patients often present for urgent evaluation of a palpable abnormality in the scrotum and while a comprehensive discussion of testicular and paratesticular masses is beyond the scope of this text, familiarity with the imaging appearance of common lesions can be helpful. The majority of extratesticular lesions are of benign etiology, such as lipomas, adenomatoid tumors, epididymal cysts, and spermatoceles. The majority of intratesticular masses are malignant. Approximately 95% of malignant testicular neoplasms are of germ cell origin, of which seminoma is the most common histologic subtype.

4.7.2 Imaging

The first line imaging modality for characterizing scrotal masses is US, which is up to 99% accurate in

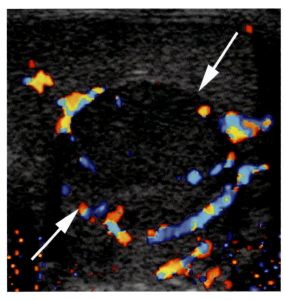

Fig. 23 Color Doppler US of a testicular seminoma demonstrates intralesional vascularity. This feature can allow differentiation from intratesticular hematomas, which may be well circumscribed and relatively homogeneous in appearance but lack internal vascularity

differentiating between intratesticular and extratesticular disease (Rifkin et al. 1985). Seminoma typically appears as a homogeneous hypoechoic, vascular mass (Fig. 23). Cystic areas and calcification are less common than in non-seminomatous germ cell tumors. The presence of any non-seminomatous cell type in a testicular germ cell tumor classifies it as a non-seminomatous germ cell tumor (yolk sac tumor, embryonal cell carcinoma, choriocarcinoma, teratocarcinoma, and teratoma). Non-seminomatous germ cell tumors tend to occur in younger patients and sonographically are more heterogeneous in echotexture than seminomas, with cystic areas and calcifications often present (Fig. 24) (Dogra et al. 2003). In the setting of multiple solid testicular lesions, diagnostic considerations should include lymphoma, leukemia, metastases, granulomatous disease, Leydig cell hyperplasia, and bilateral primary testicular neoplasm.

4.8 Varicocele

4.8.1 Terminology and Clinical Issues

A scrotal varicocele is an abnormal dilation of the venous (pampiniform) plexus that drains the testis and epididymis along the spermatic cord. This condition is

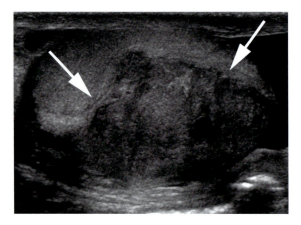

Fig. 24 In contrast to seminomatous germ cell tumors, US of non-seminomatous neoplasms typically demonstrates irregular, heterogeneous masses with cystic areas (*arrows*), as in this case of embryonal cell carcinoma. Note the general similarity in appearance to the testicular abscess in Fig. 18. Calcifications, although not evident in this case, are a relatively common feature of non-seminomatous germ cell tumors

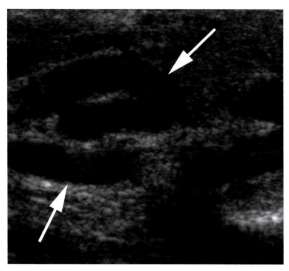

Fig. 25 Dilated pampiniform plexus veins on US, measuring 2.5 mm at rest (*arrows*) or 3 mm with a Valsalva maneuver, are diagnostic of varicoceles

present in up to 15% of asymptomatic men and is usually an incidental finding at scrotal US. The incidence is higher (approximately 40%) in patients being evaluated for decreased fertility. Varicoceles present most commonly on the left or bilaterally.

4.8.2 Imaging

Clinically significant varicocele may be accurately diagnosed at US by demonstrating two to three prominent pampiniform plexus veins, at least one of which measures ≥2.5 mm at rest or ≥3.0 mm with the Valsalva maneuver (Fig. 25) (Pilatz et al. 2011). An isolated right varicocele is relatively rare, likely because the right gonadal vein drains directly into the inferior vena cava. Evaluation of the retroperitoneum with US or cross-sectional imaging for an obstructing or compressing mass lesion may be considered in the setting of an isolated right-sided or new left-sided varicocele, particularly in older patients (>40 years) although the positive yield in otherwise asymptomatic patients is low (El-Saeity and Sidhu (2006).

4.9 Hydrocele/Hematocele/Pyocele

The tunica vaginalis surrounds a potential space in the scrotum that may fill with fluid (hydrocele), blood (hematocele), or pus (pyocele). Acquired hydroceles are often due to prior trauma and manifest

sonographically as predominantly anechoic fluid in the hemiscrotum. Hematoceles and pyoceles manifest as complex scrotal fluid collections and cannot reliably be differentiated at US. An acute hematocele may initially appear hyperechoic but subsequently evolves into complex, septated fluid collections with fluid–fluid levels and low level internal echoes (Dogra et al. 2003).

4.10 The Undescended Testis

An ovoid soft-tissue mass in the posterior abdomen or in the inguinal canal region may be incidentally noted on cross-sectional imaging. This should not be assumed to represent a mass or abnormal lymph node, and an undescended or retractile testis should be considered before initiating an evaluation for more ominous etiologies (Fig. 26).

4.11 Prostate Infection and Abscess

4.11.1 Terminology and Clinical Issues
Patients with acute prostatitis typically present with fever, dysuria, pelvic pain, and a very tender prostate on digital rectal examination. The diagnosis is made based on clinical exam, laboratory findings, and patient history. Imaging is generally reserved for

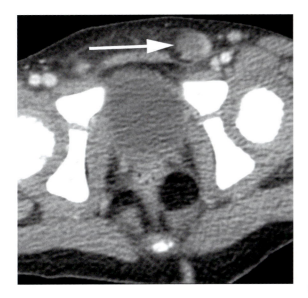

Fig. 26 An undescended or ectopic testis may appear as a soft-tissue nodule in the abdomen, pelvis, or in the inguinal canal as in this CT examination of a pediatric patient with a left-sided undescended testis (*arrow*)

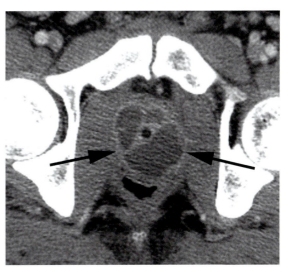

Fig. 27 Prostatic abscesses are uncommon but may be accurately identified on CECT as a complex rim enhancing fluid collection in the prostate, often with multiple septations (*arrows*)

patients who do not respond to standard antimicrobial therapy, as abscess formation in the prostate, while uncommon, is a serious complication of acute bacterial prostatitis and may be difficult to detect clinically.

Prostatic abscess is usually found in elderly or immunocompromised patients and may develop in the setting of prostatitis, urinary tract infection, or endocarditis with septic emboli (particularly in younger patients) (Barozzi et al. 1998).

4.11.2 Imaging

Transrectal US is sensitive for detecting prostatic fluid collections and directing aspiration, but in the emergency department setting, prostatic abscesses are most frequently initially diagnosed with CT, where they will appear as a low-attenuation collection within the prostate with peripheral enhancement and possible septations (Fig. 27).

4.12 Prostate Hypertrophy

Benign prostatic hypertrophy (BPH) is a frequent incidental finding on CT scans of the pelvis performed for other reasons. The prevalence increases with age, approaching 90% in patients over 90 years of age. The prostate may become quite large and the central gland may protrude into the base of the bladder. While the degree of hypertrophy may not correlate directly with lower urinary tract symptomatology, prostate volumes greater than 30 ml are significantly associated with obstructive symptoms (Girman et al. 1995). Secondary signs of significant bladder outlet obstruction in the setting of a large prostate may include a thickened, trabeculated bladder wall, bladder diverticuli, or hydronephrosis. In the absence of large peripheral or exophytic prostatic masses or extensive periprostatic lymphadenopathy, CT and routine pelvic MRI are not usually helpful in evaluating for the presence of prostate cancer.

5 Pelvic Osseous Trauma

5.1 Terminology and Clinical Issues

Pelvic ring disruptions are frequently described using the Young-Burgess classification system (Young and Resnik 1990). In the evaluation of a pelvic ring injury, the anterior component of the injury is first assigned to one of several categories: lateral compression (LC), anteroposterior compression (APC), vertical shear (VS), or combined mechanism. The posterior component of an LC or APC injury is then assessed to determine the injury subcategory for these mechanisms.

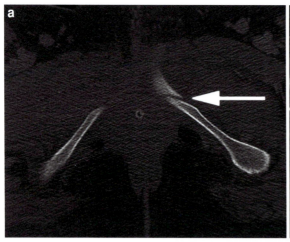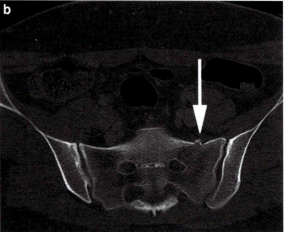

Fig. 28 Lateral compression I fracture. LC-I fractures can be subtle on radiographs, as only mild displacement of the pubic rami fractures may be evident. Subtle sacral fractures might only be visualized on CT. **a** A minimally displaced coronally oriented fracture through the left inferior pubic ramus (*arrow*); **b** a buckled compression fracture of the left sacral ala (*arrow*) caused by a lateral compression force producing injury. The sacroiliac joints are normal

In LC fractures, lateral forces to the pelvis tend to internally rotate the innominate bone. The anterior injury characterizing this group is a "transverse" (axial or coronal) fracture of the pubic rami (ipsilateral, contralateral or bilateral with respect to the applied force). LC-I injuries consist of a sacral compression fracture (Fig. 28). LC-II injuries demonstrate a crescent fracture arising from the medial portion of the iliac bone adjacent to the sacroiliac joint, with medial rotation of the remainder of the ilium. In LC-III injuries, there is an LC-I or LC-II injury on the side of impact, and an open-book type injury (see APC injuries below) on the contralateral side. This is referred to as a "windswept pelvis" as both the ipsilateral and contralateral hemipelves are rotated in the same direction, analogous to trees bent in the same direction by the wind.

Forces in the sagittal plane will result in APC fractures, such as occurs following a high-energy blow to the front of the pelvis during a motor vehicle crash. The anterior injuries characterizing this group are diastasis of the symphysis pubis or vertical (sagittal) fractures of pubic rami. In APC-I injuries, there is mild widening of the symphysis pubis (1–2 cm) without the vertical pubic rami fractures that may be seen with the other APC injuries. Posteriorly, the sacrotuberous, sacrospinous, and anterior sacroiliac (SI) ligaments may be stretched but they remain intact, resulting in at most very mild widening of one

SI joint, without pelvic ring instability on physical exam. APC-II injuries demonstrate widening of the SI joint and external rotation of the hemipelvis due to disruption of the anterior SI, sacrotuberous, and sacrospinous ligaments. This is referred to as an "open-book fracture." APC-III injuries consist of complete separation of the hemipelvis from the remainder of the pelvic ring, with disruption of both the anterior and posterior SI ligaments.

In VS injuries (Fig. 29), severe axial loading of a hemipelvis results in its vertical displacement with respect to the remainder of the pelvis. The anterior injury usually causes diastasis of the symphysis pubis or, less commonly, vertical fractures of the pubic rami. The posterior injury often leads to complete disruption of the SI joint or, less commonly, an iliac wing or sacral fracture.

Combined-mechanism injuries result from a combination of the above mechanisms, typically APC and LC.

5.2   Imaging

When initial radiographs identify hip dislocation in a patient who will subsequently obtain a pelvic CT, hip reduction is attempted prior to CT, if the patient's condition allows. This permits imaging evaluation of the post-reduction alignment as well as detection of

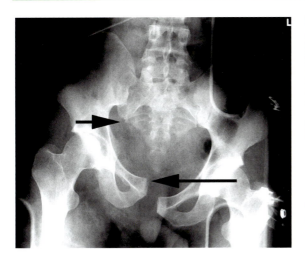

Table 1 Predictors of hemorrhage (from Blackmore et al. 2006)

Number of predictors	Probability of major hemorrhage	Sensitivity	Specificity
0	0.016	1.00	0
1	0.14	0.97	0.49
2	0.46	0.75	0.83
3 or 4	0.66	0.3	0.96

Fig. 29 Vertical shear injury. More severe pelvic ring fractures can often be clearly characterized on radiographs, although additional injuries may be present on CT. Despite the frequently present overlying artifact from the backboard, this radiograph clearly demonstrates widening of the symphysis pubis and of the right sacroiliac joint, with superior displacement of the right pubis (*long arrow*) with respect to the left, and superior displacement of the right ilium with respect to the sacrum. The inferior margin of the right sacroiliac joint is identified (*short arrow*)

unsuspected fractures and intra-articular fragments, without requiring additional radiation of the pelvis. The typical posterior hip dislocation demonstrates superior displacement of the femoral head and internal rotation of the femur, while anterior hip dislocations typically demonstrate inferior and medial dislocation of the femoral head and external rotation of the femur. More subtle dislocations may present with minor incongruency of the femoral head with respect to the acetabulum.

The diagnosis of pelvic osseous trauma is usually made on the initial portable AP pelvic radiograph. Most patients with fractures then undergo CT of the abdomen and pelvis to evaluate for internal injuries, and bone algorithm pelvic images are reconstructed from this study. Sagittal and coronal reformations are generated to improve the detection and characterization of injuries, such as subtle transverse fractures through the sacrum, which are sometimes only visualized on the sagittal images. Volume-rendered images to simulate AP, internal and external rotation Judet, and inlet and outlet radiographs of the pelvis are helpful to provide a baseline set of images that can be used for comparison with intraoperative fluoroscopy or follow-up radiographs.

6   Traumatic Pelvic Hemorrhage

Retroperitoneal hemorrhage is challenging to identify clinically or with rapid bedside tests during the acute evaluation. Rotationally (and vertically) unstable pelvic injuries can externally rotate and significantly increase the potential space for retroperitoneal hemorrhage by reducing the natural tamponade effect of an intact pelvis. When these injuries are identified, rapid stabilization or reduction of the external pelvic rotation is attempted to maintain or reduce the pelvic volume. This may be performed quickly using sheets or commercial binders tightly wrapped around the pelvis, or less rapidly with external fixation. Hemodynamically unstable patients with pelvic injuries placing them at risk for retroperitoneal hemorrhage, and without strong evidence of significant hemorrhage elsewhere that could be rapidly addressed (e.g., hemoperitoneum treated with laparotomy) are usually sent emergently for angiographic evaluation and embolization, although retroperitoneal pelvic packing is an alternative approach that has been proposed recently. Patients who are hemodynamically stable during their initial evaluation could continue to bleed and rapidly destabilize. Guidelines for predicting which patients are at risk for this transition can help direct clinical management.

A clinical prediction rule was developed to determine which patients with pelvic injuries following blunt trauma are at risk for major hemorrhage, using criteria available early in the patient's evaluation (portable AP pelvic radiograph, vital signs, and hematocrit) (Blackmore et al. 2006). The four predictors are: obturator ring fracture displaced ≥ 1 cm, symphysis pubis displaced ≥ 1 cm, heart rate ≥ 130 beats per minute, and hematocrit $\leq 30\%$. Patients with three or four predictors have a 66% chance of major pelvic fracture related hemorrhage (Table 1), and

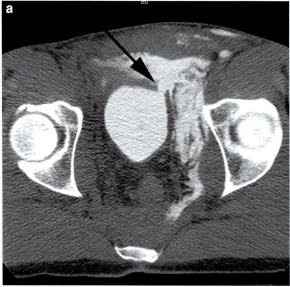 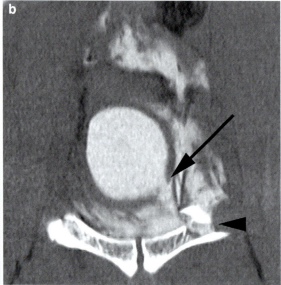

Fig. 30 Extraperitoneal bladder rupture. **a** Axial CTC image demonstrates contrast leaking through a rupture in the left anterolateral aspect of the bladder (*arrow*) and spreading in a streaky manner through the retroperitoneum and into the left anterior abdominal wall. **b** Coronal image demonstrates the inferior location of the bladder rupture (*arrow*) and a displaced left obturator ring fracture (*arrowhead*)

angiography with embolization should be one of the initial management steps considered (Blackmore et al. 2006).

7   Bladder

7.1   Bladder Trauma

7.1.1   Terminology and Clinical Issues

The most common injury of the bladder is a contusion, which may present clinically with hematuria but can be difficult or impossible to visualize on imaging studies. The most common complete tear of the bladder wall (through the entire thickness of the bladder wall) results in an extraperitoneal bladder rupture (60–90%) (Carroll and McAninch 1984, Vaccaro and Brody 2000) in which urine can leak through a defect in the bladder into the extraperitoneal space (Fig. 30). Intraperitoneal bladder ruptures (15–25%) (Carroll and McAninch 1984; Vaccaro and Brody 2000) are less common; they occur when the defect is in the dome of the bladder, allowing urine to leak into the intraperitoneal space (Fig. 31). Combined bladder ruptures (5–12%) (Carroll and McAninch 1984; Vaccaro and Brody 2000; Sandler et al. 1986) are even less common and result in urine leakage into the intraperitoneal and extraperitoneal spaces. An extremely rare injury is an interstitial rupture, consisting of a tear of the inner wall of the bladder that does not extend through the outer wall. These can be extremely difficult to identify on imaging studies.

Although less than 10% of patients with pelvic fractures have bladder ruptures (Avey et al. 2006; Corriere and Sandler 1999) more than 80% of patients with bladder ruptures have pelvic fractures (Sandler et al. 1986; Corriere and Sandler 1986) The presence of osseous pelvic trauma should prompt the radiologist to consider the possibility of bladder injury and the potential need for further imaging evaluation. Almost all cases of extraperitoneal bladder ruptures due to blunt trauma are associated with pelvic fractures. In contrast, 25% of intraperitoneal bladder ruptures occur in the absence of pelvic fractures and almost always result in gross hematuria. These may result when blunt trauma to the lower abdominal wall generates a sudden rise in intravesical pressure in a patient with a distended bladder, causing rupture of the bladder dome, which is the weakest portion of the bladder (Corriere and Sandler 1999).

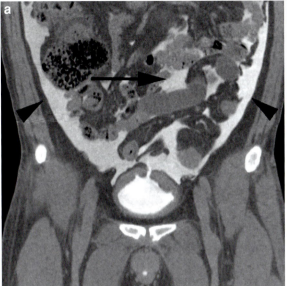 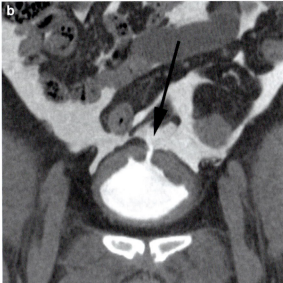

Fig. 31 **a** Intraperitoneal bladder rupture is demonstrated on CTC, with intraperitoneal contrast in the paracolic gutters (*arrowheads*) and between loops of small bowel and mesentery (*arrow*). **b** A defect in the bladder dome is clearly demonstrated (*arrow*) in this case, but the actual defect is not always visible on CTC

Table 2 Indications for obtaining a CTC following blunt abdominal trauma

Gross hematuria and free intraperitoneal fluid (which may represent urine from an intraperitoneal bladder rupture)
OR
High levels of hematuria and pelvic ring injury
>30 RBC/HPF or gross hematuria
AND
Pelvic ring fracture or disruption (excluding isolated acetabular fractures)

Table 3 CT cystography (CTC) technique

Drain urine via Foley catheter to eliminate/reduce unopacified bladder contents
Hang container of dilute water-soluble contrast ($\sim$2–3 grams iodine per 100 ml of volume) 40 cm above the bladder to generate adequate pressure
Fill the bladder with contrast until 350 ml or more have been instilled, flow of contrast stops, or bladder distension is painful to the patient
Obtain 2.5–5mm low-dose axial images through the pelvis. Coronal and sagittal reformations may help with the evaluation
If delayed images of the pelvis are being obtained for other reasons, fill the bladder with contrast and collect CTC images as part of that scan, obviating the need to further expose the patient to radiation specifically for a bladder evaluation
Otherwise, CTC is obtained following the parenchymal phase, after retrograde filling of the bladder

7.1.2 Imaging

Bladder abnormalities may be detected during specific evaluation of the urinary system by CT urography (CTU) or CT cystography (CTC), or incidentally while evaluating the abdomen and/or pelvis for other reasons with CT, US, or MRI. Conventional radiographic cystography has been replaced by CTC for the evaluation of acute traumatic bladder injury. The indications for obtaining a CTC following blunt abdominal trauma are listed in Table 2. The technique for performing a CTC is described in Table 3.

While the defect in the bladder wall may sometimes be well seen, it is often not directly visualized on CTC, especially when the defect is small, or if the bladder partially collapses as contrast leaks from it. In these cases, the presence of the relatively high density CTC contrast in the extraperitoneal and/or intraperitoneal spaces provides presumptive evidence of bladder rupture. Careful attention to prior images and other phases of the study is necessary to prevent extravasated vascular, enteric, or retrograde urethrogram contrast from being mistaken for bladder extravasation.

7.2   Bladder Fistula

Gas in the bladder in a patient who has not been recently catheterized or instrumented is presumptive evidence of a fistula (or less commonly, a gas-forming infection). CT is most commonly obtained for further evaluation, although MRI could also be considered. A fistula may develop to any of the surrounding structures, and often involves the small bowel, colon, or vagina. Clinical symptoms associated with enterovesical fistula include recurrent cystitis, abdominal pain, fever, fecaluria, and pneumaturia (Yu et al. 2004).

A fistula between the bladder and bowel often demonstrates bladder wall and bowel wall thickening, but the fistulous tract is frequently not directly visualized on standard CT performed with intravenous contrast only, and the fistula is presumed to exist based on the presence of gas in the bladder. Intraluminal administration of bladder and/or oral/rectal contrast, or delayed images in which contrast-enhanced urine is excreted into the bladder, may improve fistula visualization, if the contrast extends into the fistulous tract. (Yu et al. 2004)

7.3   Bladder Cancer

There are three primary methods to improve the evaluation of bladder lesions suspected of malignancy, all of which involve increasing the contrast between the bladder wall/lesion and the adjacent urine.

1. The unenhanced (or delayed enhancement) bladder wall can be evaluated adjacent to dense urine (Fig. 32).
2. The enhancing bladder wall can be evaluated adjacent to less dense urine.
3. The bladder wall can be evaluated adjacent to gas.

CTU images should be reviewed with narrow and wide windows, and in at least two planes (usually axial and coronal). Bladder cancers may present with asymmetric wall thickening, focal masses, or small filling defects. Diffuse, symmetric bladder-wall thickening is a rare presentation and usually is due to benign causes, such as cystitis, bladder outlet obstruction, or neurogenic bladder. While earlier studies appeared to demonstrate a high efficacy for CTU in the detection of bladder neoplasms, more

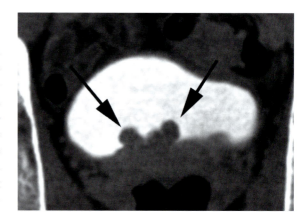

Fig. 32 Papillary bladder cancer. Bladder cancer presenting with soft-tissue density papillary projections (*arrows*) is well visualized against the contrast-filled bladder lumen on CT

recent studies obtained sensitivities of 59–74%. (Cohan et al. 2009). Cystoscopy is frequently utilized for direct evaluation of the suspected bladder lesion, with biopsy if indicated.

Bladder cancers are often unsuspected and detected incidentally during portal-venous phase CT of the abdomen and pelvis performed for other reasons. Sensitivities of up to 95% and specificities of up to 91–93% for the detection of bladder lesions has been demonstrated in portal-venous phase studies optimized to evaluate the bladder (Park et al. 2007).

A newer method is virtual CTC, in which the bladder is distended with gas to provide high contrast between the lumen and the suspected bladder-wall lesion, but this technique has yet to be widely adopted.

Regardless of the technique used, small lesions can be missed. Flat tumors that do not project into the lumen may be challenging to identify (Fig. 33), as unlike papillary tumors they do not produce filling defects and may demonstrate minimal bladder-wall thickening or abnormal enhancement. Tumors at the bladder base may be difficult to distinguish from periurethral tissue or prostatic enlargement. Thickening and scarring in radiation-treated bladders may be mistaken for tumor or may cause small tumors to be attributed to post-therapeutic changes, and thus go undiagnosed.

A posterior filling defect or apparent bladder-wall thickening, which may represent a clot, can be evaluated by re-imaging with the patient in a prone position to see whether the clot falls to the anterior bladder wall.

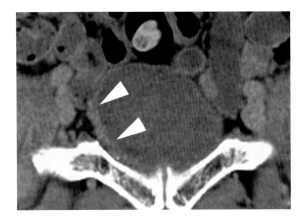

Fig. 33 Sessile bladder cancer. Bladder cancer presenting with mild focal bladder-wall thickening (*arrows*) on CT can be challenging to detect

A mass at the dome of the bladder, at or slightly offset from midline, may be seen with a urachal cancer, usually an adenocarcinoma. The classic appearance is a midline infra-umbilical soft-tissue mass (typically with mixed solid and cystic components) and calcifications (most commonly peripheral). Urachal cancers are often large. (Wong-You-Cheong et al. 2006).

The ability of CT to stage bladder cancer by evaluation of bladder-wall invasion is limited. MRI is more accurate, with extension of the intermediate T2 signal bladder mass into or through the low-signal bladder muscle, representing stage II or III disease, respectively.

References

Avey G, Blackmore CC, Wessells H, Wright JL, Talner LB (2006) Radiographic and clinical predictors of bladder rupture in blunt trauma patients with pelvic fracture. Acad Radiol 13(5):573–579

Baldisserotto M, de Souza JC, Pertence AP, Dora MD (2005) Color Doppler sonography of normal and torsed testicular appendages in children. AJR Am J Roentgenol 184(4): 1287–1292

Balen AH, Laven JS, Tan SL, Dewailly D (2003) Ultrasound assessment of the polycystic ovary: international consensus definitions. Hum Reprod Update 9(6):505–514

Barozzi L, Pavlica P, Menchi I, De Matteis M, Canepari M (1998) Prostatic abscess: diagnosis and treatment. AJR Am J Roentgenol 170(3):753–757

Bennett GL, Slywotzky CM, Giovanniello G (2002) Gynecologic causes of acute pelvic pain: spectrum of CT findings. Radiogr 22(4):785–801

Blackmore CC, Cummings P, Jurkovich GJ, Linnau KF, Hoffer EK, Rivara FP (2006) Predicting major hemorrhage in patients with pelvic fracture. J Trauma 61(2):346–352

Bree RL, Edwards M, Bohm-Velez M, Beyler S, Roberts J, Mendelson EB (1989) Transvaginal sonography in the evaluation of normal early pregnancy: correlation with HCG level. AJR Am J Roentgenol 153(1):75–79

Brosens I, Puttemans P, Campo R, Gordts S, Kinkel K (2004) Diagnosis of endometriosis: pelvic endoscopy and imaging techniques. Best Pract Res Clin Obstet Gynaecol 18(2): 285–303

Brown JM, Hammers LW, Barton JW et al (1995) Quantitative Doppler assessment of acute scrotal inflammation. Radiology 197(2):427–431

Buckley JC, McAninch JW (2006a) Use of ultrasonography for the diagnosis of testicular injuries in blunt scrotal trauma. J Urol 175(1):175–178

Buckley JC, McAninch JW (2006b) Diagnosis and management of testicular ruptures. Urol Clin North Am 33(1):111–116 vii

Buy JN, Ghossain MA, Moss AA et al (1989) Cystic teratoma of the ovary: CT detection. Radiology 171(3):697–701

Cano Alonso R, Borruel Nacenta S, Diez Martinez P, Maria NI, Ibanez Sanz L, Zabia Galindez E (2009) Role of multidetector CT in the management of acute female pelvic disease. Emerg Radiol 16(6):453–472

Carroll PR, McAninch JW (1984) Major bladder trauma: mechanisms of injury and a unified method of diagnosis and repair. J Urol 132(2):254–257

Cohan RH, Caoili EM, Cowan NC, Weizer AZ, Ellis JH (2009) MDCT Urography: exploring a new paradigm for imaging of bladder cancer. AJR Am J Roentgenol 192(6):1501–1508

Cohen-Kerem R, Railton C, Oren D, Lishner M, Koren G (2005) Pregnancy outcome following non-obstetric surgical intervention. Am J Surg 190(3):467–473

Corriere JN Jr, Sandler CM (1986) Management of the ruptured bladder: seven years of experience with 111 cases. J Trauma 26(9):830–833

Corriere JN Jr, Sandler CM (1999) Bladder rupture from external trauma: diagnosis and management. World J Urol 17(2):84–89

Dogra VS, Gottlieb RH, Oka M, Rubens DJ (2003) Sonography of the scrotum. Radiology 227(1):18–36

Durfee SM, Frates MC, Luong A, Benson CB (2005) The sonographic and color Doppler features of retained products of conception. J Ultrasound Med 24(9):1181–1186. quiz 8–9

El-Saeity NS, Sidhu PS (2006) "Scrotal varicocele, exclude a renal tumour". Is this evidence based? Clin Radiol 61(7):593–599

Funt SA, Hann LE (2002) Detection and characterization of adnexal masses. Radiol Clin North Am 40(3):591–608

Girman CJ, Jacobsen SJ, Guess HA et al (1995) Natural history of prostatism: relationship among symptoms, prostate volume and peak urinary flow rate. J Urol 153(5):1510–1515

Glantz C, Purnell L (2002) Clinical utility of sonography in the diagnosis and treatment of placental abruption. J Ultrasound Med 21(8):837–840

Hann LE, Bachman DM, McArdle CR (1984) Coexistent intrauterine and ectopic pregnancy: a reevaluation. Radiology 152(1):151–154

Kalish GM, Patel MD, Gunn ML, Dubinsky TJ (2007) Computed tomographic and magnetic resonance features of gynecologic abnormalities in women presenting with

acute or chronic abdominal pain. Ultrasound Q 23(3): 167–175

Kamaya A, Shin L, Chen B, Desser TS (2008) Emergency gynecologic imaging. Semin Ultrasound CT MR 29(5): 353–368

Levine D, Brown DL, Andreotti RF et al (2010) Management of asymptomatic ovarian and other adnexal cysts imaged at US: society of radiologists in ultrasound consensus conference statement. Radiology 256(3):943–954

Long SS, Long C, Lai H, Macura KJ (2011) Imaging strategies for right lower quadrant pain in pregnancy. AJR Am J Roentgenol 196(1):4–12

Luker GD, Siegel MJ (1994) Color Doppler sonography of the scrotum in children. AJR Am J Roentgenol 163(3):649–655

McCollough CH, Schueler BA, Atwell TD et al (2007) Radiation exposure and pregnancy: when should we be concerned? Radiogr 27(4):909–917 discussion 917–8

Nyberg DA, Laing FC, Filly RA, Uri-Simmons M, Jeffrey RB Jr (1983) Ultrasonographic differentiation of the gestational sac of early intrauterine pregnancy from the pseudogestational sac of ectopic pregnancy. Radiology 146(3):755–759

Nyberg DA, Cyr DR, Mack LA, Wilson DA, Shuman WP (1987) Sonographic spectrum of placental abruption. AJR Am J Roentgenol 48(1):161–164

Park SB, Kim JK, Lee HJ, Choi HJ, Cho KS (2007) Hematuria: portal venous phase multi detector row CT of the bladder—a prospective study. Radiology 245(3):798–805

Patel SJ, Reede DL, Katz DS, Subramaniam R, Amorosa JK (2007) Imaging the pregnant patient for nonobstetric conditions: algorithms and radiation dose considerations. Radiogr 27(6):1705–1722

Pedrosa I, Levine D, Eyvazzadeh AD, Siewert B, Ngo L, Rofsky NM (2006) MR imaging evaluation of acute appendicitis in pregnancy. Radiology 238(3):891–899

Pilatz A, Altinkilic B, Köhler E, Marconi M, Weidner W (2011) Color Doppler ultrasound imaging in varicoceles: is the venous diameter sufficient for predicting clinical and subclinical varicocele? World J Urol 29:645–650

Rifkin MD, Kurtz AB, Pasto ME, Goldberg BB (1985) Diagnostic capabilities of high-resolution scrotal ultrasonography: prospective evaluation. J Ultrasound Med 4(1): 13–19

Sahdev A (2010) Cervical tumors. Semin Ultrasound CT MR 31(5):399–413

Sandler CM, Hall JT, Rodriguez MB, Corriere JN Jr (1986) Bladder injury in blunt pelvic trauma. Radiology 158(3): 633–638

Stany MP, Hamilton CA (2008) Benign disorders of the ovary. Obstet Gynecol Clin North Am 35(2):271–284 ix

Vaccaro JP, Brody JM (2000) CT cystography in the evaluation of major bladder trauma. Radiogr 20(5):1373–1381

Vandermeer FQ, Wong-You-Cheong JJ (2009) Imaging of acute pelvic pain. Clin Obstet Gynecol 52(1):2–20

Varras M, Tsikini A, Polyzos D, Samara C, Hadjopoulos G, Akrivis C (2004) Uterine adnexal torsion: pathologic and gray-scale ultrasonographic findings. Clin Exp Obstet Gynecol 31(1):34–38

Williams PL, Laifer-Narin SL, Ragavendra N (2003) US of abnormal uterine bleeding. Radiogr 23(3):703–718

Wong-You-Cheong JJ, Woodward PJ, Manning MA, Sesterhenn IA (2006) From the Archives of the AFIP: neoplasms of the urinary bladder: radiologic-pathologic correlation. Radiogr 26(2):553–580

Yang C, Song B, Liu X, Wei GH, Lin T, He DW (2011) Acute scrotum in children: an 18-year retrospective study. Pediatr Emerg Care 27(4):270–274

Young JW, Resnik CS (1990) Fracture of the pelvis: current concepts of classification. AJR Am J Roentgenol 155(6): 1169–1175

Yu NC, Raman SS, Patel M, Barbaric Z (2004) Fistulas of the genitourinary tract: a radiologic review. Radiogr 24(5): 1331–1352

Vascular Emergencies of the Retroperitoneum

Gianpaolo Carrafiello, Monica Mangini, Anna M. Ierardi,
Chiara Recaldini, Elisa Cotta, Filippo Piacentino,
and Carlo Fugazzola

Contents

Abstract

In this chapter we review the major vascular emergencies of the retroperitoneum, including traumatic injuries of the big vessels of the retroperitoneum. We also give a brief overview of endovascular treatment in this field, with particular attention to the advantage of endovascular treatment compared to open surgical repair.

1 Abdominal Aorta

1.1 Abdominal Aortic Aneurysm

1.1.1 Terminology and Clinical Issues

Abdominal aortic aneurysm (AAA) is defined as a structural failure of the vessel wall resulting in segmental dilatation, which increases the normal vessel diameter by 50%. A dilatation of the aorta by <50% of its original diameter is called ectasia. AAA occurs in 2–9% of the population over 65 years of age, and its prevalence may be increasing. Approximately 80% of AAAs occur between the renal arteries and the bifurcation (Lederle 2009). Iliac aortic aneurysm (IAA) is seen in 2–10% of patients with abdominal aortic aneurysms (AAAs) whereas isolated IAAs are relatively rare, with an estimated prevalence of 0.03–0.08%.

Most AAAs are true aneurysms, i.e., a localized dilatation of the aorta caused by weakening of its wall. A true aneurysm involves all three layers (intima, media, and adventitia) of the arterial wall. A pseudoaneurysm (false aneurysm) is a collection of flowing blood that communicates with the arterial lumen but is not enclosed by the normal vessel wall,

G. Carrafiello (✉) · M. Mangini · A. M. Ierardi
C. Recaldini · E. Cotta · F. Piacentino · C. Fugazzola
Department of Radiology, University of Insubria,
Viale Borri 57, 21100 Varese, Italy
e-mail: gcarraf@gmail.com

M. Scaglione et al. (eds.), *Emergency Radiology of the Abdomen*,
Medical Radiology. Diagnostic Imaging,
DOI: 10.1007/174_2011_472, © Springer-Verlag Berlin Heidelberg 2012

instead contained only by the adventitia or surrounding soft tissue.

Atherosclerotic AAAs account for 90% of all AAAs. Other possible aneurysm causes are mycotic and inflammatory. A mycotic aneurysm is defined as an infectious break in the wall of an artery, with the formation of a blind, saccular outpouching that is contiguous with the arterial lumen. Inflammatory AAA is usually accompanied by a thickened wall, with infiltration of chronic inflammatory cells and dense peri-aneurysmal fibrosis. Because the fibrous tissue often adheres to adjacent structures, including ureter, duodenum, inferior vena cava, renal vein, small bowel, and colon, the condition occasionally induces severe complications (Budovec et al. 2010).

Aneurysm formation leads to progressive aortic wall degeneration over many years, culminating with rupture. The risk of rupture correlates with the amount of hemodynamic stress localized on the weakened aortic wall, because tensile strength is largely a function of aneurysm size and geometry (Laplace's law).

The annual growth rate of the aneurysm increases with its size, accelerating the time to rupture. The risk of rupture for AAAs that are <4 cm is only 1%. The annual risk of rupture increases to as much as 3% for aneurysms 4–5 cm in size, 11% for aneurysms between 5 and 7 cm, and 20% for those >7 cm (Bown et al. 2002).

Once the AAA surpasses 5.5 cm in diameter, referral to a specialist is recommended. Additional concern is required in two important circumstances. First, rapid expansion of a saccular aneurysm should alert clinical suspicion of a mycotic aneurysm, because this type tends to increase in size more rapidly than aneurysm from other causes. Second, if significant perianeurysmal fibrosis and adhesions are present, an inflammatory aneurysm should be suspected. Inflammatory aneurysms are often symptomatic and have a much higher rate of rupture that is independent of their size.

Patients with AAA rupture classically (50%) present with hypotension, back pain, and a pulsatile abdominal mass. Rupture may also present as constipation, urinary retention, urge to defecate, or syncope, as the expanding hematoma compresses the bowel, ureters, or their supplying blood vessels. In a contained rupture, patients can present with a normal hematocrit and blood pressure.

1.1.2 Imaging

Computed tomography (CT) is the modality of choice for the evaluation of acute aortic syndrome, because of the speed of the examination and the widespread availability of CT. The most common imaging finding of abdominal aortic aneurysm rupture is a **retroperitoneal hematoma** adjacent to an AAA (with a density value >50 HU). Periaortic blood may extend into the perirenal space, pararenal space, or both (Rakita et al. 2007). These findings are readily visible on non-enhanced CT (NECT) images that may have been obtained for another indication or as part of an aneurysm evaluation protocol. On CECT images, active extravasation of contrast material is frequently demonstrated.

The blood may also extend into the psoas muscle. When intraperitoneal rupture occurs, the anterior or anterolateral aortic wall is usually the source. Less commonly, rupture may be into the bowel, most often the duodenum, resulting in exsanguination. Rarely, AAA rupture into the inferior vena cava causes high-output cardiac failure, lower extremity swelling, and engorgement of the leg veins (aortocaval fistula) (Abrams 1997).

On CT, the "**drape sign**" is also specific for rupture (Halliday and Al-Kutoubi 1996). The posterior aortic wall should be sharp, and a distinct fat plane should be present between the adjacent vertebral bodies. A drape sign should be evaluated when the posterior aneurysm wall lacks sharpness or closely conforms to the vertebral body (i.e., it drapes over the vertebral body), especially if there is erosion of the vertebral body.

Findings predictive of **impending rupture** are:
- Increased aneurysm size
- Thrombus
- Crescent sign

A patient with a very large abdominal aortic aneurysm (diameter >7 cm) who presents with symptoms of acute aortic syndrome is at high risk of aneurysm rupture (Lederle et al. 2002).

Non-ruptured aneurysms generally contain more thrombus than do ruptured aneurysms, and the thrombus-to-lumen ratio decreases with increasing aneurysm size. These observations suggest that a thick circumferential thrombus is protective against rupture. In addition, enlargement of the patent lumen is indicative of partial lysis of the thrombus, which predisposes an aneurysm to rupture.

A focal discontinuity in circumferential wall calcifications is more commonly observed in unstable or ruptured aneurysms (Rakita et al. 2007).

One of the most specific signs for impending rupture is the "**crescent sign**," which is best seen on NECT images (Arita et al. 1997). This sign is most specific for rupture when a well-defined area of higher attenuation than the psoas muscle on a contrast study or an area of the aortic lumen on a non-contrast study is noted within the aneurysm wall. A crescent sign represents acute dissection into the thrombus or aneurysm wall, thereby weakening it, and signifies penetration of the protective shield supplied by the mural thrombus (Fig. 1).

1.1.3 Differentials

Occasionally, the drape sign may be confused with the duodenum, periaortic aneurysm fibrosis, or lymph nodes.

Likewise, a thrombus filled saccular aortic aneurysm compressing a vertebral body should not be confused with a periaortic malignant mass, such as multiple myeloma or plasmacytoma (Rakita et al. 2007; Halliday and Al-Kutoubi 1996).

1.2 Dissection, Intramural Hematoma, and Penetrating Atherosclerotic Ulcer

1.2.1 Terminology and Clinical Issues

One of the most common acute emergency condition of the aorta is the **aortic dissection**, defined as a disruption of the aortic wall, with separation of the intima and inner medial layer of the aorta from the outer medial layer and serosa. The intimal tear allows blood to enter the media from the vessel lumen. The blood-filled space within the medial layer becomes the false lumen. This results in two lumina—a true lumen and a false lumen—with the false lumen having pressures greater than or equal to those in the true lumen (McMahon and Squirrell 2010; Hagan et al. 2000).

The most common cause for **nonfocal dissection** of the abdominal aorta and iliac arteries is a thoracoabdominal dissection, either type A or B.

Focal dissection of the abdominal aorta is rare, occurring in 1.3% of all aortic dissections. It is associated most strongly with hypertension and with smoking, diabetes, previous aneurysm surgery, and hypercholesterolemia. Focal abdominal aortic dissections most often occur spontaneously, but trauma and iatrogenic causes (such as cardiac catheterization) also contribute. Proximally, the abdominal aortic dissection tends to occur either between the renal arteries and the internal mammary artery (33%) or the celiac trunk and the renal arteries (23%). The involvement of peripheral or splanchnic vessels is one of the principle conditions that determine dissection as an emergency condition. The distal extent of the dissection almost always terminates before the common iliac artery (Fig. 2).

Clinical manifestations of aorto-iliac dissection relate to stenoses or occlusion of abdominal visceral branch vessels resulting in mesenteric ischemia, renovascular hypertension, or iliac dissection and extremity ischemia.

Two types of branch-vessel obstruction are described in the literature: static and dynamic obstruction. With **static obstruction**, the intimal flap enters the branch-vessel origin without a re-entry point. **Dynamic obstruction** affects vessels arising from the true lumen. The intimal flap spares the branch vessel but prolapses and covers the branch-vessel origin like a curtain, causing a pressure deficit in the true lumen that results in ischemia.

Rupture of the vasa vasorum and haemorrhage into the media of the aortic wall leads to weakening of the aortic wall, resulting in **aortic intramural hematoma (IMH)**. As described in the literature, an IMH is an atypical aortic dissection because it is thought to represent either early-stage limited dissection or thrombosis of the false lumen in dissection. A nontraumatic cause of IMH is determined in 94% of these cases (Chao et al. 2009).

Penetrating atherosclerotic ulcer (PAU) is an ulcerating atherosclerotic lesion that penetrates the elastic lamina and is associated with hematoma formation within the media of the aortic wall. It was described for the first time by Stanson et al in 1986. Most commonly, the PAU occurs in the descending thoracic aorta, but it can also arise in the abdominal aorta. PAU can cause an IMH, extend along the media, or, rarely, may progress into frank dissection or rupture through the adventitia. The embolization of material from the ulcer to the distal arterial circulation is an additional recognized complication. The clinical presentation is very similar to aortic dissection and

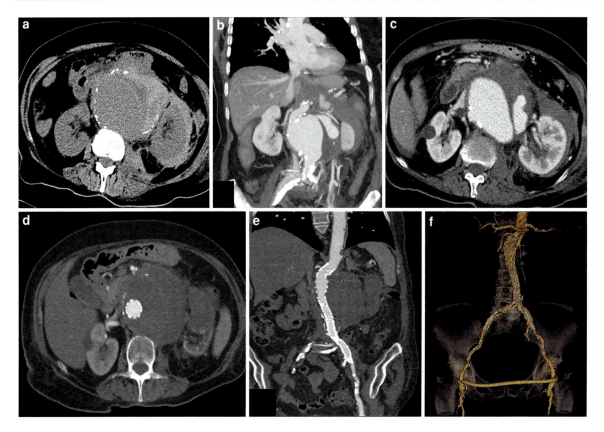

Fig. 1 **a** Aortic aneurysm rupture in an 80-year-old woman with hypotension and abdominal pain. Axial NECT image depicts an abdominal aortic aneurysm (AAA) with a hyperattenuating crescent sign, which represents an acute hematoma within the *left* aneurysm wall. **b** Coronal CECT image demonstrates active extravasation of contrast material into the thrombosed portion of an AAA, as well as extensive retroperitoneal haemorrhage. **c** Axial art CT view of the same case shows a peri-renal *left* hematoma surrounding the homolateral kidney. **d** Axial art CT phase, **e** coronal, and **f** 3D volume-rendering CT image demonstrate complete exclusion of the AAA following aorto-iliac endoprothesis deployment

IMH: severe chest pain frequently radiating to the back.

Pain is believed to be one of the most important variables in determining the appropriateness of surgical intervention (Batt et al. 2005; Bosma et al. 2009).

1.2.2 Imaging

Chest radiographic findings may be normal in 10–40% of aortic dissections. In the study by Hagan et al. (2000) a widened mediastinum was noted in 61.1% of the patients with aortic dissection. The displacement of calcifications in the aorta was reported in 14.1% of patients, with an abnormal cardiac contour noted in 25.8%. Marked enlargement of the heart, indicating a pericardial effusion or the presence of a new pleural effusion, is suggestive of complications from aortic dissection (Hagan et al. 2000).

Modern multisection CT allows rapid image acquisition and data reconstruction and aids in treatment planning. It helps differentiate type A from type B dissection, may localize the intimal entry site, and helps assess branch-vessel involvement and compromise as well as the relationship of the branch vessels to the true or false lumen. This information aids in treatment planning.

The classic intimal flap is seen in approximately 70% of the cases of aortic dissection. It occurs when blood enters the medial layer through an intimal tear, giving rise to a true lumen and a false lumen, with the flap separating the two lumina.

Rarely, a three-channel dissection develops if a secondary dissection occurs within one of the channels, with the resultant intimal flaps giving rise to the "Mercedes-Benz sign" (Williams et al. 1994; LePage et al. 2001).

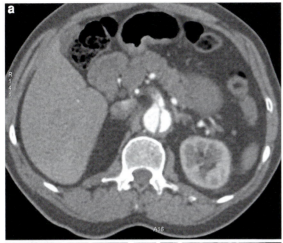

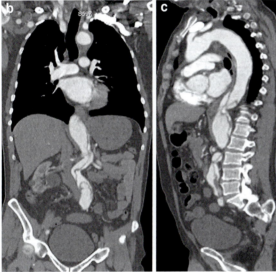

Fig. 2 Dissection of the abdominal aorta in a 64-year-old man with abdominal pain and a history of hypertension. Axial art CECT (**a**) shows the intimal flap at the level of the emergency of mesenteric artery with thrombosis at the origin. Coronal (**b**) and sagittal (**c**) maximum intensity projection (MIP) reconstruction of the arterial phase better depicts the intimal flap along the abdominal aorta up to the level of iliac axis

A narrow true lumen with a filiform shape may be seen and an intimo-intimal intussusception can subsequently occur, giving rise to a "windsock" appearance. Differentiation of the true lumen from the false lumen is important for planning endovascular interventional procedures. Important signs that indicate the false lumen include a larger cross-sectional area, the "cobweb sign," and the "beak sign."

Secondary findings of aortic dissections include internal displacement of intimal calcification, delayed enhancement of the false lumen, widening of the aorta and mediastinum, and pleural or pericardial hematoma.

For diagnosis of IMH, NECT is performed first because the presence of contrast material may obscure a subtle IMH. On NECT axial images, a crescentic, eccentric, hyperattenuating region of aortic-wall thickening (diameter, >7 mm; attenuation, 60–70 HU) is considered diagnostic of acute IMH. This is in contrast to the multilayered pattern of increasing attenuation seen in aortic dissection, in which there is partial or complete thrombosis of the false lumen (Hayter et al. 2006; Hayashi et al. 2000); displacement of intimal calcification is visible too. On CECT axial images, the intramural fluid collection appears as a non-enhancing, smooth, crescentic region of aortic-wall thickening that extends partially or entirely around the opacified aortic lumen, without spiraling of an intimal flap. It is important to document the maximal aortic diameter, the maximal axial thickness of the hematoma, and the minimum and maximum transverse diameters of the aortic lumen at the level of maximal IMH thickness. These characteristics are useful for predicting the outcome of an IMH (Fig. 3).

Both type A and type B IMHs may progress to overt aortic dissection; a fusiform or saccular aneurysm may develop at the site of an IMH.

On NECT, PAU appears as an IMH; it can be seen only if accompanied by aortic dissection or IMH.

On CECT, a localized ulceration penetrating the aortic intima into the aortic wall may be considered the characteristic finding for a PAU. Focal thickening or high attenuation of the adjacent aortic wall suggests associated IMH (Fig. 4).

Transesophageal echocardiography (TEE) is another important diagnostic tool. In particular, TEE sometimes shows a large echo-free space within the IMH, characterized by focal contrast enhancement at CT. This may suggest a small-flow communication through the intimal microtear, indicating an initial dissection (Bozzani et al. 2009).

1.2.3 Differentials

A number of findings can mimic an aortic dissection flap, and it is important to be aware of them in practice: aortic motion artifacts, pericardial recess,

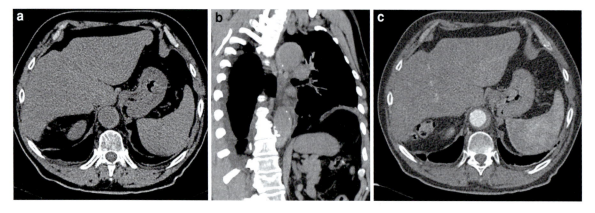

Fig. 3 Abdominal IMH. **a** Axial NECT shows a peripheral rim of increased attenuation of the abdominal aorta. **b** In the sagittal NECT image, the IMH extends along the aortic arch and the abdominal aorta, with displacement of intimal calcification.

c Axial art CECT image shows that the haematoma does not enhance after contrast administration, the aortic lumen is not compromised, and no intimal flap is seen

Fig. 4 PAU of the abdominal aorta. Axial art CECT (**a**) and coronal MPR reconstruction (**b**) show an image of "endoluminal plus" along the aortic border; the axial image evidences the IMH as a focal thickening of the aortic wall

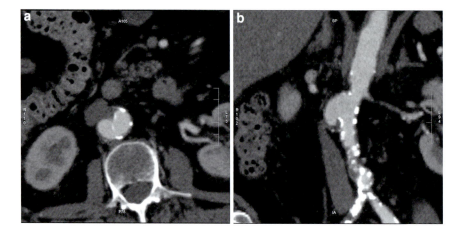

mural thrombus in a fusiform aneurysm, aortic sinus, left brachiocephalic vein, and left superior intercostal vein.

The distinguishing feature of IMH is an absence of the intimal disruption that characterizes classic aortic dissection.

1.3 Acute Leriche Syndrome

1.3.1 Terminology and Clinical Issues

Classic Leriche Syndrome describes a complex of clinical symptoms (claudication, decreased femoral pulses) attributed to the obstruction of the infrarenal aorta (Sebastia et al. 2003). An acute form of the disease is rare and mostly seen in pre-existing, severe atherosclerosis of the distal abdominal aorta and the iliac arteries (Fig. 5).

1.3.2 Imaging

Multisection CT can be used to evaluate the location of aortic stenosis and occlusion, the presence of concomitant occlusive disease affecting visceral arteries, the type and extent of collateralization, and the level of the most proximal and distal arterial segments amenable to stent-graft placement (Sebastia et al. 2003; Laganà et al. 2006).

2 Retroperitoneal Vascular Trauma

Retroperitoneal injuries are seen in a significant minority of abdominal trauma cases (12% of hemodynamically stable patients). Vascular retroperitoneal injuries are rare. Imaging, particularly, CT, plays a

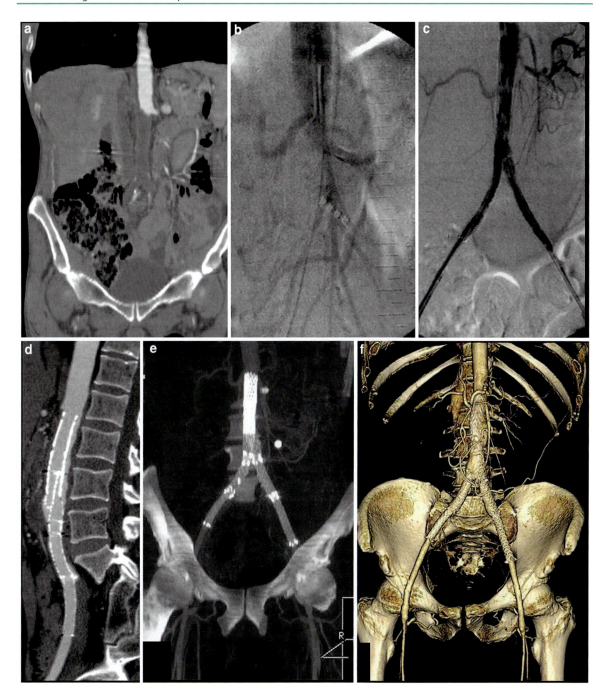

Fig. 5 Coronal art CECT image shows a complete aorto-bi-iliac thrombosis (**a**). Pre-treatment intraoperative digital subtraction angiography (DSA) demonstrates the complete occlusion of the distal tract of the abdominal aorta and of the two iliac branches (**b**). After the procedure, intraoperative DSA shows a complete recanalization of the treated vessels (**c**). Post-procedure sagittal art CECT after stent graft deployment shows patency of abdominal aorta and iliac arteries (**d**); the same findings in coronal MIP (**e**) and 3D volume rendering reconstructions (**f**)

central role in the assessment of retroperitoneal structures following blunt trauma (Daly et al. 2008).

Major retroperitoneal vascular structures include the abdominal aorta, inferior vena cava, renal vessels, proximal celiac axis and superior mesenteric arteries, superior mesenteric vein, lumbar arteries and veins, and iliac vessels within the pelvis.

2.1 Abdominal Aorta and its Branches

2.1.1 Terminology and Clinical Issues

The deep retroperitoneal position of the abdominal aorta in front of the lumbar spine protects it from blunt and penetrating injuries. Blunt injury to the abdominal aorta is uncommon, while injuries to the thoracic aortic occur 20 times more frequently, according to several autopsy series, and involve the infrarenal abdominal aorta in almost all cases (98%) (Steenburg and Ravenel 2007). The degree of injury may include subtle intimal injuries, with creation of an intimal flap, pseudoaneurysm, and transection; thrombus formation may occur with partial or total aortic occlusion.

The proposed mechanisms for traumatic rupture of the abdominal aorta include direct forces on the abdominal aorta, such as between a lap belt and the lumbar spine, as well as indirect forces generated by transmission of the pressure of the initiating force through adjacent organs to the aortic wall.

Rupture and pseudoaneuysms of the renal artery usually develop after penetrating trauma, but may also present after blunt trauma as the result of sudden anterior displacement of the relatively mobile kidneys and stretching of the renal artery and vein or by direct vessel wall contusion against the vertebral bodies (Cura et al. 2011). The extraparenchymal or intraparenchymal renal artery and its branches may be involved. Stretching of the artery with only intimal discontinuation may result in renal artery thrombosis. Subcapsular and perinephric renal haematomas are frequently associated.

Dissection of the right renal artery due to blunt abdominal trauma is a rare but important complication because it can be the cause for the sudden onset of renovascular hypertension. Sudden deceleration of the body or a contusion between the abdominal wall and spine results in subintimal tears, which mostly affect the left renal artery. This may lead to a subintimal dissection, with thrombosis and either a consecutive stenotic lesion or the total occlusion of the renal artery (Harris et al. 2001).

Pelvic arterial hemorrhage is rarely a result of bleeding from large vessels, such as the common and external iliaca artery. Iliac artery injury is seen in 0.4% of arterial traumas. More often, arterial disruption occurs from smaller hypogastric arterial branches. Vascular damage may be caused by a laceration or the angulation of an artery or vein by a fragment of pelvic bone, or by a contusion or tear due to direct application of the external force, which causes sudden stretching and twisting of the vessels. In penetrating trauma, the vessels are directly damaged by the contact with the assaulting object, such as a sharp weapon or a bullet (Sangthong et al. 2006). Commonly, the involved arteries are the superior gluteal artery and the lateral sacral artery. Posterior dislocation of the pelvic ring (open book fractures) normally involves injury of the internal iliac arteries or their branches; a "butterfly" fracture is defined as a rupture of the inferior pudendal artery; anterior compressive forces may damage the external iliac artery or the femoral arteries.

Traumatic lesions of the lumbar artery are rare in the medical literature and are usually described after penetrating injuries. They are also reported following blunt trauma.

Spinal fractures caused by blunt abdominal trauma are associated with significant mortality and morbidity and they represent the most important mechanisms for traumatic lesions of the lumbar arteries (Yoon et al. 2004).

2.1.2 Imaging

Ultrasound in most cases allows the study of the abdominal aorta but in trauma patients is frequently difficult.

In case of dissection, CT identifies the intraluminal flap and double lumen, which is usually more limited in extension in traumatic than in non-traumatic dissection; pseudoaneurysm, periaortic hematoma, or the extravasation of contrast media are detected in aortic-wall rupture.

Angiography is performed only in case endovascular treatment is planned.

In traumatic injury of the renal arteries, active contrast extravasation after a contrast-enhanced study is noted as an intensely enhancing area within a hematoma in the arterial phase that enlarges into an irregular dense collection in delayed scanning (Harris et al. 2001).

CT is the imaging method of choice to study the pelvic arteries. Extravasation of contrast material in the pelvis at CECT is an accurate indicator of ongoing arterial hemorrhage in patients with pelvic fractures (Sangthong et al. 2006; Yoon et al. 2004). On CECT scan, the extravasation of contrast material is a reliable indicator of arterial hemorrhage, with a sensitivity of 66–90%, specificity of 85–98%, and accuracy of 87–98% reported. Dissection and thrombosis are relatively rare lesions that involve the common and external iliac arteries.

In lumbar-artery injury, CT scan shows the same features reported for pelvic arteries; in particular, pseudoaneurysm and contrast media extravasation. Pseudoaneurysm of the lumbar artery can present as an increased density or as soft-tissue thickening in the psoas muscle region on NECT scans. The lumen of the aneurysm can be demonstrated on CT scan following bolus contrast injection. CT angiography is very helpful in depicting the extension of the aneurysm, its relation to the feeding vessel, the level and diameter of the feeding artery of the pseudoaneurysm, and in treatment planning.

2.1.3 Differentials

Retroperitoneal hematoma can be secondary to vertebral or pelvic ring fracture, trauma to the pancreas or genito-urinary organs, or vascular injuries.

Traumatic retroperitoneal haematoma must be differentiated from a neoplastic mass and from an abscess. Hematoma does not enhance after contrast administration unlike abscess; after some time, a peripheral ring of enhancement, due to reabsorption of the hemorrhage, can be seen but it must not be confused with a suprainfection, the only sign of which is the presence of air bubbles in patients who have not undergone interventional procedures (Fig. 6).

2.2 Inferior Vena Cava

2.2.1 Terminology and Clinical Issues

Due to its location, the IVC is rarely involved in traumatic injuries, with only a few published reports in the literature. IVC injury can include contusion, small or large lacerations, complete transection and, rarely, dissection (Huerta et al. 2006; Netto et al. 2006).

2.2.2 Imaging

The CT findings of blunt IVC injury vary depending on the location of the injury: retroperitoneal hematoma with a paracaval epicenter, irregular IVC contour, and extravasation of contrast material have been described with infrahepatic IVC injury. With retrohepatic IVC injuries, severe associated liver trauma is often seen. The CT finding of IVC dissection is a crescent-shaped, contrast-filled lumen displaced and compressed by a non-opacified thrombus beneath the intimal flap, somewhat similar to the CT appearance of aortic dissection (Kandpal et al. 2008).

3 Inferior Vena Cava Thrombosis

3.1 Terminology and Clinical Issues

Thrombosis is a major cause of IVC acute obstruction and typically is an acquired condition. Common causes of IVC thrombosis are idiopathic thrombophlebitis in the lower extremities or pelvis, general conditions such as dehydration, sepsis, localized inflammation, pelvic inflammatory disease, coagulopathy, congestive heart failure, immobility, and tumor invasion (Kandpal et al. 2008).

3.2 Imaging

Ultrasound, including color Doppler flow imaging, is a useful modality for the initial evaluation of thrombosis. However, it is operator dependent, and visualization of the IVC (especially the infrahepatic portion) may be hampered due to bowel gas or obesity. Thus, in emergency situations, CT is essential for diagnosis, staging, and treatment planning. On NECT images, the fresh thrombus can be hyperattenuating.

The IVC is typically evaluated in the portal-venous phase of a CT study (60–70 s after the injection of 100–150 ml of non-ionic contrast material at a rate of 3–5 ml/s), and dynamic multi-phasic imaging is performed only if indicated (e.g., in renal cell carcinoma). In the portal-venous phase, there is denser contrast material in the renal and suprarenal IVC than in the infrarenal portion due to venous return from the kidneys (Fig. 7).

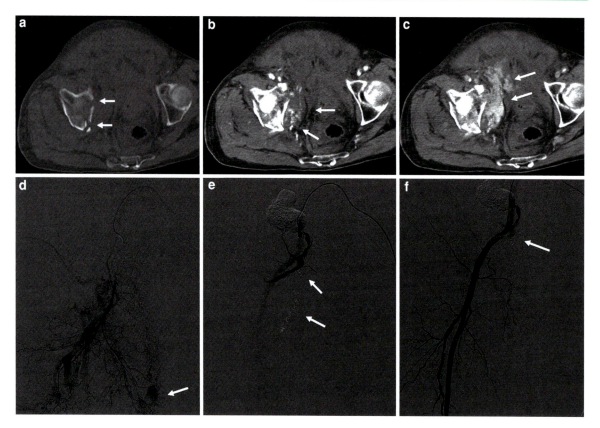

Fig. 6 Polytrauma patient (male, 81 years old) with obturator artery injury. **a** Axial NECT scan shows a right acetabular fracture (*arrows*). **b** Axial art CT scan: hematoma with active bleeding at the level of the medial acetabular wall and the right perineal region (*arrows*). **c** Axial pv CT scan demonstrates a substantial increase in the spreading of contrast medium, due to obturator artery injury (*arrows*). **d** Selective angiogram of the right internal iliac artery shows active contrast medium extravasation from the distal branches of right obturator artery (*arrow*). **e** Superselective embolization of an injured vessel, obtained with multiple steel coils (3-mm diamond shaped) followed by a Gelfoam suspension embolization (*arrows*). **f** Post-procedural selective angiogram of the right internal iliac artery shows the complete exclusion of bleeding (*arrow*)

3.3 Differentials

Expansion of the vessel lumen and enhancement of the filling defect help differentiate malignant from bland thrombus. Malignant thrombi in the IVC are often clinically asymptomatic, although occasionally they can embolize into the pulmonary circulation.

4 Iliopsoas Hemorrhage

4.1 Terminology and Clinical Issues

The iliopsoas compartment consists of all of the muscles covered by the iliopsoas fascia, including the greater psoas, smaller psoas, and iliac muscles.

The iliopsoas muscle passes beneath the inguinal ligament to insert on the lesser trochanter of the femur via the psoas tendon. Hemorrhage confined within the iliopsoas compartment may be caused by a bleeding diathesis or anticoagulant therapy or it may be spontaneous. Hemorrhage may occur secondary to trauma, tumor, recent surgery or biopsy, and by extension from adjacent bleeding organs and vessels (Kwon et al. 2009).

4.2 Imaging

On CT scans, fresh hemorrhage is seen as a discrete mass of high density. A fluid-fluid level may be present owing to the hematocrit effect. Fresh primary

Fig. 7 A 67-year-old woman
with acute IVC thrombosis.
Pv CECT scans in the coronal
view (**a**) and coronal MIP
(**b**) of the focal deep vein
thrombosis of the ICV
continuing to the proximal
left iliac vein. Transjugular
vein access DSA shows
the IVC thrombosis (**c**);
post-procedural DSA
after caval-filter
positioning (**d**)

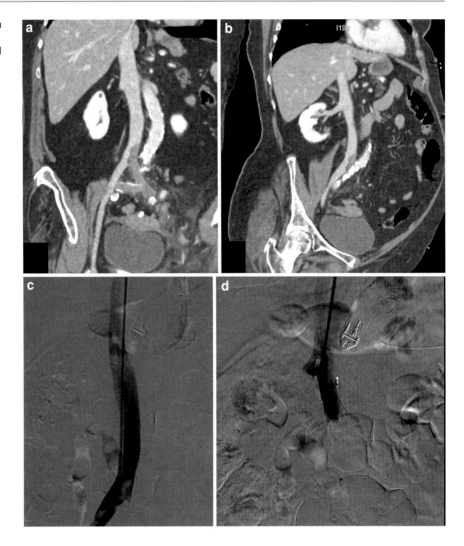

iliopsoas hemorrhage has a hyperattenuating appearance at NECT scans. After constrast media administration, an active blush is seen during arterial phase,
enlarging in the venous and late phases (Muttarak and
Peh 2000) (Fig. 8).

4.3 Differentials

Hemorrhage must be differentiated from an abscess or
a mass of unknown origin, usually malignant. In case
of spontaneous hemorrhage in the retroperitoneum or
pelvis, a ruptured AAA must be ruled out first;
another frequent cause of spontaneous retroperitoneal
hemorrhage is anticoagulant therapy or bleeding
tumor (e.g., renal angiomyolipoma).

5 Interventional Treatment of Vascular Emergencies of the Retroperitoneum

5.1 Terminology and Clinical Issues

5.1.1 Abdominal Aortic Aneurysm

In the treatment of AAA, endovascular aneurysm
repair (EVAR) has been confirmed as an effective
alternative to open surgery due to its lower invasiveness and reduced morbidity and mortality and the
lower overall treatment cost (Greenhalgh et al. 2004;
Prinssen et al. 2004). Since its first introduction into
clinical practice, in 1991, endovascular stent grafting
has gained wide acceptance, with satisfactory results

achieved. Indeed, with the continued success of elective EVAR, this procedure has been extended to treat ruptured AAA (rAAA) in selected patients because of its lower mortality rate (Hinchliffe et al. 2006; Hoornweg et al. 2007). The two largest randomized trials of endovascular and open surgery for rAAA (Hinchliffe et al. 2006; Hoornweg et al. 2007) underlined the importance of CT scan to confirm the suitability of endovascular repair of rAAA, without delaying treatment. A meta-analysis reported the possibility of EVAR in 47% of the patients with rAAA (Mastracci et al. 2008). The systematic review of Visser et al reported a lower intra-operative and 30-day mortality in patients with rAAA treated with EVAR (Visser et al. 2007). The 30-day mortality after elective surgical repair in major randomized trials ranges from 2.7 to 5.8% and is influenced by the volume of procedures performed at the hospital and the expertise of the surgeon (Greenhalgh et al. 2004; Lederle et al. 2009). Other benefits of endovascular repair are reduced hospital stay, shorter recovery time and return to baseline functional capacity, and less blood loss (Sadat et al. 2008).

An important role in the management of a patient with rAAA is that of the logistics; in fact, the impossibility of an endovascular repair can be related to the inability to perform CT-angiography immediately after the patient's arrival in the emergency unit, the lack of an adequate operating room, and of an experienced staff (Hinchliffe et al. 2006).

Endovascular rAAA repair remains experimental, it is an evolving technique but seems to offer the potential for improved outcomes in patients who otherwise have a high morbidity and mortality. A multidisciplinary approach that involves the vascular surgeon, emergency department physicians, anesthesiologists, operating room staff, and radiology technicians, the availability of a variety of off-the-shelf stent-grafts, and an operating room that is adequately equipped to perform endovascular procedures are crucial in obtaining better outcomes.

5.1.2 Aortocaval Fistula (ACF)

Open surgical repair of this rare complication of AAA is associated with high morbidity and mortality; there are considerable difficulties with the open repair of central abdominal fistulae related to the arterialization of venous structures and perivascular inflammation, resulting in an increased risk of significant blood loss.

Additionally, there is an increased risk of pulmonary embolization.

Endovascular stent-graft treatment has also been proposed as an attractive therapeutic alternative. According to the literature review reported by Antoniou et al. (Antoniou et al. 2009), the technical success rate is 96%. However, the mean follow-up in this review was only 9 months, with only one study reporting a follow-up of 24 months. Therefore, no conclusions can yet be reached regarding the long-term efficacy of the endovascular repair of major abdominal ACF.

5.1.3 Abdominal Aortic Traumatic Injury

Here too, endovascular repair is an effective form of treatment (Gunn et al. 2007). The reasons for non-operative management are generally refusal of surgery, do-not-resuscitate order, diffuse brain injury, small intimal tear, and technical difficulty an endovascular stent graft provides a less invasive method of repair in this population. Some reports suggest a conservative treatment in stable patients. For example, in the series of Aladham et al. (2010), 29 of the 48 patients had early or delayed aortic repair; the other 19 were closely followed.

5.1.4 Isolated Dissection of the Abdominal Aorta

The indications for operative intervention in these patients include aortic rupture, lower extremity ischemia, unremitting pain, associated aortic aneurysm, and prevention of future aneurysmal degeneration. Operative intervention consists of open or endovascular repair of the abdominal aorta, with decision-making greatly influenced by the anatomical condition together with the surgeon's experience. As dissection may extend to the iliac arteries, aortobifemoral grafting is the procedure of choice. Endovascular treatment of isolated dissection has been associated with a high rate of technical and clinical success, with reduced morbidity and mortality rates, in experienced centers (Dake et al. 1999; Berthet et al. 2003).

5.1.5 Penetrating Atherosclerotic Ulcer

The treatment of PAU is still controversial. Although some authors believe immediate surgical treatment is not always required—because most PAU have a benign clinical course—early intervention has been

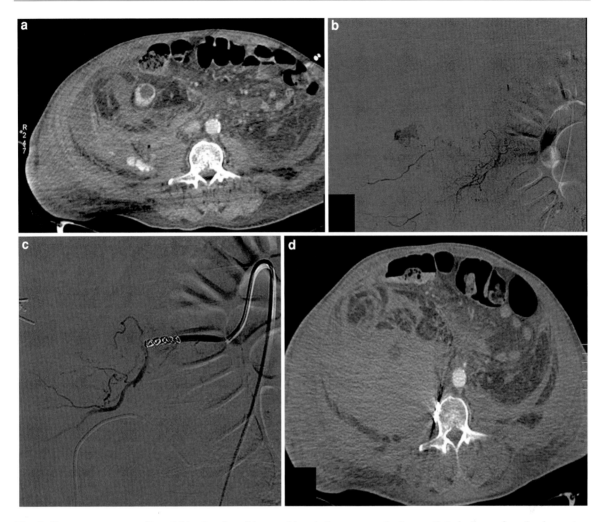

Fig. 8 Spontaneous retroperitoneal bleeding in a 74-year-old man receiving warfarin. **a** The art CECT scan shows enlargement of the right psoas muscle and an active blush of contrast material causing a peripheral area of higher attenuation, suggestive of active bleeding of retroperitoneal origin. **b** DSA during super-selective catheterization of a lumbar artery demonstrates the active extravasation of contrast material. **c** DSA after lumbar artery embolization with coils shows the complete exclusion of active bleeding. **d** Axial art CT shows the complete resolution of iliopsoas bleeding

recommended when PAU is complicated by aneurysm expansion, regardless of size, rupture, embolic symptoms, or uncontrolled pain. Open surgical repair with graft interposition has been used traditionally, but patients with PAU are generally not ideal candidates for open repair because of advanced age and poor general status. An aortic stent-graft could probably change the strategy for the treatment of PAU. This less-invasive procedure is suitable for high-risk patients and can also be used in cases of rupture. As a less-invasive treatment, endovascular stent grafting has been advocated and several reports of the endovascular treatment of PAU have been published (Piffaretti et al. 2007).

5.1.6 Infrarenal Aortic Occlusive Disease

The usual management of this condition involves endarterectomy for focal lesions or surgical bypass for more extensive aorto-iliac disease. Since 1980, endovascular treatment has been proposed as a feasible and safe alternative to open surgery in these patients. The available data have established the safety and effectiveness of PTA, with an 85% primary and a 90% secondary patency rate, together with a low (3%) risk of major complications, such as vessel-wall rupture and distal and visceral embolism.

The endovascular approach can be considered valid for the acute or the chronic presentation of this disease (Fig. 5). Primary or direct stenting has been proposed based on the favorable results obtained in the iliac arteries, including higher patency rates than obtained with PTA, and has been employed selectively in complex stenotic lesions (ulcerated, eccentric, irregular and/or calcific plaques) and, more rarely, in total occlusions (Schedel et al. 2004; Badiola et al. 1999). The rationale for direct stenting is based on the frequent early post-PTA elastic recoil due to the extensive presence of elastic fibers in the aortic wall and to the risk of rupture due to the large diameter of the aorta, according to Laplace's law. Moreover, stent deployment without pre-dilation (direct stenting), reduces the risk of distal embolism of atherothrombotic debris. The choice of a balloon-expandable stent for aortic lesions is based on its superior radial force and the fact that it can be further dilated after the initial expansion in order to achieve a hemodynamically satisfying diameter.

Among the complications, the most feared, aortic wall rupture, is quite rare and only sporadic cases have been reported after PTA and stenting. This complication too can be treated with stent-grafts. Among the causes of late clinical failure, intimal hyperplasia is the most frequent; it may cause restenosis and lead, when highly critical, even to thrombotic reocclusion of the stent. The endovascular approach does not interfere with sexual function which, especially in men, may be compromised in up to 30% of cases after surgery. Finally, the endovascular strategy does not preclude open surgical management in case of procedural failure or disease progression.

5.1.7 Arterial Hemorrhage

This is one of the most serious problems associated with pelvic fractures and it remains the leading cause of death in pelvic fracture. The high morbidity (40–50%) and mortality (5–30%) rates are due to the inability to surgically control pelvic retroperitoneal bleeding. Among patients with closed pelvic fractures and hemodynamic instability, mortality rises to approximately 27% and it increases to approximately 55% for open pelvic fractures.

Post-traumatic pelvic bleeding can be of arterial, venous, or bone origin. Arterial injures are the most common and the most severe. The most important aspect in the management of pelvic hemorrhage associated with pelvic fractures is its detection and subsequent treatment, as death due to the hemorrhage of a pelvic fracture frequently occurs within the first 24 h of injury. Several authors have suggested that the external fixation is not likely to be sufficient to stop arterial bleeding. Surgical control of pelvic arterial hemorrhage often fails as a result of uncontrolled hemorrhage from inaccessible vessels.

Urgent angiography and subsequent transcatheter embolization are currently accepted as the most effective methods for controlling ongoing arterial bleeding in pelvic fractures. As a result, since first reported in the 1972 by Margolies et al., pelvic angiography has become the gold standard for the treatment of pelvic arterial hemorrhage (Fig. 6).

The efficacy of transcatheter arterial embolization (TAE) in the management of arterial hemorrhages caused by pelvic fractures has been demonstrated (Papakostidis et al. 2011). The success rate, expressed in terms of hemorrhage control and reduction in transfusion requirement, ranges from 85 to 100%. TAE should be performed as early as possible, because effective embolization must be achieved before severe systemic coagulopathy and multiple organ failure develop.

Active bleeding due to a lesion of a small distal vessel responds well to embolization using particles such as those of polyvinylalcohol (150–300 μm), embospheres (300–500 μm), or Gelfoam in small segments (1 mm). Gelfoam is inexpensive and easy to use; however, it is not permanent and re-bleeding may occur in cases of pseudoaneurysms or fissurations, a potentially effective embolization agent is microcoils, placed distally and proximally to the pseudoaneurysm. Microcoils have to be customized to the vessel diameter.

In conclusion, percutaneous control of pelvic hemorrhage is a valuable therapeutic option: TAE is a rapid, safe, effective, and minimally invasive technique.

5.1.8 Traumatic Injuries of the Suprarenal IVC or the Iliocaval Bifurcation

Emergency surgical repair of these vessel segments remains a technical challenge, with high morbidity and mortality rates (50–100%). Interventional vascular techniques are an important alternative approach in the armamentarium of trauma and vascular

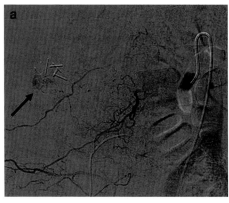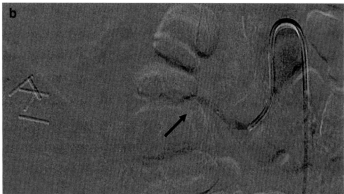

Fig. 9 A 58-year-old patient, on anticoagulation therapy for kidney transplantation. **a** DSA shows active bleeding from a right lumbar artery (*arrow*). **b** Post-procedural angiogram after deployment of the vascular plug (*arrow*) shows complete exclusion of the bleeding

surgeons for the treatment of many different vessel districts. The key to the successful management of abdominal vascular injuries lies in the immediate control of the hemorrhaging vessel. Watarida et al. (2002) reported the successful use of a fenestrated stent-graft to manage a traumatic rupture of the juxtahepatic IVC. In these cases, proper facilities, radiological expertise and experience, and an assortment of devices must be available.

5.1.9 Retroperitoneal Vascular Emergency

Management of, retroperitoneal vascular emergency, especially in unstable patients, is both difficult and highly challenging, and it requires multidisciplinary protocols. The control of bleeding can be accomplished by either surgical or endovascular approaches. The results of surgical exploration and primary repair in hemodynamically unstable patients are well known. This strategy is associated with a high mortality rate, ranging from 30 to 80%, regardless of the lesion's localization. The high mortality rate is linked to the opening of the retroperitoneum space, which leads to suppression of the tamponade effect, disruption of the hematoma, and destabilization of the patient.

Thus, the treatment of retroperitoneal hematoma remains controversial. Regardless of the etiology of the retroperitoneal bleed, all patients should initially be managed in a high dependency or intensive care unit, with careful monitoring, fluid resuscitation, blood transfusion, and normalization of coagulation factors.

There are no specific guidelines to suggest when an endovascular or open surgical intervention to stop the bleeding is best performed. If the patient is hemodynamically stable with no evidence of on-going bleeding, conservative management is recommended. There is a growing trend in the use of endovascular techniques as an alternative to open surgery in the management of retroperitoneal hemorrhage. The main options are selective intra-arterial embolization or stent-grafts to stop the bleeding.

In the case of spontaneous retroperitoneal hemorrhage, the mainstay of management remains a conservative approach, with withdrawal of anticoagulation therapy, correction of coagulopathy, volume resuscitation, and supportive measures.

Intra-arterial embolization is being used with increasing frequency in patients whose angiogram shows active bleeding sites (Isokangas and Perala 2004). Coils are probably the safest agent, but Isokangas and Perala (2004). commented that proximal coiling of the bleeding artery may not be sufficient in the retroperitoneum, where there is a rich network of collateral arteries and new arterial pathways may develop after obliteration of the lumbar arteries. It is important to place embolic agents both proximally and distally to the bleeding site to prevent re-bleeding. The indications for embolization are based on the hemodynamic stability of the patient and the degree of blood loss. Embolization is becoming more common as an alternative to open surgery in the treatment of retroperitoneal bleed following iatrogenic injuries, after procedures such as percutaneous lumbar sympathectomy, renal biopsy, and percutaneous nephrostomy, or following iatrogenic iliofemoral vessel injuries.

A relatively new system for definitive embolization is the Amplatzer vascular plug (AVP); this versatile device has been successfully used in the closure of arteries (internal iliac and subclavian), pulmonary arteriovenous malformations, hemodialysis fistulae, and gastric varices (Ferro et al. 2007). It is a cylindrical, self-expandible system made of 144 nitinol mesh wires secured on both ends with platinum marker bands. Once the release site has been reached, the catheter is withdrawn to expose the plug and the metallic guide turned counterclockwise to release the device (Fig. 9).

Open surgery is indicated if the patient remains unstable despite adequate fluid and blood product resuscitation, or if interventional radiology is either not successful or unavailable.

References

Abrams HL (ed) (1997) Aneurysms of the abdominal aorta. In: Abram's angiography: vascular and interventional radiology. 4th edn. Little, Brown, Boston

Aladham F, Sundaram B, Williams DM, Quint LE (2010) Traumatic aortic injury: computerized tomographic findings at presentation and after conservative therapy. J Comput Assist Tomogr 34(3):388–394

Antoniou GA, Koutsias S, Karathanos C et al (2009) Endovascular stent-graft repair of major abdominal arteriovenous fistula: a systematic review. J Endovasc Ther 16(4):514–523

Arita T, Matsunaga N, Takano K et al (1997) Abdominal aortic aneurysm: rupture associated with the high-attenuating crescent sign. Radiology 204:765–768

Badiola CM, Scappaticci F, Scoppetta DJ (1999) Primary stenting in complete aortic occlusion. AJR Am J Roentgenol 172:501–503

Batt M, Haudebourg P, Planchard PF et al (2005) Penetrating atherosclerotic ulcers of the infrarenal aorta: life-threatening lesions. Eur J Vasc Endovasc Surg 29:35–42

Berthet JP, Marty-Ane CH, Veerapen R et al (2003) Dissection of the abdominal aorta in blunt trauma: endovascular or conventional surgical management? J Vasc Surg 38:997–1004

Bosma MS, Quint LE, Williams DM et al (2009) Ulcerlike projections developing in noncommunicating aortic dissections: CT findings and natural history. AJR Am J Roentgenol 193(3):895–905

Bown MJ, Sutton AJ, Bell PR et al (2002) A meta-analysis of 50 years of ruptured abdominal aortic aneurysm repair. Br J Surg 89(6):714–730

Bozzani A, Palmieri P, Arici V, Ragni F, Odero A (2009) Echo-free space and intimal micro-tear: initiating event or decompression rent of intramural haematoma? Eur J Vasc Endovasc Surg Extra 17:17–19

Budovec JJ, Pollema M, Grogan M (2010) Update on multidetector computed tomography angiography of the abdominal aorta. Radiol Clin North Am 48(2):283–309

Chao CP, Walker TG, Kalva SP (2009) Natural history and CT appearances of aortic intramural haematoma. Radiographics 29(3):791–804

Cura M, Elmerhi F, Bugnogne A et al (2011) Renal aneurysms and pseudoaneurysms. Clin Imaging 35(1):29–41

Dake MD, Kato N, Mitchell RS et al (1999) Endovascular stentgraft placement for the treatment of acute aortic dissection. N Engl J Med 340:1546–1552

Daly KP, Ho CP, Persson DL, Gay SB (2008) Traumatic retroperitoneal injuries: review of multidetector CT findings. RadioGraphics 28:1571–1590

Ferro C, Petrocelli F, Rossi UG et al (2007) Vascular percutaneous transcatheter embolisation with a new device: amplatzer vascular plug. Radiol Med 112:239–251

Greenhalgh RM, Brown LC, Kwong GP, Powell JT, Thompson SG (2004) Comparison of endovascular aneurysm repair with open repair in patients with abdominal aortic aneurysm (EVAR trial 1), 30-day operative mortality results: randomised controlled trial. Lancet 364:843–848

Gunn M, Campbell M, Hoffer EK (2007) Traumatic abdominal aortic injury treated by endovascular stent placement. Emerg Radiol 13:329–331

Hagan PG, Nienaber CA, Isselbacher EM et al (2000) The international registry of acute aortic dissection (IRAD): new insights into an old disease. JAMA 283(7):897–903

Halliday KE, Al-Kutoubi A (1996) Draped aorta: CT sign of contained leak of aortic aneurysms. Radiology 199:41–43

Harris AC, Zwirewich CV, Lyburn ID et al (2001) CT findings in blunt renal trauma. Radiographics 21(Spec No): S201–S214

Hayashi H, Matsuoka Y, Sakamoto I et al (2000) Penetrating atherosclerotic ulcer of the aorta: imaging features and disease concept. RadioGraphics 20:995–1005

Hayter RG, Rhea JT, Small A et al (2006) Suspected aortic dissection and other aortic disorders: multi–detector row CT in 373 cases in the emergency setting. Radiology 238:841–852

Hinchliffe RJ, Bruijstens L, MacSweeney ST, Braithwaite BD (2006) A randomized trial of endovascular and open surgery for ruptured abdominal aortic aneurysm—results of a pilot study and lessons learned for future studies. Eur J Vasc Endovasc Surg 32:506–513

Hoornweg LL, Wisselink W, Vahl A et al (2007) The amsterdam acute aneurysm trial: suitability and application rate for endovascular repair of ruptured abdominal aortic aneurysms. Eur J Vasc Endovasc Surg 33:679–683

Huerta S, Bui TD, Nguyen TH et al (2006) Predictors of mortality and management of patients with traumatic inferior vena cava injuries. Am Surg 72(4):290–296

Isokangas JM, Perala JM (2004) Endovascular embolization of spontaneous retroperitoneal haemorrhage secondary to anticoagulant treatment. Cardiovasc Interv Radiol 27:607–611

Kandpal H, Sharma R, Gamangatti S et al (2008) Imaging the inferior vena cava: a road less traveled. Radiographics 28(3):669–689

Kwon OY, Lee KR, Kim SW (2009) Spontaneous iliopsoas muscle haematoma. Emerg Med J 26(12):863

Laganà D, Carrafiello G, Mangini M et al (2006) Endovascular treatment of steno-occlusions of the infrarenal abdominal aorta. Radiol Med 111:949–958

Lederle FA (2009) In the clinic. Abdominal aortic aneurysm. Ann Intern Med 150(9):ITC5-1–ITC5-15

Lederle FA, Johnson GR, Wilson SE et al (2002) Rupture rate of large abdominal aortic aneurysms in patients refusing or unfit for elective repair. JAMA 287:2968–2972

Lederle FA, Freischlag JA, Kyriakides TC et al (2009) Outcomes following endovascular vs open repair of abdominal aortic aneurysm: a randomized trial. JAMA 302:1535–1542

LePage MA, Quint LE, Sonnad SS et al (2001) Aortic dissection: CT features that distinguish true lumen from false lumen. AJR Am J Roentgenol 177(1):207–211

Mastracci MT, Garrido Olivarese L, Cinà CS, Clase CM (2008) Endovascular repair of ruptured abdominal aortic aneurysms: a systematic review and meta-analysis. J Vasc Surg 47:214–221

McMahon MA, Squirrell CA (2010) Multidetector CT of aortic dissection: a pictorial review. Radiographics 30(2):445–460

Muttarak M, Peh WC (2000) CT of unusual iliopsoas compartment lesions. Radiographics 20(Spec No):S53–S66

Netto FA, Tien H, Hamilton P et al (2006) Diagnosis and outcome of blunt caval injuries in the modern trauma center. J Trauma 61(5):1053–1057

Papakostidis C, Kanakaris N, Dimitriou R, Giannoudis PV (2011) The role of arterial embolization in controlling pelvic fracture haemorrhage: a systematic review of the literature. Eur Radiol Mar 24 [Epub ahead of print]

Piffaretti G, Tozzi M, Lomazzo C et al (2007) Endovascular repair of abdominal infrarenal penetrating aortic ulcers: a prospective observational study. Int J Surg 5(3):172–175

Prinssen M, Verhoeven EL, Buth J et al (2004) A randomized trial comparing conventional and endovascular repair of abdominal aortic aneurysms. N Engl J Med 351:1607–1618

Rakita D, Newatia A, Hines J et al (2007) Spectrum of CT findings in rupture and impending rupture of abdominal aortic aneurysms. RadioGraphics 27:497–507

Sadat U, Boyle JR, Walsh SR et al (2008) Endovascular vs open repair of acute abdominal aortic aneurysms—a systematic review and meta-analysis. J Vasc Surg 48:227–236

Sangthong B, Demetriades D, Martin M et al (2006) Management and hospital outcomes of blunt renal artery injuries: analysis of 517 patients from the national trauma data bank. J Am Coll Surg 203(5):612–617

Schedel H, Wissgott C, Rademaker J, Steinkamp HJ (2004) Primary stent placement for infrarenal aortic stenosis: immediate and midterm results. J Vasc Interv Radiol 15:353–359

Sebastia C, Quiroga S, Boye R et al (2003) Aortic stenosis: spectrum of diseases depicted at multisection CT. Radio-Graphics 23:S79–S91

Steenburg SD, Ravenel JG (2007) Multi-detector computed tomography findings of atypical blunt traumatic aortic injuries: a pictorial review. Emerg Radiol 14(3):143–150

Visser JJ, van Sambeek MR, Hamza TH, Hunink MG, Bosch JL (2007) Ruptured abdominal aortic aneurysms: endovascular repair versus open surgery–systematic review. Radiology 245:122–129

Watarida S, Nishi T, Furukawa A et al (2002) Fenestrated stent-graft for traumatic juxtahepatic inferior vena cava injury. J Endovasc Ther 9:134–137

Williams DM, Joshi A, Dake MD et al (1994) Aortic cobwebs: an anatomic marker identifying the false lumen in aortic dissection—imaging and pathologic correlation. Radiology 190(1):167–174

Yoon W, Kyu Kim J, Yeon Jeong Y et al (2004) Pelvic arterial haemorrhage in patients with pelvic fractures: detection with contrast-enhanced CT. RadioGraphics 24:1591–1606

MRI of the Acute Abdomen and Pelvis

Garry Choy, Ajay K. Singh, and Robert A. Novelline

Contents

G. Choy (✉) · A. K. Singh · R. A. Novelline
Department of Radiology, Division of Emergency
Radiology and Teleradiology,
Massachusetts General Hospital,
55 Fruit Street, Founders 210,
Boston, MA 02114, USA
e-mail: gchoy@partners.org

Abstract

Acute abdominal and pelvic conditions require rapid and accurate diagnosis in the emergency department setting. While the imaging modalities of ultrasound, CT, and radiography play a significant role, magnetic resonance imaging (MRI) offers a distinct number of advantages in certain conditions and situations. MRI is often a diagnostic problem solver and can be used in selected patients. With increasing vigilance regarding ionizing radiation dose, MRI will likely play an increasing role in the emergency department. This chapter provides an overview of MR imaging of the abdomen and pelvis in the emergency setting including the descriptions of facility logistics and design, imaging protocols, and a review of imaging features of common acute abdominopelvic conditions.

M. Scaglione et al. (eds.), *Emergency Radiology of the Abdomen*,
Medical Radiology. Diagnostic Imaging,
DOI: 10.1007/174_2011_473, © Springer-Verlag Berlin Heidelberg 2012

1   Introduction

Acute abdominal and pelvic conditions require rapid and accurate diagnosis in the emergency department setting. While the imaging modalities of ultrasound (US), computed tomography (CT), and radiography play significant roles, magnetic resonance imaging (MRI) offers a distinct number of advantages in certain conditions and situations. These include its the lack of ionizing radiation, vascular imaging without intravenous contrast, and better soft-tissue discrimination (Tkacz et al. 2009; Pedrosa and Rofsky 2003; Erturk et al. 2005; Singh et al. 2007, 2009). However, the relatively high cost of MRI, the lengthy exam times, and its limited availability in most hospitals have hindered its widespread use in emergency settings. Nonetheless, MRI is often a diagnostic problem solver and is appropriate in selected patients (for example, pregnant or pediatric patients). With the increasing societal vigilance regarding ionizing radiation exposure, MRI will likely play an increasing role in the emergency department.

This chapter provides an overview of MRI of the abdomen and pelvis in the emergency setting, including descriptions of facility logistics and design, imaging protocols, and a review of the imaging features of common acute abdomino-pelvic conditions.

2   Facility, Logistics, and Design of an MRI Suite in the Emergency Department

2.1   Capacity and Workflow

Given the high volume of patients in busy emergency departments, magnetic resonance scanning protocols need to be optimized to increase patient throughput. Fast sequences should be implemented whenever possible. In addition, fast breath-hold sequences should be obtained, unless patients are too ill or unable to cooperate, in which case free-breathing protocols should be followed. The availability of an additional scanner will allow sudden increases in demand for MRI scanner time to be met when the emergency department is busy.

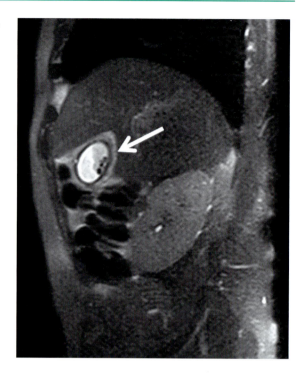

Fig. 1 Acute cholecystitis. Post-contrast enhanced T1-weighted sagittal image that demonstrates pericholecystic fluid, cholelithiasis, and gallbladder wall thickening (*arrow*)

2.2   Layout and Planning

The convenience of a magnetic resonance scanner inside or adjacent to the emergency department can dramatically improve the level of patient care. The basics of MRI safety must be adhered to. Hospital staff must be properly trained prior to granting them access to the scanner area. Controlled access must be maintained in order to ensure safety and security. For example, access to the MRI suite and control room could be restricted by electronic-key-card-based entry (Fig. 1).

2.3   Technologist Staffing

It is critical to have qualified MRI technologists providing round-the-clock, 24-h coverage. The technical skills of MRI technologists working in the emergency radiology facility of the emergency department should include imaging of the abdomen and pelvis as well as knowledge about the imaging requirements of the brain, spine, and musculoskeletal system. Furthermore, the technological staff must be well versed in patient care, with an awareness of the needs of acutely ill patients, pregnant patients, etc. The staff must also be highly skilled at workflow management and operational efficiency, given the high volume and urgency of emergency department cases. There should be two technologists for each shift as this will expedite efficient throughput and workflow.

3 Protocols for MRI of the Acute Abdomen

The protocols used in MRI should be tailored to minimize acquisition time, to accommodate patients who may not be able to cooperate with breath-hold instructions. As a result, MRI protocols should be carefully designed, considering the patient's acute clinical condition. Oral contrast use should be optional, since, for example, patients who are unconscious are unable to ingest oral contrast in addition to being at risk for aspiration. However, in patients who can tolerate oral contrast, identification of the pathology provoking the acute abdomen and pelvis, whether drainable fluid collections, abnormal bowel loops, ovarian torsion, etc., will be more reliable. Recommended oral contrast materials includes ferumoxsil (Gastromark; Mallinckrodt Medical, St. Louis, Missouri) and dilute barium sulfate (Readi-Cat 2; E-Z-Em Canada, Westbury, New York) (Singh et al. 2007, 2009), based on their minimal susceptibility to artifacts on MRI (Singh et al. 2007). While many centers have different protocols and mixtures, oral contrast doses are fairly consistent, ranging from 300 to 750 ml.

MRI protocols can be classified generally into those for breath-hold and free-breathing. For patients presenting acutely, the use of free-breathing protocols is preferred. However, if patients are able to follow instructions and hold their breath for longer than 15–25 s, then breath-hold protocols will offer superior image quality. With the use of free breathing, most image acquisition is focused at the end-expiratory phase (Erturk et al. 2005; Singh et al. 2007, 2009).

T1-weighted and T2-weighted sequences are the protocols mainly used for imaging the acute abdomen. T1-weighted sequences will facilitate the detection of

hemorrhage, which demonstrates high signal intensity on these sequences. Furthermore, artifacts from air, metal, or hemosiderin are more visible on T1-weighted images with long echo times. Fat-suppressed T1 sequences or STIR (short inversion time recovery) sequences are utilized to eliminate the fat signal, resulting in improved identification of pathologic findings with high signal intensity on T1. Single-shot fast spin echo (SS FSE) T2-weighted images allow the characterization and detection of ascites, abscess collections, pancreatic or biliary ductal abnormalities, fluid-filled bowel, and hydronephrosis (Singh et al. 2007, 2009).

Intravenous contrast-enhanced T1 sequences with gadolinium chelates such as gadopentetate dimeglumine (Magnevist; Berlex Laboratories, Wayne, New Jersey, USA) are recommended to evaluate inflammatory or infectious processes, the parenchyma of abdominal organs, and the vasculature (Singh et al. 2007). Dynamic contrast-enhanced MRI can be performed to evaluate the liver and abdomen in arterial, portal-venous, and delayed-venous phases.

The most common indications for imaging the acute abdomen include suspected inflammatory, infectious, or ischemic conditions (e.g., in case of ovarian torsion). As a result, the standard MRI protocol for the acute abdomen and pelvis consists of axial and coronal SS FSE, STIR, and axial T1-weighted images, and possibly contrast-enhanced T1-weighted images if there are no contraindications. Intravenous contrast should not be used either in patients with severe renal insufficiency or in pregnant patients (Pedrosa and Rofsky 2003; Erturk et al. 2005; Singh et al. 2007, 2009; Lam et al. 2008; Barger and Nandalur 2010).

4 Cholecystitis and Biliary Duct Obstruction

4.1 Terminology and Clinical Issues

While US is very effective in the detection of acute cholecystitis and in identifying biliary obstruction, further characterization by MRI is often helpful. MRI increases sensitivity of detecting gallbladder wall edema and pericholecystic fluid and in soft tissue discrimination. MRCP is a non-invasive alternative to

Table 1 MRI findings of cholecystitis

- T2 hyperintensity correlating with edema surrounding the gallbladder and wall
- Gallbladder-wall thickening
- Pericholecystic fluid
- Gallstones (T1 and T2 hypointense)
- Dilated biliary ducts and gallbladder
- T1-weighted post-gadolinium enhancement of gallbladder mucosa and wall

endoscopic retrograde cholangiopancreatography (ERCP) in the assessment of biliary obstruction, cholecystitis, pancreatitis, duodenal perforation, and biliary or pancreatic ductal tears. MRCP relies on heavily T2-weighted based sequences in order to maximize the contrast between fluid filled structures, such as ducts, compared to adjacent soft tissues. MRCP allows for maximal visualization of the biliary ductal and pancreatic ductal systems. It can be performed in the coronal and axial planes with thin-slice acquisitions along with maximal intensity projection (MIP) images that can be utilized to visualize small stones or small tears. MRCP techniques rely on breath-hold or free breathing 2D or 3D T2-weighted sequences, including SS FSE or half-Fourier acquisition single-shot turbo spin-echo (HASTE) techniques.

4.2 Imaging

The imaging findings of cholecystitis consist of gallbladder-wall thickening, edema (on T2-weighted images) surrounding the gallbladder, and T1/T2 hypointense intraluminal stones in the biliary tree or gallbladder (Table 1, Fig. 2) (Catalano et al. 2008; Watanabe et al. 2007). In the case of biliary obstruction from choledocholithasis, stones can appear as filling defects of low signal intensity in the dilated biliary ducts (Table 2, Fig. 3). Stones typically have a round, oval, or angular shape on MRI. It is important to note that air bubbles, sludge, and neoplasm can also be of low signal intensity on MRI sequences (Singh et al. 2007; Catalano et al. 2008; Watanabe et al. 2007). Any equivocal filling defect can be further evaluated with a histologic diagnosis via ERCP.

4.3 Differentials

The differential diagnosis for gallbladder thickening mimicking cholecystitis includes hepatitis, liver cirrhosis, congestive heart failure, renal failure, adenomyomatosis, and pancreatitis. However, these diagnostic considerations typically lack surrounding edema and signs of infection clinically. Gallbladder carcinoma should also be considered in the differential diagnosis if there is apparent invasion or involvement of adjacent liver or lymph nodes.

Filling defects in a dilated bile duct suggest a differential diagnosis of ampullary stenosis and obstructing bile duct or a neoplasm in the pancreatic head. The neoplastic causes of biliary-duct obstruction typically have an irregular and infiltrative appearance. Furthermore, if intravenous contrast is administered, enhancement of filling defects can be seen on MRI or CT. ERCP can be performed for tissue diagnosis.

5 Inflammatory Bowel Disease

5.1 Terminology and Clinical Issues

While multiple centers typically utilize CT for the evaluation of inflammatory bowel disease such as Crohn's disease, MRI is gaining ground based on its lack of ionizing radiation. Moreover, the fact that Crohn's disease is often seen in the pediatric age group provides further support for MRI in the evaluation of inflammatory bowel disease. CT is still more sensitive and specific, but MRI has demonstrated improved diagnostic accuracy and performance in recent years. It provides excellent contrast resolution and detects with high sensitivity extraluminal disease complications such as fistulas and abscess collections.

5.2 Imaging

The MRI features of Crohn's disease are mucosal enhancement, bowel-wall thickening, hypervascularity, abscess collections, fistulas, and strictures (Figs. 3, 4) (Gee and Harisinghani 2011). Ulcerative colitis can also be evaluated with MRI in pediatric

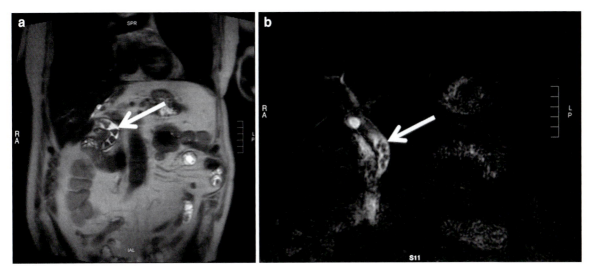

Fig. 2 Two patients with choledocholithiasis. **a** Coronal T2-weighted HASTE sequence shows dilated and curved extrahepatic biliary duct (*arrow*) filled with obstructing stones. **b** MRCP from heavily T2-weighted sequence in another patient shows numerous stones in a dilated biliary duct (*arrow*)

Table 2 MRI findings of obstructive choledocholithasis

- T2 hyperintense dilated biliary tree
- Stones in gallbladder and/or biliary ducts (T1 and T2 hypointense)
- Possible concurrent cholecystitis

patients. Diffuse mural thickening and mucosal enhancement primarily involving the colon are seen (Gee and Harisinghani 2011) (Table 3).

5.3 Differentials

The differential diagnosis of mural thickening and enhancement involving the bowel includes infection, ischemia, and neoplasm. Enteritis from infectious causes may be indistinguishable from inflammation in the acute phase. Ischemic causes of bowel-wall abnormalities may be localized to certain patterns, such as in the watershed regions of the hepatic and splenic flexures of the colon. Other signs of ischemia such as extensive atherosclerotic disease may be present. Neoplasms of the bowel may include a primary colon malignancy, small-bowel carcinoma, metastatic disease, or lymphoma. Secondary findings of lymphadenopathy and marked irregularity due to bowel-wall thickening are potential signs of malignancy.

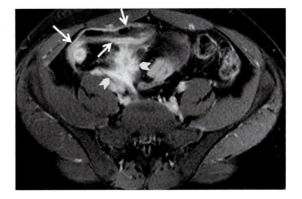

Fig. 3 Crohn's disease. Post-intravenous contrast enhanced T1-weighted axial image shows significant enhancement of the thickened bowel wall of the terminal ileum (*white arrows*). There is also marked hyperemia of the adjacent mesenteric vessels (space between *arrowheads*)

6 Appendicitis in Pregnant and Pediatric Patients

6.1 Terminology and Clinical Issues

Acute appendicitis is the most common surgical emergency. According to the American College of Radiology (ACR) Appropriateness Criteria®, MRI, when available, rather than CT is the preferred imaging modality because it does not involve exposure of the

Fig. 4 Fistula formation in complicated Crohn's disease. Pre- and post-contrast enhanced T1-weighted fat-suppressed sagittal images illustrate severe enhancement of two fistulas (*arrows*) in the perirectal region in a patient with active Crohn's disease

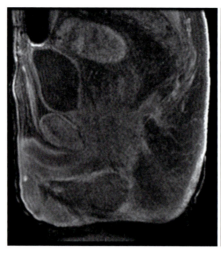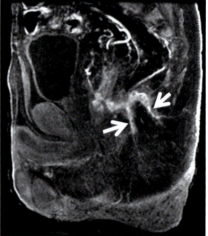

Table 3 MRI findings of inflammatory bowel disease

- Crohn's disease: mural thickening, mural enhancement, hypervascularity, abscess, stricture, or fistulas, most visible on T2-weighted images
- Ulcerative colitis: diffuse mural thickening, mucosal enhancement, diffusely involving the colon

Table 4 MRI findings of appendicitis

- Enlarged appendix >6 mm in diameter
- T2 hyperintensity correlating with edema surrounding the appendix
- T2 hyperintense fluid collections in case of ruptured or complicated appendicitis
- Periappendiceal and wall enhancement
- Low-signal-intensity wall on fat-suppressed T1-weighted images

patient to ionizing radiation (Andreotti et al. 2009). In the diagnosis of appendicitis in pregnancy, MRI has a high sensitivity and specificity and may permit the visualization of a normal appendix in approximately 83–90% of all patients (Andreotti et al. 2009; Long et al. 2011; Birchard et al. 2005; Pedrosa et al. 2006). It is also useful for patients in the pediatric age group, in which radiation is a concern because of the increased risk of malignancy.

In addition, MRI has two notable advantages over CT, the traditionally used imaging modality for suspected appendicitis in pregnant patients: (1) MRI does not require intravenous contrast material, minimizing possible adverse reactions; (2) CT exposes the fetus to ionizing radiation. As a result, in the pregnant patient in whom acute appendicitis is suspected, MRI is the optimal diagnostic modality of choice. No currently known risks to the fetus are associated with MRI (Andreotti et al. 2009; Long et al. 2011; Birchard et al. 2005; Pedrosa et al. 2006).

6.2 Imaging

The diagnostic imaging work-up for pregnant patients and pediatric patients with suspected appendicitis typically may begin with US. However, US is

user-dependent and is often limited by overlying bowel gas. Furthermore, in a pregnant patient, the enlarged uterus can alter the position of the abdominal contents, making the appendix difficult to identify. MRI may also facilitate the identification of other acute conditions that can mimic symptoms of acute appendicitis, such as abscess, colitis, ovarian torsion, fibroid degeneration, hydronephrosis, and bowel obstruction.

MRI findings of appendicitis are dependent mainly on periappendiceal inflammatory changes, as these result in increased edema which can be detected on T2-weighted sequences (Erturk et al. 2005; Singh et al. 2007, 2009; Long et al. 2011; Birchard et al. 2005; Pedrosa et al. 2006) (Table 4, Figs. 5, 6). Fat-suppressed sequences are also important to detect the low-signal-intensity thickened wall in an appendix with inflammatory changes. As with CT, an abnormally enlarged appendix is defined as >6 mm in diameter (Long et al. 2011; Birchard et al. 2005; Pedrosa et al. 2006).

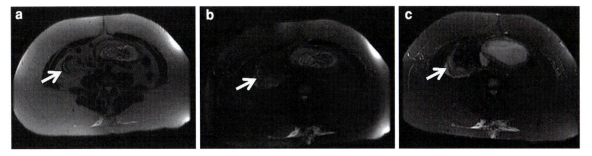

Fig. 5 Appendicitis in a first-trimester pregnancy. **a** T1 non-fat-suppressed axial image demonstrates a dilated appendix (*arrow*). **b** T2 SS-FSE fat-suppressed image demonstrates dilated appendix with edema (*arrow*). **c** T2 STIR image further illustrates edema related to peri-appendiceal inflammation (*arrow*)

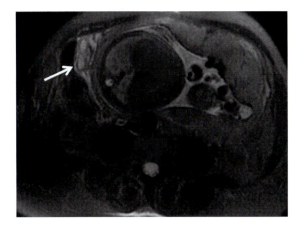

Fig. 6 Appendicitis in a second-trimester pregnancy. Fat-suppressed SS-FSE T2-weighted image demonstrates a dilated appendix (*arrow*) with thickened walls and surrounding free fluid. The gravid uterus is also shown adjacent to the appendix

Table 5 MRI findings of ruptured hemorrhagic cysts

- T1-hyperintense cystic components
- T1-hyperintense free fluid containing blood products
- T2 hyperintense inflammatory changes in adnexal region correlating to the rupture site

6.3 Differentials

The differential diagnosis for infectious acute appendicitis mainly includes an appendiceal neoplasm (mucinous adenocarcinoma, non-mucinous adenocarcinoma, and carcinoid). Other manifestations may also suggest neoplasm, such as pseudomyxoma peritonei which can be seen in the setting of mucinous adenocarcinoma of the appendix. The presence of intussusception should raise concern for an underlying pathologic mass in the appendix.

Table 6 MRI findings of endometriosis

- T1 homogeneous hyperintensity (utilize fat-suppressed images)
- T2 "shading"
- Variable enhancement patterns on post-contrast sequences

7 Endometriosis and Rupture of Hemorrhagic Ovarian Cysts

7.1 Terminology and Clinical Issues

Ruptured ovarian cysts and endometriosis can produce abdominal pain that may mimic a variety of acute abdominal conditions. The imaging characteristics specific for a ruptured hemorrhagic cyst and endometriomas are best identified using MRI.

7.2 Imaging

Hemorrhagic cysts and endometriomas alike may lead to hemorrhage, resulting in blood containing ascites in the intraperitoneal space and usually manifesting in the cul-de-sac. While CT and US may demonstrate fluid suggestive of hemorrhage, MRI is superior in characterizing the contents of the fluid as blood is T1 hyperintense. Furthermore, MRI is also superior to CT and US in more definitively characterizing the adnexal lesions of hemorrhagic cysts or endometriomas (Tables 5, 6).

On T2-weighted images, endometriomas may demonstrate homogeneous low signal or "shading" (Fig. 7a, b). On T1-weighted images, they show homogeneously high "light-bulb" signal hyperintensity, unlike cysts and abscesses, which have low signal

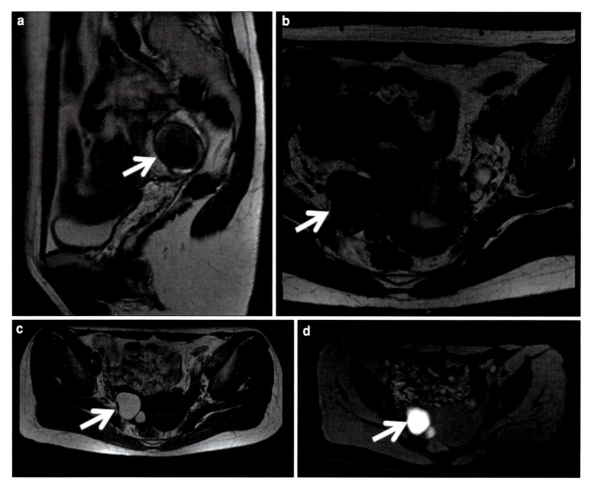

Fig. 7 Endometrioma. T2-weighted sagittal (**a**) and axial (**b**) images show endometrioma with low signal intensity and a "shading" effect. T1 (non-fat-suppressed) axial image demonstrates endometrioma in right ovary with homogeneous hyperintensity reflecting hemorrhagic contents (**c**) T1 (fat-suppressed) axial image of the same endometrioma demonstrates "light-bulb" bright hyperintensity, a characteristic finding (**d**)

intensity on these sequences (Fig. 7c, d). Hemorrhagic cysts also have high T1 signal intensity but a much higher homogeneous T2 signal intensity, distinct from endometriomas in most cases. Fluid–fluid levels may be present within the hemorrhagic cyst (Fig. 8).

7.3 Differentials

Cystic lesions in the adnexal region may indicate a tubo-ovarian abscess in pelvic inflammatory disease (PID) or a cystic-appearing ovarian neoplasm. Tubo-ovarian abscess are characterized by marked rim enhancement and are possibly associated with dilated fallopian tubes. Ovarian neoplasms may demonstrate cystic components with enhancing mural nodules. Lymphadenopathy,

peritoneal carcinomatosis, and ascites may also be seen in advanced-stage ovarian malignancies.

8 Fibroid Degeneration

8.1 Terminology and Clinical Issues

Patients with fibroid degeneration often present to the emergency department with symptoms of focal pain, tenderness, fever, and leukocytosis, which mimic many other acute pelvic conditions. Fibroid degeneration is an ischemic process in which fibroids outgrow their vascular supply, resulting in infarction or degeneration (Singh et al. 2009). US may be helpful in correlating a fibroid in the region of clinical concern, where pain is

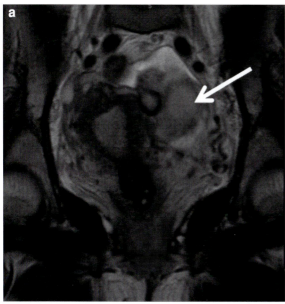

Fig. 8 Hemorrhagic cyst of the left ovary with rupture. **a** Coronal T2-weighted non-fat-suppressed image demonstrates a left ovarian hemorrhagic cyst with intrinsic T2 hyperintensity with surrounding fluid consistent with rupture. **b** Axial T1 axial image shows an irregular fluid–fluid level in a hemorrhagic cyst in the left adnexa with a dependent blood clot

Table 7 Imaging findings of fibroid degeneration on MRI

- T1-weighted images showing diffuse or peripheral high signal intensity, indicating hemorrhagic components
- T2 hyperintense rim around the fibroid due to obstructed veins at the periphery
- T2 weighted images indicating significant diffuse or heterogeneous edema from a pre-degeneration state and/or as a sequel of venous congestion
- Contrast-enhanced images demonstrating the heterogeneous appearance and less enhancement than seen in non-degenerating cellular fibroids

maximal, with areas of heterogeneous echogenicity. However, MRI is more specific and sensitive for the detection of fibroid degeneration (Table 7).

8.2 Imaging

Diffuse or heterogeneous edema, either in the pre-degeneration state or after venous congestion has occurred, is well seen on MRI. A T2 hyperintense rim around the fibroid may be present due to obstructed veins at the periphery (Singh et al. 2009). T1-weighted images demonstrate diffuse or peripheral high signal intensity indicating the development of hemorrhagic components (Singh et al. 2009). Furthermore, following gadolinium

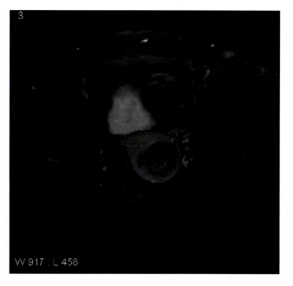

Fig. 9 Fibroid degeneration. Images demonstrate large myometrial mass with low signal intensity (post intravenous contrast) consistent with fibroid degeneration. Just anterior to the uterus, note increased signal due to the presence of bladder contrast

administration, contrast-enhanced images may show a heterogeneous appearance and areas of decreased enhancement due to poor blood supply, versus more cellular and non-degenerating fibroids (Fig. 9).

8.3 Differentials

The differential diagnosis of degenerating fibroids commonly includes non-degenerating fibroids that have a mild to moderate heterogeneously enhancing pattern. A less common diagnostic consideration is the uterine neoplasm leiyomyosarcoma. This tumor demonstrates rapid interval growth, large-mass lesions at the time of diagnosis, and markedly heterogeneous enhancement patterns.

9 Ovarian Torsion

9.1 Terminology and Clinical Issues

Ovarian torsion is caused by a partial or complete rotation of the adnexal structures. It can involve the fallopian tube or ovary, but likely both. Risk factors for torsion include an ipsilateral adnexal mass such as a large cyst or dermoid (Jain 1995; Rha et al. 2002); in fact, torsion is infrequent without an adnexal mass. Adnexal torsion most commonly occurs in the first three decades of life and can lead to ischemia and potentially irreversible infarction of both the fallopian tube and the ovary (Jain 1995; Rha et al. 2002). Early diagnosis is important to preserve ovarian function, particularly in young women.

According to the ACR Appropriateness Criteria®, US is the imaging modality of choice for the initial evaluation of suspected adnexal torsion (Andreotti et al. 2009). However, US may be non-diagnostic in patients with large body habitus or in pregnant patients due to displacement of adnexal structures by the gravid uterus. MRI is considered by the ACR Appropriateness Criteria® to be superior to CT in the case of torsion in the setting of a concomitant adnexal mass (Andreotti et al. 2009). Furthermore, MRI may enable the evaluation of acute and non-acute causes of pelvic pain mimicking ovarian torsion (Fig. 10).

9.2 Imaging

The MRI features of ovarian torsion include unilateral ovarian enlargement with an edematous stroma of increased T2 hyperintensity. Twisting and thickening of structures including the fallopian tube are common

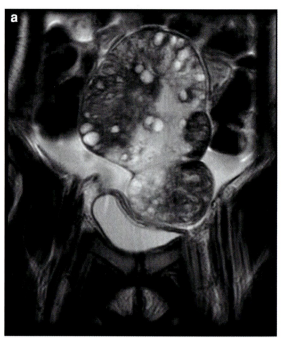

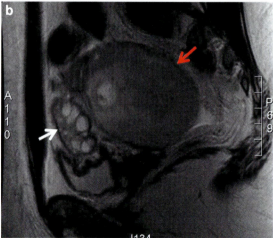

Fig. 10 a Ovarian torsion. Coronal T2-weighted images demonstrate markedly enlarged left ovary located at the midline and with areas of T2 hyperintensity consistent with edema. Peripheralization of follicles is also demonstrated in this image. There is also T2-hyperintense free fluid. **b** Sagittal T2-weighted image shows a severely enlarged and heterogeneous left ovary (*red arrow*). A normal right ovary is shown (*white arrow*)

findings. Heterogeneous enhancement and hemorrhagic components with hyperintense T1 appearance should be expected. The identification of an adnexal mass, most commonly a benign neoplasm, may also be identified, as such lesions predispose patients to adnexal torsion (Table 8).

Table 8 MRI findings of ovarian torsion

- T1 hyperintense hemorrhagic components of cyst, fallopian tube, or vascular pedicle
- T2 hyperintense, edematous, enlarged ovary
- Heterogeneous enhancement of ovary and adnexal components
- Thickening and twisting of structures in the adnexal region
- Displaced location of the ovary to the midline
- Adnexal mass predisposing to torsion, such as large endometrioma, hemorrhagic cyst, or dermoid

Table 9 MRI findings of PID

- Round or oval, possibly septated lesion
- Layering debris (in some cases)
- T1 hypointense and T2 hyperintense
- Lesions of high protein content seen as intermediate or high T1 signal intensity
- Rim and/or surrounding enhancement

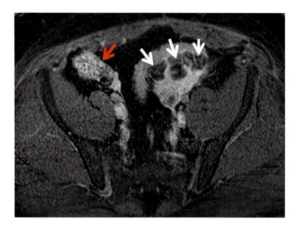

Fig. 11 Pelvic inflammatory disease. T2 fat-suppressed axial image demonstrates multiple dilated fallopian tubes with surrounding edema (T2 hyperintensity) (*white arrows*). The normal right adnexa is shown (*red arrow*)

9.3 Differentials

The main diagnostic consideration for an enlarged ovary is a benign or malignant neoplasm. Frequently, torsion is associated with an underlying pathologic mass in the ovary. For benign neoplasms, dermoid or fibromas should be considered. Dermoids tend to have multiple tissue types including fat (hyperintense on T1-weighted images and hypointense on fat-suppressed images) and calcification (hypointense on all sequences). Fibromas do not enhance significantly, in addition to demonstrating components that are hypointense on T1- and T2-weighted images. Malignant neoplasms may feature cystic components with mural nodules or a markedly heterogeneous enhancement pattern.

10 Pelvic Inflammatory Disease

10.1 Terminology and Clinical Issues

Pelvic inflammatory disease (PID) is an acute condition commonly encountered in the emergency department. It arises from an infection that ascends into the fallopian tubes and may extend into the intraperitoneal cavity. Patients present with low abdomino-pelvic pain and possibly also significant localizing pain due to complications of abscess formation, hydrosalpinx, or pyosalpinx. A rapid diagnosis is essential for proper triage to medical versus surgical treatment. Appropriate treatment includes immediate antibiotic therapy or surgical intervention, in the case of tubo-ovarian abscess. While US is the first line of diagnostic study, MRI has a high specificity and sensitivity in evaluating the complications

of PID (Singh et al. 2007, 2009; Andreotti et al. 2009; Long et al. 2011). CT is another imaging option but its ionizing radiation poses a risk for young patients. Instead, MRI is an attractive alternative that offers superior definition of the pelvic, uterine, and adnexal anatomy.

10.2 Imaging

Superior characterization of adnexal lesions, edema, and tubal abnormalities is achieved with MRI. The imaging characteristics of tubo-ovarian abscess are associated with mid to high signal hyperintensity on T1-weighted images. The high signal of T2-weighted images is related to the presence of edema and cystic components (Fig. 11). Post-gadolinium images demonstrate wall thickening and rim enhancement. Hydrosalpinx, which can produce severe pain, is also readily identified on T2 weighted MRI sequences (Table 9).

10.3 Differentials

The differential diagnosis for abscesses in the adnexal region includes simple ovarian cysts, hemorrhagic ovarian cysts, and endometriomas. Fluid–fluid levels may be present in hemorrhagic cysts. Characteristic findings such as T2 shading and a light-bulb bright appearance on T1-weighted images can assist in the identification of endometriomas.

11 Summary

In the emergency department, MRI is useful in evaluating a number of acute conditions of the abdomen and pelvis. When US findings are non-diagnostic for appendicitis in pregnant patients or pediatric patients, MRI is a powerful and appropriate imaging modality. Protocols should be tailored to minimize acquisition time and customized to effectively assess each patient's acute presentation. Acute pathology in the pelvis, including ruptured cysts, degenerating fibroids, and ovarian torsion, may also be detected with MRI. As an alternative that does not rely on ionizing radiation in the assessment of inflammatory bowel disease, MR enterography can assist in characterizing the acute processes of Crohn's disease and ulcerative colitis. Proper planning and resource utilization will minimize the high cost and maximize the availability of MRI for patients presenting to the emergency department with an acute abdomen or pelvis.

References

Andreotti RF, Lee SI, Choy G, DeJesus Allison SO, Bennett GL, Brown DL, Glanc P, Horrow MM, Javitt MC, Lev-Toaff AS, Podrasky AE, Scoutt LM, Zelop C (2009) ACR appropriateness criteria on acute pelvic pain in the reproductive age group. J Am Coll Radiol 6(4):235–241

Barger RL Jr, Nandalur KR (2010) Diagnostic performance of magnetic resonance imaging in the detection of appendicitis in adults: a meta-analysis. Acad Radiol 17(10):1211–1216 Epub 2010 Jul 15

Birchard KR, Brown MA, Hyslop WB, Firat Z, Semelka R (2005) MRI of acute abdominal and pelvic pain in pregnant patients. AJR Am J Roentgenol 184(2):452–458

Catalano OA, Sahani DV, Kalva SP, Cushing MS, Hahn PF, Brown JJ, Edelman RR (2008) MR imaging of the gallbladder: a pictorial essay. Radiographics 28(1):135–155 quiz 324

Erturk SM, Mortelé KJ, Oliva MR, Barish MA (2005) State-of-the-art computed tomographic and magnetic resonance imaging of the gastrointestinal system. Gastrointest Endosc Clin N Am 15(3):581–614

Gee MS, Harisinghani MG (2011) MRI in patients with inflammatory bowel disease. J Magn Reson Imaging 33(3):527–534

Jain KA (1995) Magnetic resonance imaging findings in ovarian torsion. Magn Reson Imaging 13:111–113

Lam M, Singh A, Kaewlai R, Novelline RA (2008) Magnetic resonance of acute appendicitis: pearls and pitfalls. Curr Prob Diag Radiol 37:57–66

Long SS, Long C, Lai H, Macura KJ (2011) Imaging strategies for right lower quadrant pain in pregnancy. AJR Am J Roentgenol 196(1):4–12

Pedrosa I, Rofsky NM (2003) MR imaging in abdominal emergencies. Radiol Clin North Am 41(6):1243–1273

Pedrosa I, Levine D, Eyvazzadeh AD, Siewert B, Ngo L, Rofsky NM (2006) MR imaging evaluation of acute appendicitis in pregnancy. Radiology 238(3):891–899

Rha SE, Byun JY, Jung SE, Jung JI, Choi BG, Kim BS, Kim H, Lee JM (2002) CT and MR imaging features of adnexal torsion. Radiographics 22(2):283–294

Singh A, Danrad R, Hahn PF, Blake MA, Mueller PR, Novelline RA (2007) MR imaging of the acute abdomen and pelvis: acute appendicitis and beyond. Radiographics 27(5):1419–1431

Singh AK, Desai H, Novelline RA (2009) Emergency MRI of acute pelvic pain: MR protocol with no oral contrast. Emerg Radiol 16(2):133–141 Epub 2008 Jul 23

Tkacz JN, Anderson SA, Soto J (2009) MR imaging in gastrointestinal emergencies. Radiographics 29(6):1767–1780

Watanabe Y, Nagayama M, Okumura A, Amoh Y, Katsube T, Suga T, Koyama S, Nakatani K, Dodo Y (2007) MR imaging of acute biliary disorders. Radiographics 27(2):477–495

Imaging the Acute Abdomen Within the Pediatric Population

Fred E. Avni, Nasroolla Damry, and Marie Cassart

Contents

Abstract

The authors propose a clinico-radiologic decision tree approach to solve the problem of a chid with acute abdominal. This approach is based on clinical conditions, age and gamuts of differential diagnosis. The couple US + plain film of the abdomen should solve most of the cases. Ultrasound examinations should be optimized using high resolution transducers with settings, fitted to the child size and weight. The entire abdominal cavity should be examined. In selected cases, CT (dosis fitted to children) and MR imaging provide useful information. Most frequent diagnosis include appendicitis and its mimickers. Once appendicitis and other intestinal diseases are excluded, extra digestive (i.e. gynaecologic diseases) conditions and extra abdominal conditions should be considered (i.e. pneumonia).

1 Introduction and Imaging Techniques

Dealing with abdominal emergencies patients is one of the largest components of the workload in a pediatric radiology department. Emergencies encompass a very wide spectrum of diseases and entities, some of which are life-threatening while other are more benign or even "psychological." In this setting, the role of imaging is of utmost importance as in many cases, especially in young children, the origin of the disease is not obvious. Furthermore, among the various entities, non-accidental trauma and child abuse are conditions that the examining physician must not forget.

F. E. Avni (✉) · M. Cassart
Radiology, Erasme Hospital,
Route de Lennik 808, 1070 Brussels, Belgium
e-mail: Freddy.Avni@erasme.ulb.ac.be

N. Damry
Pediatric Imaging, Children's Hospital Queen Fabiola,
Avenue J.J. Crocq 15, 1020 Brussels, Belgium

M. Scaglione et al. (eds.), *Emergency Radiology of the Abdomen*,
Medical Radiology. Diagnostic Imaging,
DOI: 10.1007/174_2011_474, © Springer-Verlag Berlin Heidelberg 2012

In abdominal emergencies, ultrasound (US) plays a central role in the differential diagnoses. Appropriate patient management requires a clinico-radiological triage based on age, sex, symptoms, medical history, and sonographic findings (Strouse 2006). For instance, in newborns, one should expect to find (consequences of) congenital anomalies or diseases related to premature birth. In older children, intussusceptions or appendicitis need to be considered first. Gynecological diseases are a possibility in adolescents girls whereas a history of trauma will orient the work-up accordingly. Also, one should certainly not forget that any disease can occur at any age. Some diseases will present with obvious symptoms, and others with tricky ones. Laboratory findings may orient the diagnosis but in other cases can hide it. Finally, priorities are very important, as frequent diseases should be placed at the top of the list comprising the differential diagnosis but rarer diseases must be included as well.

The advantage of US and the basis of its central role among imaging techniques is that it is non-irradiating, easy to perform (although operator-dependent), and inexpensive. Nonetheless, the US examination has to be optimized and tailored to the size and age of the patient. High-resolution linear transducers should be used in the examination of superficial and digestive structures. Sectorial or curvilinear transducers are intended for deeper structures or for use in older children. Whatever the purpose of the study, the entire abdomen should be scanned. Knowledge of the normal appearances of all abdominal structures according to patient age is essential for distinguishing normal from abnormal cases. Finally, in many cases, color Doppler will provide additional information, differentiating between vascular and non-vascular structures or defining the nature of a lesion's vascularization (De Bruyn 2005).

Depending on the US findings, complementary examinations will be necessary. In a few cases a plain film of the abdomen will be needed to visualize calcifications or foreign bodies. In others, a computed tomography (CT) scan provides additional information useful for proper management. The CT settings should be adapted to the child's age and size in order to ensure the lowest irradiation possible, according to ALARA principles (Vorona et al. 2011).

Magnetic resonance imaging (MRI) is rarely performed as an emergency procedure, unless an abdomino-pelvic mass is detected and a secondary epidural compression suspected. The most useful sequences will be used as indicated by the clinical inquiry (Pedrosa and Rofsky 2003).

Finally, fluoroscopy has limited indications in emergency abdominal imaging, reserved mainly in the treatment of intussusceptions. There are other indications for barium follow-through, i.e., imaging of the digestive tract, and enema, but not as emergency procedures (Applegate 2009).

2 Acute Non-Traumatic Abdominal Conditions

The primary approach towards acute abdominal conditions should be to initiate the work-up on the basis of patient age. Four groups are typically considered: (a) around birth to 6 months; (b) between 6 months and 2 years; (c) between 2 and 12 years; (d) above 12 years.

2.1 Around Birth to 6 Months

2.1.1 Terminology and Clinical Issues

Entities to consider are mainly congenital anomalies (and their complications), those related to premature birth, and hypertrophic pyloric stenosis.

2.1.2 Imaging

Congenital anomalies are being increasingly detected during obstetrical US examinations (i.e., intestinal atresia). In most cases, the anomaly has been recognized by the time of birth so that the proper management can be applied immediately afterwards, if necessary. However, some malformations will escape antenatal diagnosis and instead detected only after birth. For instance, in intestinal (sub)obstruction, bowel loops will appear obviously dilated on scout views of the abdomen (Fig. 1a). Complementary US will confirm the presence of dilated loops filled with fluid and meconium. US is also able to differentiate between distended and empty bowel loops and to determine the level of obstruction. Other complications, such as meconium peritonitis, can be suggested by the presence of peritoneal calcification, ascites, or meconium pseudocyst. The technique can also demonstrate an associated congenital mass, such as a duplication (Fig. 1b), responsible for the obstruction. After US, and if necessary, an enema using

Fig. 1 Neonate with intestinal obstruction due to duplication cyst. **a** Plain film of the abdomen shows obvious signs of intestinal obstruction. **b** US of the abdomen demonstrates a cystic mass with echogenic content and a typical layered wall

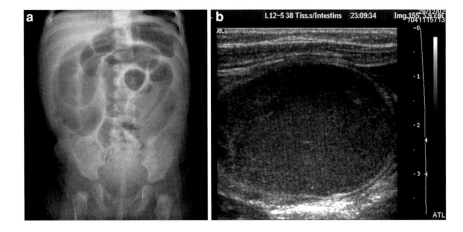

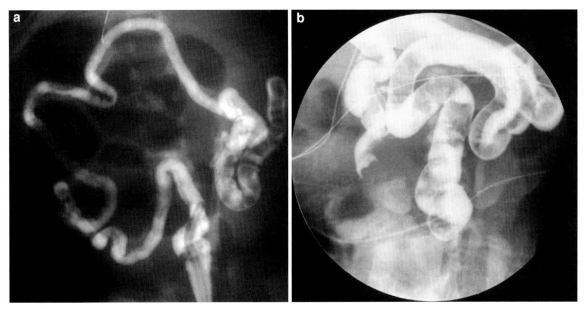

Fig. 2 The use of enema to differentiate between causes of neonatal obstruction. **a** Typical unused small colon associated with a meconium ileus; the obstruction is located above the terminal ileus (prone view). **b** Typical meconial plug (sub-obstruction). The colon is of normal caliber and contains hypodense meconium plugs (decubitus view)

hydrosoluble contrast can be administered in order to differentiate between meconium ileus with complete obstruction and a small unused colon from a meconium plug, in which case the colon is of normal caliber (Fig. 2) (Laje et al. 2010).

Premature infants are at risk for developing digestive complications, such as necrotizing enterocolitis. The severity of the disease depends upon the degree and extent of digestive involvement. At an early stage, the bowel loops appear distended on a scout view of the abdomen, and US may demonstrate bowel wall thickening and a small amount of free fluid. As the disease progresses, peristalsis may become absent, intestinal pneumatosis may develop (Fig. 3a), and the amount of fluid increases. These findings are seen on US. In such cases, intraparietal gas may then dissect the intestinal wall and progress into the portal vein system, evidenced by hyperechoic dots diffused within the liver (Fig. 3b). In poorly evolving cases, a pneumo-peritoneum may develop due to perforation. In these patients, surgery becomes mandatory (Epelman et al. 2007).

In a 6-week-old vomiting baby boy, hypertrophic pyloric stenosis is the most probable diagnosis. US is confirmatory as it demonstrates the thickened pyloric

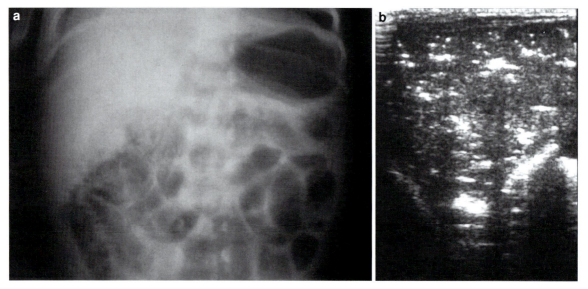

Fig. 3 Necrotizing enterocolitis. **a** Plain film of the abdomen (focused view) shows the mottled appearance of the air-filled bowel loops in the right upper quadrant, corresponding to air dissecting the bowel wall. **b** US of the liver shows a multitude of hyperechoic spots, indicating free air in the portal vein system

Fig. 4 US of hypertrophic pyloric stenosis. **a** Sagittal view of the hypertrophied pylorus; **b** transverse view of the stenosis, appearing as a doughnut

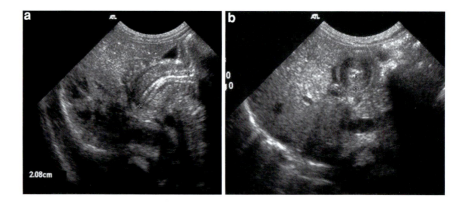

muscle, appearing as a doughnut on a transverse scan and as a sandwich pattern on a longitudinal scan (Fig. 4). The stomach is usually fully elongated after meals and hyperperistaltic. Measurements include a diameter of the "doughnut" >12 mm, a muscle length >20 mm, and a muscle thickness >4 mm (Maheshwari et al. 2009).

2.2 Between 6 Months and 2 Years

2.2.1 Terminology and Clinical Issues

In this age group, the main diagnoses to consider are acute intestinal intussusception, volvulus, and inguinal hernia.

2.2.2 Imaging

Intussusception has a classical clinical and sonographic appearance. According to the symptoms of acute intestinal intussusception, which include signs of intestinal obstruction, vomiting and reddish gelatinous stools, at US, a large doughnut pattern is visualized (>2.5 cm diameter). The intussusceptions may be demonstrated anywhere in the abdomen, but are typically seen in the mid abdomen (Fig. 5). Many small ganglions are usually visualized around or within the intussuceptum. Intestinal obstruction, trapped fluid within the intussuceptum (Fig. 6), reduced peristalsis, and reduced intestinal wall vascularization on color Doppler are elements of severity and contraindicate an attempt to reduce the acute

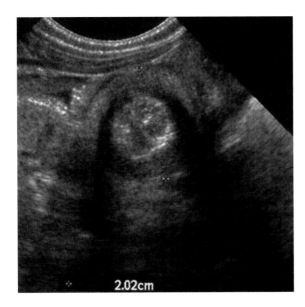

Fig. 5 Acute intestinal intussusception, showing the cockade appearance of a typical mass

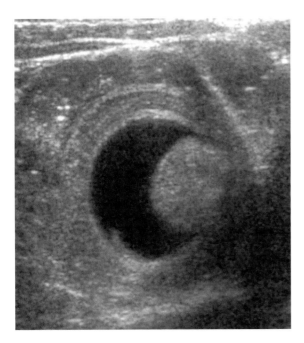

Fig. 6 Trapped fluid and acute intestinal intussusception. A crescent-shaped fluid collection is visible; this finding is an element of severity. (Image courtesy of Baud)

intestinal intussusception under radiological control. A normal location of the ileo-cecal valve indicates a small bowel or colo-colic intussusception.

The reduction procedure, which can be either hydrostatic or pneumatic, must be performed in the presence of a surgeon, with the child under sedation (or general anesthesia in some institutions) and subsequently monitored. For hydrostatic enema, a saline solution placed in a bag at a maximum height of 120 cm can be used. The procedure is guided by US. For pneumatic reduction, air is administered with a maximum pressure of 108 mm Hg. Here too, the procedure is guided by fluoroscopy or US. The criteria of complete reduction are disappearance of the intussusception and reflux into the small bowel. These can also be demonstrated by US (Fig. 7).

Most intussusception are primary. Some (usually those encountered before 6 months or after 2 years) are secondary to leading lesions (duplications, Meckel's diverticulum, lipoma, lymphoma) that are easier to demonstrate by US after therapeutic reduction (Bateni et al. 2011; Gartner et al. 2011).

Intestinal volvulus is an acute condition that complicates intestinal malrotation and induces acute intestinal obstruction. On US examination of the epigastric area, the mesenteric vein lies to the right of the mesenteric artery. A volvulus will cause the bowel loops to circle the mesenteric vessels, accounting for the "whirlpool sign," which is characteristic of the condition (Fig. 8). A volvulus is a surgical emergency (Applegate 2009; Lampl et al. 2009; Epelman 2006).

An inguinal hernia corresponds to bowel loops entrapped within the inguinal canal. On US, intra-intestinal air and bowel loop peristalsis are visualized (Fig. 9a). The inguinal hernia can usually be reduced, but in some instances obstruction develops and the infant will present with acute symptoms. Noteworthy, in girls, an ovary can be entrapped within the hernia. This condition should be operated on rapidly (Fig. 9b) (Laing et al. 2007).

2.3 Between 2 and 12 Years

2.3.1 Terminology and Clinical Issues

The spectrum of conditions occurring within this age group is wide and the differential diagnosis is accordingly a challenge. Two conditions outnumber all others and should be considered first: constipation and appendicitis.

Constipation is by far the commonest cause for abdominal pain in children. The diagnosis will be achieved through a careful interrogation of the child (if possible) and his/her parents. If necessary, a plain

Fig. 7 Pneumatic reduction. Three sequences showing the progression of the air column and reflux in the small bowel. (Image courtesy of C. Baud, MD)

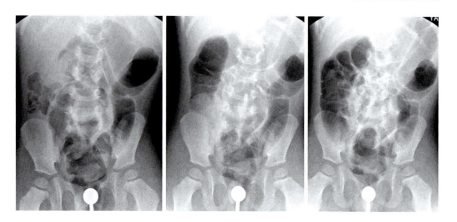

Fig. 8 Volvulus as seen on US. **a** Typical whirlpool sign; bowel loops and vessels circle the mesenteric vessels; **b** color Doppler confirmation

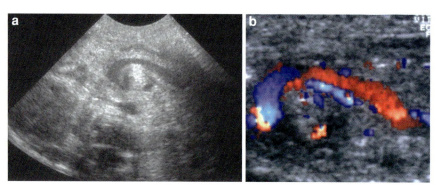

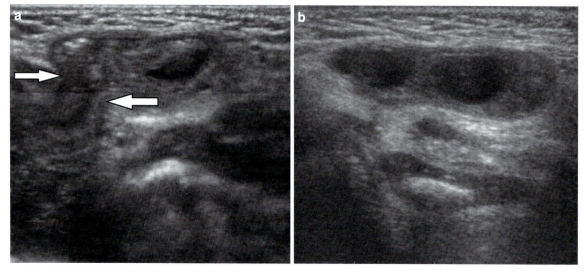

Fig. 9 Inguinal hernia as seen on US. **a** In this baby boy. US demonstrates the hole (*arrows*) of the hernia with the herniated bowel containing air. **b** In this baby girl. The hernia contains an ovary with characteristic cystic follicles

film of the abdomen may confirm the condition, showing the abnormal amount of stools. In such cases, no other imaging examination is necessary (Fig. 10) (Rajindrajih and Devanarayana 2011).

Acute appendicitis is the second most common reason for acute pain in children of this age group and accordingly is the one most often suspected by the emergency room physician. In children under the age

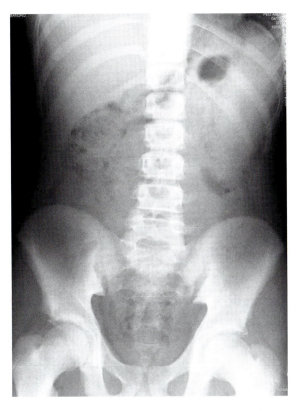

Fig. 10 Constipation, as seen on a plain film of the abdomen. Stools predominate in the right flank

Table 1 Ultrasound signs of acute appendix in children

Diameter of the appendix >6 mm
Swollen, non-depressible appendix
Painful under US compression
Hypertrophied mesenteric fat
Hypervascularization on color Doppler
Small ganglions
Echogenic appendicolith

of 4, it is the most frequent indication for surgery; however, 30–50% of these operations end by excluding appendicitis.

2.3.2 Imaging

In children, the evaluation should always begin with US, even in somewhat obese children. There is no rationale to start with CT.

The sonographic diagnosis of acute appendicitis is based on a thickened, swollen, non-compressible appendix (>6 mm diameter) and other specific signs (Table 1) (Figs. 11, 12). A notable finding is the presence of free fluid in an amount that does not correspond to the degree of perforation. Whenever the disease progresses, perforation may develop and evolve towards peritonitis. On imaging, the amount of free fluid will be significantly increased, with one or multiple abscesses distributed throughout the peritoneal cavity (Fig. 13). At this stage, the disease may be difficult to characterize and complimentary CT may be necessary. The indications of CT in case of acute appendicitis should be as limited as possible in order

to reduce radiation exposure. Clearly, CT is useful in unusual clinical presentations (i.e., younger age), clinico-imaging discrepancies, and complicated cases (multiple abscesses) (Fig. 14). In the future, MRI may replace CT for these indications (Fig. 15) (Hennelly and Bachur 2011; Wan et al. 2009; Park et al. 2011; Yigiter et al. 2011; Rosendahl et al. 2004; Garcia-Pena Cook and Maudl 2004).

As mentioned above, not all conditions or diagnoses are obvious on imaging. False-negative diagnoses may result from a non-compressible right lower quadrant, from localized inflammation, or non-visualization of an appendix located in an unusual site (i.e., retrocecal or retrohepatic). False-positive cases include non-inflammatory causes of appendiceal infiltrations (carcinoïd tumor, cystic fibrosis, Crohn's disease, etc.) (Figs. 16, 17) (Schmittenbecher 2001; Sung et al. 2006).

2.3.3 Differentials

Once acute appendicitis has been excluded directly by the demonstration of a normal appendix (Fig. 18), the list of differential diagnosis widens; all potential diagnoses have to be considered and, if possible, excluded progressively (Table 2).

Other diseases of the digestive tract. The digestive tract can be involved by various diseases, localized or diffuse. For instance, the terminal ileum may be affected by infectious or inflammatory processes that can lead to a thickening of the bowel loop (usually thicker than in appendicitis), as in some adenopathies. On color Doppler, the segment will be hypervascularized. The area will invoke pain at compression. Also, as mentioned, inflammatory bowel diseases such as Crohn's may completely mimic appendicitis as the appendix itself can be involved (Fig. 17).

In other diseases (Henoch-Schonlein purpura, hemolytic and uremic syndrome), the entire digestive

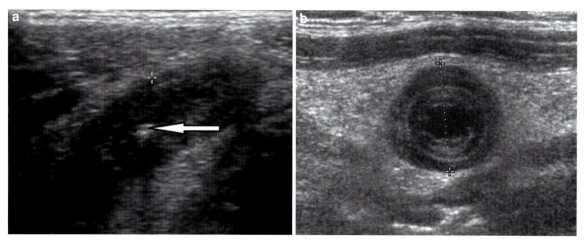

Fig. 11 Acute appendicitis. **a** Sagittal view of the inflamed appendix shows a small appendicolith (*arrows*). **b** Transverse scan demonstrates the Increased hyperechogenicity of mesenteric fat around the inflamed appendix. (Image courtesy of Baud)

Fig. 12 Acute appendicitis (role of Doppler). **a** Sagittal view of the inflamed appendix shows hypervascularization; **b** transverse scan highlights the increased peri-appendicular vascularization

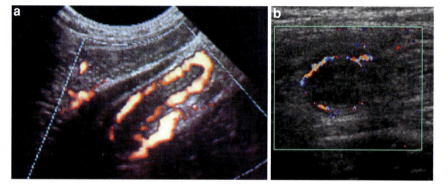

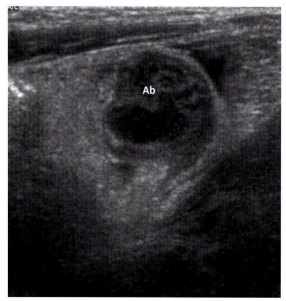

Fig. 13 Appendicular abscess. US of the right lower quadrant demonstrates the abscess (*Ab*) and a small amount of free fluid

tract can be involved. Henoch-Schonlein purpura is characterized by thickening of the bowel walls, hypervascularization of the thickened walls, a large amount of ascites, and ileo-ileal intusssuceptions (Fig. 19). Hemolytic and uremic syndrome associates oligo-anuria related to acute renal failure, bloody diarrhea, and acute abdominal pain. During the acute phase of the disease, the renal parenchyma will appear hyperechoic, diastolic flow disappears (RI = 1), and the bowel walls are hypovascularized; during the healing phase, diastolic flow resumes (predicting normal urine production) and the bowel loops appear hypervascularized (Baud et al. 2004; Chang et al. 2004; De Buys Roessingh et al. 2007).

The differential diagnosis includes Meckel's diverticulum and its complications, such as secondary intestinal intussuception and diverticulitis (Fig. 20), possibly ruptured and with abscess formation. Complicated Meckel's has to be differentiated from complicated urachal cyst; the latter connects the umbilicus to the

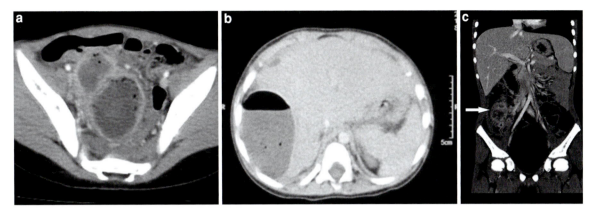

Fig. 14 A complicated appendix as seen on CT. **a** Multiple abscesses in the pelvic cavity are demonstrated on this contrast-enhanced CT. **b** Retrohepatic abscess resulting from perforation of a retrohepatic appendicitis. **c** Pericecal abscess (*arrow*) resulting from a perforated acute appendix

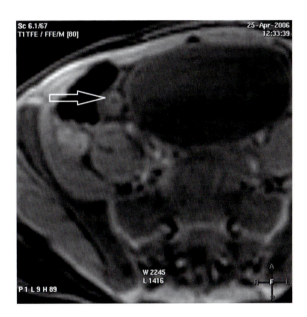

Fig. 15 Acute appendicitis as seen on MRI. T1-weighted sequence with an incidental finding of an inflamed appendix (*arrow*), subsequently confirmed surgically

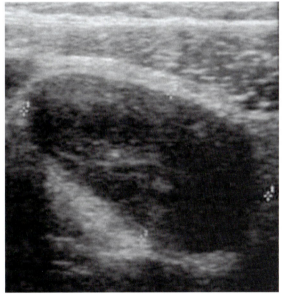

Fig. 16 Carcinoid tumor of the appendix, as seen on US. Sagittal view of the thickened and tumoral appendix (>15 mm diameter)

dome of the bladder (Fig. 21, whereas Meckel's diverticulum is an omphalo-mesenteric remnant (Levy and Hobbs 2004; Darge and Anupindi 2009).

Hepato-biliary disease. Biliary lithiasis may develop under various favorable conditions (sickle cell disease, infections, post-surgery, underlying malformations of the biliary tract, etc.). They are often but not always associated with cholecystitis. Conversely, acute cholecystitis may develop under the same favorable conditions, with or without the presence of a lithiasis. Lithiasis and cholecystitis in most cases display the classical US features (Fig. 22). Congenital choledochal cysts may first be detected in this age group due to their complications, such as inflammation or lithiasis. MRI provides additional important information for their proper management (Fig. 23) (Rozel et al. 2011; Lowe 2008).

Pancreatic diseases. In children, the pancreas may be affected by acute conditions secondary to viral diseases (mumps), medications, congenital anomalies, or

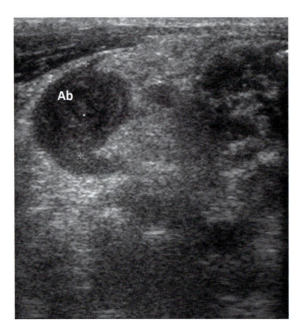

Fig. 17 Crohns's involvement of the appendix, as seen on US. Transverse view of the right lower quadrant. Abscess (*Ab*) around the inflamed appendix, with hyperechoic mesenteric fat

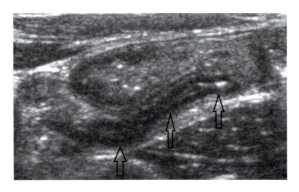

Fig. 18 A normal appendix as seen on US. Sagittal view of the appendix (*arrows*)

Table 2 Conditions mimicking acute appendicitis

Mesenteric adenitis
Inflammatory bowel disease
Infectious ileitis
Tumoral involvement of the appendix
Autoimmune diseases involving the digestive tract
Meckel's diverticulitis
Urachal cyst
Abdominal tumors
Gynecological diseases
Acute pyelonephritis
Hepatitis
Cholecystitis
Pancreatitis
Pneumonia
Skeletal diseases

complementary diagnostic and therapeutic procedures (Darge and Anupindi 2009).

Mesenteric adenitis. Small and middle-size adenopathies are frequent findings during an abdominal US examination. Once all other differential diagnoses of acute appendicitis have been excluded, the diagnosis of mesenteric adenitis can be evoked especially if an ear/nose/throat (ENT) inflammation has preceded the abdominal symptoms (Fig. 25).

Abdominal and ovarian tumors. Benign or malignant abdominal tumors may occur at any age and involve every organ. The role of imaging in an emergency setting will be to demonstrate the presence of a mass, the organ of origin, and the probable diagnosis. The demonstration of complications, such as hemorrhage developing within the tumor or torsion (Fig. 26) provides important additional information (Wootton-Gorges et al. 2005; Hernon et al. 2010; Kaste et al. 1995). The most common tumors in girls involve the ovaries, with teratoma (or dermoïd cyst) as the most frequent histologic type encountered. Due to their fatty content and calcifications, these tumors have very typical imaging features on every modality (US, CT, MRI) (Fig. 27). They can be bilateral. In some cases, torsion is the presenting symptom (Fig. 26).

Other typical tumors in children include cystic lymphangioma and teratoma. Either one can be

trauma (Fig. 24). Furthermore, an acute bout may complicate chronic conditions (cystic fibrosis, familial chronic pancreatitis). On US, in acute pancreatitis, the gland appears swollen and hypoechoic. In cystic fibrosis, the underlying pancreas is small and hyperechoic; macrocysts will progressively develop. In case of chronic (familial) pancreatitis, the underlying pancreas is diffusely calcified; the pancreatic duct may appear distended and obstructed by lithiasis. Such cases will mandate magnetic resonance and endoscopic cholangiopancreatography (MRCP, ERCP, respectively) as

Fig. 19 Henoch-Schonlein purpura. **a** The thickened bowel wall as seen on US, transverse scan. **b** Ileo-Ileal intussusception, with a typical cockade appearance and a maximum diameter of 20 mm

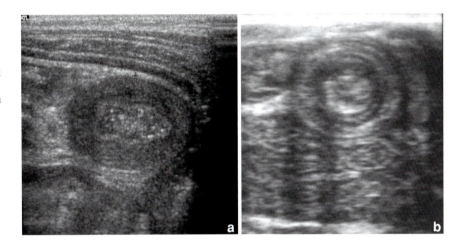

Fig. 20 Acute Meckel's diverticulitis. **a** US shows the distended inflamed diverticulum (*M*), directed towards the umbilicus. **b** Contrast-enhanced CT, reformatted sagittal view, demonstrates the fluid-filled diverticulum (*arrow*). (Images courtesy of L. Rausin, MD)

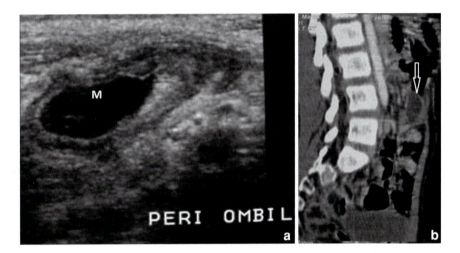

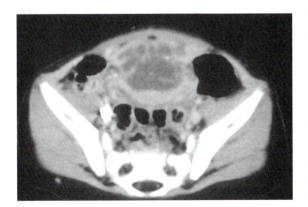

Fig. 21 Urachal abscess. Contrast-enhanced CT shows a heterogeneous, partially cystic mass lying just above the bladder, as seen along its midline

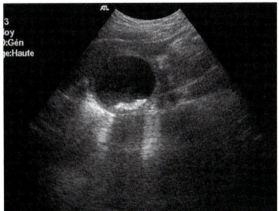

Fig. 22 Biliary lithiasis in a patient with sickle cell disease. Transverse view of the gallbladder displays the typical lithiasis and sludge

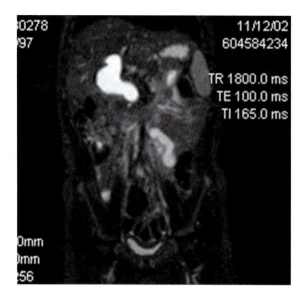

Fig. 23 Typical choledochal cyst. As seen on a T_2-weighted sequence

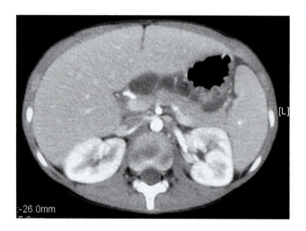

Fig. 24 Pancreatitis following pancreatic trauma. Contrast-enhanced CT shows the free fluid collections in Morrison's pouch

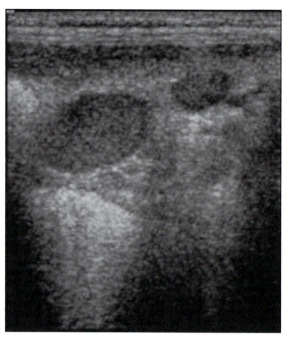

Fig. 25 Typical US appearance of mesenteric adenitis

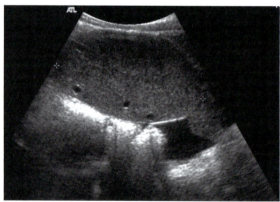

Fig. 26 Torsion of an ovary (involved by lymphoma). US show a swollen ovary with peripheral follicles

retro- or intraperitoneal. Cystic lymphangioma appears as a large multiseptated cystic tumor whereas teratoma is usually more complex, including echogenic solid components, cystic parts, as well as calcifications. These tumors may bleed or be complicated by infection (Wootton-Gorges et al. 2005; Kaste et al. 1995).

Non-peritoneal diseases. Once peritoneal diseases have been excluded, other entities that may manifest as acute abdominal pain include pneumonia (Fig. 28), acute pyelonephritis, testicular torsion, psoas abscess, and skeletal diseases (Papagelopoulos et al. 1998).

2.4   Above 12 Years

The list of diseases to be considered in children over the age of 12 years resembles that of in adults and includes gastritis, gastro-duodenal ulcers, bowel inflammatory diseases, and their respective complications.

In adolescent girls, gynecological pathologies have to be additionally considered, as they constitute the commonest group of diseases. Ovarian cysts or

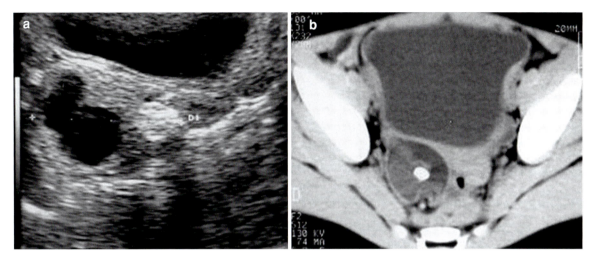

Fig. 27 Dermoid cyst of the right ovary. **a** Transverse US scan of the pelvis shows the mass, with a mixed pattern of fluid and highly echogenic areas. **b** CT scan confirms the various different patterns typical of this tumor

large follicles develop frequently, with torsion as a classical complication. In such cases, US typically demonstrates a swollen ovarian stroma and the follicles shifted peripherally. Doppler findings may or may not be abnormal. At menarche, previously unrecognized gynecological malformations will become symptomatic due to the hematocolpos distending an obstructed or malformed vagina (Fig. 29). Furthermore, pelvic inflammatory disease and extra-uterine pregnancy must be included in the differential diagnosis of lower abdominal pain in an adolescent girl (Lurie et al. 2000; Ziereisen et al. 2005; Anders and Powell 2005).

3 Acute Traumatic Abdominal Conditions

Abdominal trauma occurs often in young children. The liver, spleen, and, less commonly, the intestines can be injured. US may depict the lesions and their consequences, although more definitive findings are obtained with CT (Figs. 30, 31). The presence of a small amount of peritoneal fluid does not imply parenchymal lesions necessitating surgery (Simanovsky et al. 2011).

Trauma to the liver classically results in a hematoma. When isolated, conservative treatment and a clinico-radiological follow-up are sufficient. Yet in some cases, the hepatic artery or part of the biliary tree may be ruptured and a biloma will develop.

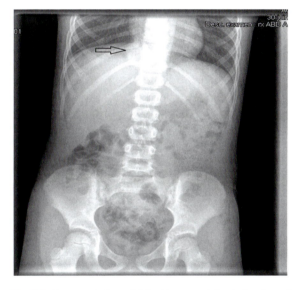

Fig. 28 Pneumonia in a child with acute abdominal pain and right lower lobe pneumonia (*arrow*)

For such lesions, therapeutic interventional imaging or surgery may be necessary.

For the spleen, regardless of the lesion, conservative treatment is usually advised in order to reduce the number of splenectomies.

Traumatic rupture of the digestive tract occurs most often at the level of the duodenum. Free air will be visualized around the duodenum but also in the retroperitoneum. Surgery is mandatory.

Fig. 29 Obstructed left-hemi-uterus in a patient with duplex vagina and uterus.
a Sagittal oblique scan of
a the normal right horn and
b the obstructed left horn with its distended lumen (*arrows*)

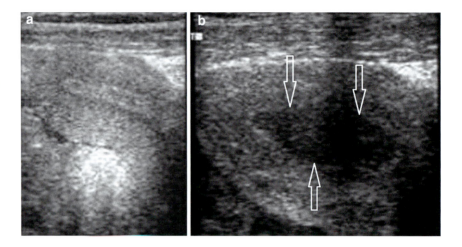

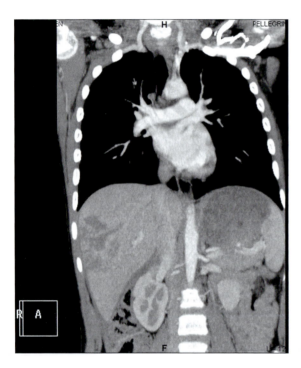

Fig. 30 Post-traumatic hepatic hematoma. Frontal reformation of a contrast-enhanced CT shows a typical hematoma in the right lobe. (Image courtesy of JF. Chateil, MD)

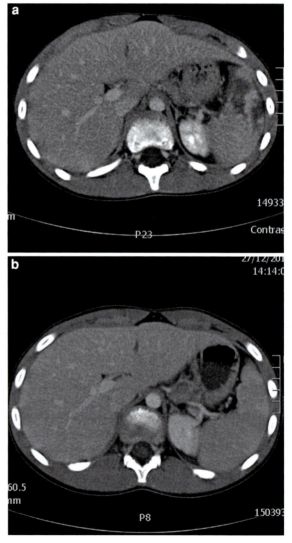

It should be stressed that, in children, traumatic lesions may occur following child abuse (non-accidental trauma). Imaging patterns of the traumatic lesions in such cases are similar to those of the usual forms of trauma. Therefore, a meticulous inquiry within and around the family circle is mandatory in order to identify suspicious cases (Ruess et al. 1995; Resende et al. 2002; Hilmes et al. 2011).

Fig. 31 Evolution of a post-traumatic spleen (contrast-enhanced CT). **a** Acute stage: typical splenic hematoma; **b** Follow-up: complete healing

References

Anders JF, Powell EC (2005) Urgency of evaluation and outcome of acute ovarian torsion in pediatric patients. Arch Pediatr Adolesc Med 159:532–535

Applegate K (2009) Evidence-based diagnosis of malrotation and volvulus. Pediatr Radiol 39(Suppl 2):S140–S143

Bateni C, Stein-Wexter R, Wootton-Gorges SL, Li CS (2011) Radiology resident's experience with intussusception reduction. Pediatr Radiol 41:721–726

Baud C, Saguintaah M, Veyrac C, Couture A, Ferran JL, Barneon G, Veyrac M (2004) Sonographic diagnosis of colitis in children. Eur Radiol 14:2105–2119

Chang WL, Yang YH, Lin YT, Chiang BL (2004) Gastro-intestinal manifestations in Henoch-Schönlein purpura: a review of 261 patients. Acta Pediatr 93:1427–1431

Darge K, Anupindi S (2009) Pancreatitis and the role of US, MRCP and ERCP. Pediatr Radiol 39(Suppl 2):S153–S157

De Bruyn R (2005) General issues of methods and equipment in pediatric ultrasound, 2nd edn. Churchill Livingstone, Oxford, pp 1–14

De Buys Roessingh AS, de Lagausie P, Baudoin V, Loirat C, Aigrain Y (2007) Gastro-intestinal complications of post-diarrheal hemolytic uremic syndrome. Eur J Pediatr Surg 17:328–334

Epelman M (2006) The whirpool sign. Radiology 240:910–911

Epelman M, Daneman A, Navarro OM, Moraq I, Moore I, Moore AM, Kim JH, Faingold R, Taylor G, Gerstle JT (2007) Necrotizing enterocolitis : review of state-of-the art imaging findings with pathologic correlation. Radio Graphics 27:285–305

Garcia-Pena Cook EF, Maudl KD (2004) Selective imaging strategies for the diagnosis of appendicitis in children. Pediatrics 113:24–28

Gartner RD, Levin TL, Borenstein SH, Han BK, Blumfield E, Murphy R, Freeman K (2011) Interloop fluid in intussusception: what is its significance? Pediatr Radiol 41:727–731

Hennelly KE, Bachur R (2011) Appendicitis update. Curr Opin Pediatr 23:281–285

Hernon M, McKenna J, Busby G, Sanders C, Garden A (2010) The histology and management of ovarian cysts found in children and adolescents. BJOG 117:181–184

Hilmes MA, Hernanz-Schulman M, Greeley CS, Piercey LM, Yu C, Kan JH (2011) CT identification of abdominal injuries in abused pre-school-age children. Pediatr Radiol 41:643–651

Kaste SC, Young CW, Holmes TP, Baker DK (1995) Imaging pediatric oncologic emergencies of the abdomen. AJR 173:729–736

Laing FC, Townsend BA, Rodriguez JR (2007) Ovary-containing hernia in a premature infant US findings. J Ultrasound Med 26:985–987

Laje P, Flake AW, Adzick NS (2010) Prenatal diagnosis and post-natal resection of intraabdominal enteric duplications. J Pediatr Surg 45:1554–1558

Lampl B, Levin TL, Berdon WE, Cowles RA (2009) Malrotation and midgut volvulus: a historical review and current controversies in diagnosis and management. Pediatr Radiol 39:359–366

Levy AD, Hobbs CM (2004) Meckel's diverticulum: radiological features with pathologic correlation. Radio Graphics 24:565–587

Lowe HL (2008) Imaging hepato-biliary disease in children. Semin Roentgenol 43:39–49

Lurie S, Feinstein M, Mamet Y (2000) Unusual presentation of acute abdomen in a syndrome of double uterus, unilaterally imperforated double vagina, and ipsilateral renal agenesis. Acta Obstet Gynecol Scand 79:152–153

Maheshwari P, Abograra A, Sharman O (2009) US evaluation of GI obstruction in infants: a pictorial essay. J Pediatr Surg 44:2037–2042

Papagelopoulos PJ, Currier BL, Shaughnessy WJ, Sim FH, Ebersold MJ, Bond JR, Unni KK (1998) Aneurysmal bone cyst of the spine management and outcome. Spine 23:621–628

Park NH, OH HE, Park HJ, Park JY (2011) US of normal and abnormal appendix in children. World J Radiol 3:85–91

Pedrosa I, Rofsky NM (2003) MR Imaging in abdominal emergencies. Radiol Clin N Am 41:1243–1273

Rajindrajih S, Devanarayana NM (2011) Constipation in children: novel insight into epidemiology, pathophysiology and management. J Neurogastroenterol Motil 17:35–47

Resende V, Tavares WC Jr, Drumond DA (2002) Helical computed tomography characteristics of splenic and hepatic trauma in children subjected to nonoperative treatment. Emerg Radiol 9:309–313

Rosendahl K, Aukland SM, Fosse K (2004) Imaging strategies in children with suspected appendicitis. Eur Radiol 14:2138–2145

Rozel C, Garel L, Rypens F, Viremouneix L, Lapierre C, Decarie JC, Dubois J (2011) Imaging of biliary disorders in children. Pediatr Radiol 41:208–220

Ruess L, Sivit CJ, Eichelberger MR, Taylor GA, Bond SJ (1995) Blunt hepatic and splenic trauma in children: correlation of a CT injury severity scale with clinical outcome. Pediatr Radiol 25:321–325

Schmittenbecher PP (2001) Carcinoid tumours of the appendix in children-epidemiology, clinical aspects and procedures. Eur J Pediatr Surg 11:428–432

Simanovsky N, Hiller N, Lubashevsky N, Rozovsky K (2011) US evaluation of the free intraperitoneal fluid in asymptomatic children. Pediatr Radiol 41:732–735

Strouse PJ (2006) US evaluation of the child with lower abdominal or pelvic pain. Radiol Clin North Am 44:911–923

Sung T, Callahan MJ, Taylor GA (2006) Clinical and imaging mimickers of acute appendicitis in the pediatric population. AJR 186:67–74

Vorona GA, Ceschin RC, Clayton BL, Sutcavage T, Tadros SS, Panigraphy A (May 19, 2011) Reducing abdominal CT dose with the adaptative statistical iterative reconstruction technique in children. Pediatr Radiol

Wan MJ, Krahn M, Ungar WJ, Caku E, Sung L, Medina LS, Doria AS (2009) Acute appendicitis in young children:

cost-effectiveness of US versus CT in diagnosis—a Markov decision analytic model. Radiology 250: 378–386

Wootton-Gorges SL, Thomas KB, Harned RK, Wu SR, Stein-Wexler R, Strain D (2005) Giant cystic abdominal masses in children. Pediatr Radiol 35:1277–1288

Yigiter M, Kantarci M, Yalçin O, Yalçin A, Salman AB (2011) Does obesity limit the sonographic diagnosis of appendicitis in children? J Clin Ultrasound 39:187–190

Ziereisen F, Guissard G, Damry N, Avni EF (2005) Sonographic imaging of the paediatric female pelvis. Eur Radiol 15:1296–1309

The Role of Interventional Radiology

Stefan Wirth and Marcus Treitl

Contents

S. Wirth (✉)
Department of Clinical Radiology, Clinical Center of the
Ludwig-Maximilians-University of Munich,
Nussbaumstrasse, 20, 80336 Munich, Germany
e-mail: swirth@med.uni-muenchen.de

M. Treitl
Department of Clinical Radiology, Clinical Center of the
Ludwig-Maximilians-University of Munich,
Pettenkoferstrasse, 8a, 80336 Munich, Germany

Abstract

Over the past decades technical developments have highly influenced the field of interventional radiology. High-speed, sub-millimetric resolution has triggered increasing indications for cross-sectional imaging with highest diagnostic and thus therapeutic value. From the interventional point of view this results in two major effects. First, in angiography a shift in daily routine working from diagnostic to therapeutic procedures is evident. Second, CT is taking over many procedures, which were formerly performed using ultrasound or fluoroscopic guidance. However, due to its minimal-invasive nature, the cardinal benefit of interventional radiology is to speed up therapy with lower risks for the patients and shortened hospitalization.

1 Introduction

In recent decades, technical developments have highly influenced the field of interventional radiology. High-speed, sub-millimetric resolution has triggered increasing indications for cross-sectional imaging with highest diagnostic and thus therapeutic value. From the interventional point of view, this has had two major effects. First, in angiography, a shift in daily routine, from diagnostic to therapeutic procedures, is evident. Second, in many procedures, CT is replacing ultrasound (US) or fluoroscopic guidance. However, due to its minimally invasive nature, the cardinal benefit of interventional radiology is to speed up the initiation of therapy, thus reducing adverse patient outcome and shortening hospitalization.

M. Scaglione et al. (eds.), *Emergency Radiology of the Abdomen*,
Medical Radiology. Diagnostic Imaging,
DOI: 10.1007/174_2011_476, © Springer-Verlag Berlin Heidelberg 2012

2   DSA-Guided Interventions

The use of digital subtraction angiography (DSA) in the treatment of vascular pathologies has evolved enormously during the past decade. Today, the interventionalist can choose from a wide-ranging armamentarium of materials for vessel occlusion, stabilization, and recanalization. The availability of an endovascular-trained staff and a well-sorted selection of endovascular materials and catheters should be a precondition at every first-line trauma center. The technical aspects of DSA and its clinical indications are discussed in the following sections.

2.1   Materials and Basic Principles of DSA-Guided Interventions

Conservation of as much of the native vessel as possible should be the goal of any endovascular approach to vascular pathologies. This will allow the preservation of organ function, avoid additional patient morbidity, and reduce the risk of complications. In the following section, some general aspects of endovascular therapy and a short overview of the currently available catheters and materials are given.

2.2   General Aspects and Vascular Access

Careful selection of the best vascular access site is crucial for planning an endovascular procedure. For abdominal endovascular interventions, retrograde inguinal access, typically from the right groin, is suitable in most cases, especially those involving the treatment of organ injuries and spinal or pelvic bleedings. For the latter, probing the internal iliac artery might be easier from the contralateral side. In rare cases, e.g., the treatment of gastrointestinal ischemia due to stenosis of the superior mesenteric artery, a transbrachial access might be the better choice. However, in order to keep the risk of cerebral embolization to a minimum, transbrachial access should be from the left arm only!

A 4F sheath is applicable for most routine interventions. This is of particular interest since an access-site hematoma can contribute to an aggravation of the patient's clinical state and should thus be avoided whenever possible. However, for placement of larger occlusion balloons, vascular plugs, or covered stents, larger sheaths, typically 6F or 7F, are necessary.

Use of puncture closing devices is advisable to seal the access site after the intervention, since this facilitates patient mobilization and eases further treatment, especially in polytrauma patients.

In many cases, super-selective catheterization according to the co-axial technique is necessary. The interventionalist should be familiar with this technique and especially with the use of micro-catheters. In addition, the compatibility of all chosen materials, e.g., diagnostic catheters and co-axial micro-catheters, should be confirmed when planning the endovascular armory for emergency procedures. All members of the team should be familiar with the properties of the stored materials.

Embolization therapy, especially with flow-directed materials such as gelatin sponge particles or microspheres, should be monitored with frequent control angiograms to avoid unintentional embolization of non-target vessels. In addition, some embolization procedures may be painful, e.g., due to the material, such that analgo-sedation will be required to reduce the procedural stress for the patient.

2.3   Materials and Methods for Embolization

For embolo-therapy, mechanical, particulate, and liquid embolic agents are available. Table 1 provides a short overview of the different classes of embolic agents (Landwehr et al. 2008).

2.3.1   Occlusion Balloons
Standard PTA balloons or compliant low-pressure balloons such as those made of latex are typically used for temporary vessel occlusion, e.g., to plan further endovascular treatment, to control bleeding until definitive surgical repair of the traumatized area can be accomplished, or to reduce blood flow during the use of liquid embolic agents.

2.3.2   Coils
While there is a broad variety of commercially available coils, basically two types can be distinguished. Push coils are not wire bound and have to be injected

Table 1 Embolic agents (from Landwehr et al. 2008)

Mechanical embolic agents	Occlusion balloons
	Detachable balloons
	Coils
	Plugs (e.g., Amplatzer Vascular Plug)
Particulate embolic agents	Gelatin sponge (e.g., Gelfoam)
	Polyzene-coated hydrogel particles (e.g., Embozene, Fig. 2)
	Starch microspheres (e.g., Embocept)
	PVA particles (e.g., Contour/Contour SE)
	PVA-hydrogel particles (e.g., Bead Block)
	Gelatin microspheres (e.g., Embospheres)
Liquid embolic agents	Ethylene vinyl alcohol copolymer (e.g. Onyx)
	Oily contrast agent (e.g., Lipiodol)
	Cyanoacrylate (e.g., Histoacryl)
	Thrombin
	Sclerosing agents (e.g., Polydocanol)

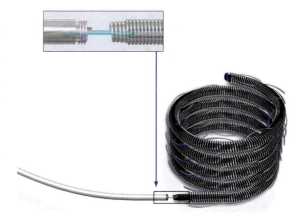

Fig. 1 Mechanically detachable fibered coil (Concerto coil; with the kind permission of ev3 Endovascular, Plymouth, MN, USA). The small filament within the delivering hypotube can be retracted to release the coil after its correct placement

into the target vessel by a small bolus of sterile saline or contrast agent. Their use requires a very stable position of the delivery catheter within the target vessel since the liquid bolus can expel the delivery catheter from the target vessel by repulsion, leading to coil loss and non-target vessel embolization. In addition, the final position of these coils cannot be precisely guided or predicted. However, they are inexpensive and useful for "packing" a larger vessel to achieve fast occlusion, as long as the precautions are considered. If a more precise positioning of the coils is necessary or if it is not possible to achieve a stable catheter position within the target vessel, then detachable coils are an alternative (Fig. 1). The different systems include mechanical detachable coils and electrolytic detaching mechanisms.

Furthermore coils differ in size. For use with standard diagnostic catheters, 0.035-inch coils are available, and for co-axial micro-catheters 0.018-inch coils.

Some coils are fibered with small Dacron fibers, which increases thrombogenicity. However, when used in more sensitive vascular beds, e.g. for organ bleedings, fibered coils might have a slightly higher risk for thromboembolism and non-target vessel embolization.

For larger-vessel or aneurysm treatment, additional 3D coils are an option.

Coil embolization requires the packing of coils of different diameters in order to achieve complete vessel occlusion. Usually, coils with larger diameters are used to establish an anchor within the target vessel, which is then filled with coils of smaller caliber, until complete hemostasis is reached.

2.3.3 Vascular Plugs

Vascular plugs (e.g., the Amplatzer Vascular Plug family) are available in different sizes (3–22 mm, depending of the type of plug) and shapes (I–IV). They are typically used as the sole embolic agent to achieve complete vessel occlusion with a single device. Like detachable coils, they can be repositioned before final detachment, but in contrast to coils they require slightly larger (5F–9F) vascular access and delivery catheters. However, newer developments, such as the Vascular Plug IV, exhibit more flexible delivery systems, allowing even tortuous vessel areas to be crossed. Accordingly, the Vascular Plug family is a feasible tool for emergency embolization in case of bleedings, since the need for only a single device reduces intervention time dramatically.

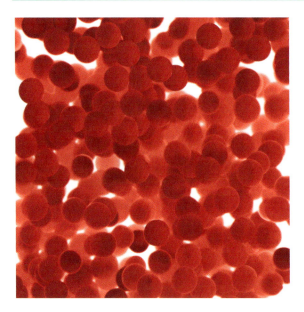

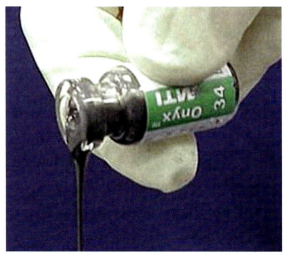

Fig. 3 The liquid embolic agent Onyx (with the kind permission of ev3 Endovascular, Plymouth, MN, USA)

Fig. 2 Embozene microspheres, 500 μm in size. The particles are colored to distinguish the different sizes. The magnified image demonstrates the precise sizing of the particles (with the kind permission of CeloNova BioSciences, Ulm, Germany)

2.3.4 Particulate Embolic Agents

Temporary or permanent vascular occlusion can be achieved with particulate embolic agents (Landwehr et al. 2008). For temporary embolization, gelatin sponge particles that have been ground and then suspended in, e.g., contrast material (CM), can be used. Starch microspheres are a commercially available alternative, offering more-defined particle sizes. For permanent embolization, different types of industrial particles, in sizes ranging from 45–1200 μm, are an option (see Table 1 and Fig. 2 for details). Particulate embolic agents are useful in the presence of more diffuse bleedings, but have the risk of non-target vessel embolization. They should thus be used with caution and with frequent angiographic control of the extent of vascular occlusion, since the immediate stoppage of blood flow can induce particle reflux. Typically, the particles are resuspended in CM, which allows better control of their action. The interventionalist should refer to the recommendations of the particle manufacturer since the preparation scheme will depend on both the size and quantity of particles used.

2.3.5 Liquid Embolic Agents

Liquid embolic agents are useful for the rapid occlusion of smaller vascular beds in case of more diffuse bleedings. In the past, oily contrast agents were used. Today, cyanoacrylate or the ethylene vinyl alcohol copolymer Onyx is preferred. Oily contrast agents are useful to occlude larger vascular beds, e.g., in case of tumor embolization. Cyanoacrylate offers immediate vessel occlusion but has the disadvantage of potential catheter encasement since it is adhesive to all catheter materials. In addition, its use requires training and considerable experience, including exactly how to prepare the material for intravascular application.

Currently, the copolymer Onyx is the most sophisticated liquid embolic agent available (Fig. 3). It is non-adhesive but cohesive, reducing the risk of catheter encasement to a minimum, and is available in several predefined viscosities (Onyx-18, -20, -34, and -500) suitable for a range of blood-flow velocities in the target vessel. Higher viscosities are used for high-flow situations and in large vessels, and lower viscosities in low-flow situations and small vascular beds if the diffuse filling of small capillaries is necessary. The principle of Onyx is the precipitation of the copolymer when the substance leaves the catheter tip while its organic solvent dimethyl sulfoxide (DMSO) dissolves in the blood stream. The resulting soft spongy cast that

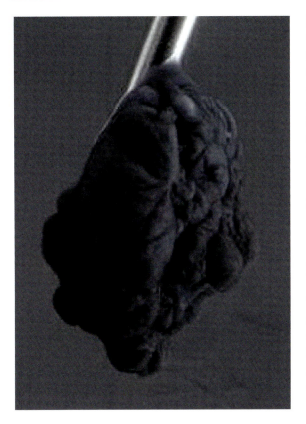

Fig. 4 Precipitation of the Onyx cast at the tip of an injection needle in a liquid environment (with the kind permission of ev3 Endovascular, Plymouth, MN, USA)

forms at the tip of the catheter (Fig. 4) remains shapeable for a few minutes. As for any liquid embolic agent, training is required prior to its first use. The interventionalist must especially keep in mind that Onyx has to be prepared by vortexing for about 20 min prior to use since it contains tantalum powder, for fluoroscopic visualization (since the copolymer alone is not visible under fluoroscopy), which has to be re-suspended completely prior to its injection in order to avoid nontarget vessel embolization. In addition, the solvent DMSO is quite aggressive in its reaction with several kinds of plastic materials. Therefore, only DMSO-compatible catheters should be used with this embolic agent. However, since this product seems to have gained relatively broad acceptance, most manufacturers will be sure to clearly indicate the DMSO compatibility of their catheters.

If used appropriately, Onyx is a fast-acting, well controllable liquid embolic agent, exhibiting the lowest recanalization rates of all products now on the market.

For larger vessels, the combination of Onyx with coils, which act as an anchoring mesh for the Onyx cast, is advisable. It should be noted that DMSO can be angiotoxic and will cause the patient remarkable pain during injection. Therefore, patients will require analgo-sedation prior to treatment. In addition, to avoid the risk of angio-necrosis, the injection rate of Onyx should not exceed 0.3 ml/min but it must be >0.05 ml/min in order to avoid precipitation within the catheter.

2.4 Other Endovascular Materials for Emergency Situations: Stents and Stent Grafts

In sealing aneurysms or vascular bleedings, it is sometimes necessary to preserve the target vessel. This can be achieved with covered stent grafts or the newly developed multilayer stents, which are based on the principle of flow diversion (see below). In general, self-expanding stents have to be distinguished from balloon-expandable stents. The latter exhibit greater radial force and are significantly less flexible. They are generally used in vascular segments without significant movement (bending or compression), e.g., the proximal iliac vessels, or when a high radial force is required, e.g., to recanalize atherosclerotic vessel segments such as the ostia of the splanchnic arteries in case of atherosclerotic ostial stenosis. In high flexion zones, typified by the distal segments of the iliac arteries or the mid and distal segments of the splanchnic arteries, or in case of severe bending or kinking of the vessel, self-expanding stents made of nitinol are preferred. Vascular leakage, either traumatic, iatrogenic, or due to erosion, is typically sealed with a covered stent graft. Today, both self-expanding and balloon-expandable covered stent grafts are available. These fulfill all of the potential demands for abdominal endovascular intervention.

Recently, a new type of stent was introduced for the treatment of arterial aneurysms. These so-called multilayer stents consist of multiple tightly woven layers of thin nitinol or cobalt chromium wires that form a thin mesh permeable to blood and blood cells. However, the placement of a multilayer stent in an aneurysmic vessel will lead to the homogenization of blood flow within the stent and thus to stasis in the aneurysm, inducing thrombosis and slow occlusion of the aneurysm. This effect is known as flow diversion, and to date it is frequently exploited in the treatment of cerebral aneurysms. The great advantage of this type of stent is, besides its high flexibility, the fact that side branches originating from the target vessel in the proximity of the aneurysm can be covered but will remain patent, since the stent's wire mesh is permeable to blood and blood cells. Animal studies have shown that endothelialization of the stent will stop at the margins of a side-branch ostium, leaving this vessel segment patent.

2.5   Pharmacological Treatment

Pharmacological treatment can be adjunctive or stand-alone and is based on either spasmolysis or fibrinolysis. Spasmolysis may be necessary especially after the treatment of splanchnic vessels, which tend to become more spastic after catheter manipulation than other vessel areas. Typically, glycerol-trinitrate at a dose of 100–200 µg is intra-arterially administered directly, injected over the diagnostic catheter or the super-selective micro-catheter.

Fibrinolysis makes use of urokinase or recombinant tissue plasminogen activator (rt-PA) The latter is more specific for fibrin and faster-acting, but with greater systemic effects, even if used locally. For all fibrinolytic agents, direct application into the thrombus is essential; this is also true for a combination of fibrinolysis with systemic heparinization, with a target partial thromboplastin time (PTT) of 60–70 s.

A detailed scheme for intra-arterial fibrinolysis is provided in Sect. 2.8.1.2.

2.6   Post-Interventional Treatment

Following the completion of an endovascular procedure, adequate hemostasis at the access site is required. Puncture closing devices are favored since they confer immediate hemostasis and allow a more flexible mobilization of the patient during post-interventional aftercare or follow-up surgery.

While after vascular embolization no specific treatment is required, treatment with stents or stent-grafts necessitates sufficient anticoagulation with acetylsalicylic acid (ASA) in combination with clopidogrel. Heparinization is an alternative to

clopidogrel for patients who require surgery in the post-interventional phase, since the drug dramatically increases the surgical risk of severe bleedings. ASA (100 mg per day) is typically administered life-long, even for patients requiring surgery. For non-surgical patients, clopidogrel is administered at a loading dose of 300 mg immediately after the interventional procedure, followed by 75 mg per day for the next 4 weeks. Patients under anticoagulation with cumarin derivatives should receive cumarin again, accompanied by 100 mg ASA per day instead of clopidogrel. The reader should note that the above suggestions are based on their successful use at the authors' institution; they are not supported by clinical trials.

2.7   Organ Injuries

The non-surgical treatment of organ injuries after blunt abdominal trauma is well accepted for hemodynamically stable patients. This approach can be divided into observation, on the one hand, and endovascular treatment with angiography and embolization, on the other. Patient observation requires his or her admission to a ward and monitoring of vital signs, strict bed rest, frequent determination of the red blood cell count, and serial abdominal examinations (van der Vlies et al. 2010). In carefully selected cases, the success rates of endovascular treatment of injury-induced organ bleedings can reach 90% (Malhotra et al. 2000; Pachter et al. 1998; Holden 2008). The endovascular approach has been widely evaluated and is now well-established for the treatment of splenic and hepatic injuries; experience with these techniques for other organ injuries continues to evolve (Holden 2008). However, still unsolved is the question whether and when they should be applied in the hemodynamically less stable patient.

2.7.1   Splenic Injury

Splenic injury is the most often observed organ injury after blunt abdominal trauma, occurring in up to 32% of abdominal injuries and frequently associated with injuries to other organs. Preservation of the spleen is important in order to avoid serious complications such as the overwhelming post-splenectomy syndrome (OPSI) and impaired immune system function (Holden 2008). Accordingly, many strategies have been developed to preserve the spleen after injury.

2.7.1.1 Patient Selection

The decision whether a patient is a good candidate for non-surgical treatment after splenic injury is mainly based on his or her hemodynamic status. Today, conditions such as active bleeding, as demonstrated on imaging by contrast extravasation, pseudoaneurysm formation, and arterio-venous fistula can be treated endovascularly and are no longer considered to be absolute contraindications for the endovascular treatment of splenic injury. In addition, simple observation alone has a failure rate of up to 34%, and even higher in patients with high-grade splenic injuries (Haan et al. 2005). On the other hand, recent studies have demonstrated that even high-risk lesions can in many cases be successfully treated by endovascular embolization (Haan et al. 2005; Nix et al. 2001).

2.7.1.2 Endovascular Procedure

The combination of intensive patient monitoring and angiographic evaluation of the vasculature of the spleen followed by embolization is the minimally invasive treatment modality of choice (Holden 2008). Recent studies recommend endovascular treatment in the presence of the following CT findings: active contrast extravasation, pseudoaneurysm or arterio-venous fistula, large hemoperitoneum, and a higher grade of injury (grades III–V) (van der Vlies et al. 2010; Haan et al. 2005). The endovascular approach can significantly lower the requirement for blood products. The interventionalist can choose between proximal and distal embolization of the splenic artery. In all cases of diffuse organ injury or in hemodynamically unstable patients, proximal embolization is the method of choice (Fig. 5). The procedure consists of proximal occlusion of the main stem of the splenic artery prior to its branching, e.g., with a vascular plug or the implantation of multiple coils (packed). This leads to a significant reduction in the perfusion pressure of the splenic parenchyma, thus allowing hemostasis. Since this procedure is indirect, it may take some time until hemostasis is complete. However, blood loss is reduced immediately, promoting rapid hemodynamic stabilization of the patient. In addition, the risk of splenic infarction is reduced because collateral perfusion is preserved (Holden 2008). In patients in whom splenic bleeding can be attributed to a single arterial lesion, distal embolization is preferred since the loss of parenchyma is kept

to a minimum. A single branch or segment artery feeding a bleed is embolized, e.g., by packing with multiple coils. Nevertheless, the reported outcomes for the two techniques are similar (Holden 2008; Haan et al. 2004). Some authors suggest the use of Gelfoam pledgets since the action of the embolizing agent is only temporarily necessary and dissolution of the pledgets may lead to the reperfusion of the occluded artery, additionally conserving organ function (Holden 2008).

2.7.1.3 Results

The failure rate for endovascular treatment of splenic injury necessitating surgical repair is <10% (Haan et al. 2004). Today, this approach is accepted even for high-grade injuries (grade IV) and should be implemented whenever allowed by the patient's hemodynamic condition.

2.7.1.4 Complications

Failure of the endovascular approach leads to open conversion with surgical treatment (Holden 2008). This mainly occurs in patients with high-grade injuries with large blood loss, and in those with multi-organ injuries. In rare cases, the endovascular approach can result in splenic infarction, abscess formation, and coil migration (Holden 2008; Haan et al. 2005, 2004). Splenic infarcts are mainly observed with distal embolization and in up to 20% of the cases (Haan et al. 2004), but normally resolve completely.

2.7.2 Hepatic Injury

Similar to splenic injuries, non-surgical treatment of hepatic injuries is well accepted for hemodynamically stable patients and is being increasingly used for unstable patients as well (Holden 2008).

2.7.2.1 Patient Selection

The endovascular approach can be performed either alone or in combination with surgical techniques such as debridement and packing of the injured liver segment (Velmahos et al. 2003). In contrast to splenic injuries, arterial hepatic bleeding must be differentiated from central portal venous injury or caval injury, either of which always requires surgical repair. Ongoing hemorrhage is the main reason for immediate intervention.

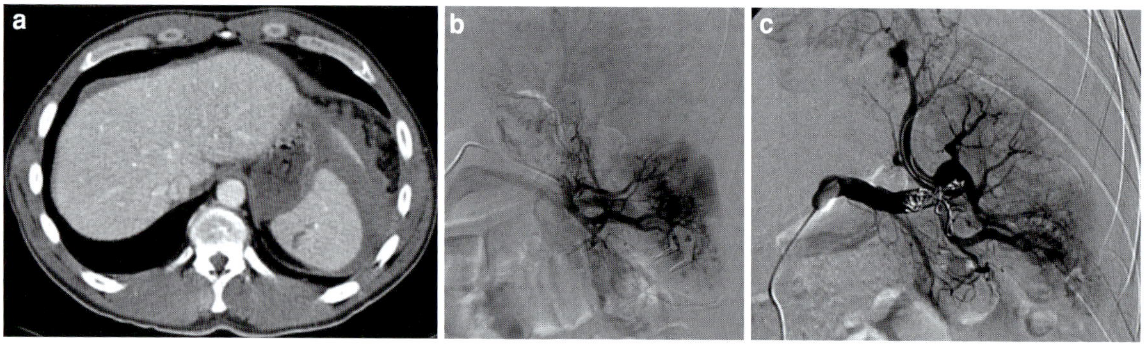

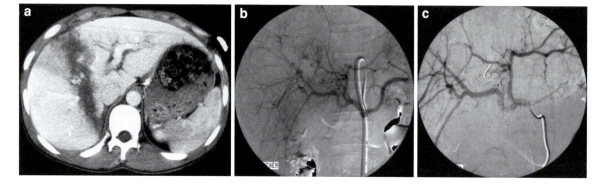

Fig. 5 Splenic injury successfully treated by proximal embolization. **a** Post-traumatic CT scan in the axial plane demonstrating splenic laceration with perisplenic hematoma. **b** Splenic angiogram prior to treatment reveals diffuse bleeding. **c** Splenic angiogram after proximal embolization and placement of an additional occlusion balloon. Pseudoaneurysm formation and diffuse blush indicate the persisting diffuse splenic trauma

Fig. 6 Hepatic injury with super-selective embolization. **a** CT scan in the axial plane demonstrating hepatic laceration; **b** non-selective angiogram of the hepatic artery; **c** super-selective embolization with a push-coil

2.7.2.2 Endovascular Procedure

Angiographic evaluation of hepatic injuries requires selective and super-selective depiction of the right and left hepatic artery branches. In contrast to splenic injury, distal embolization, as close to the vessel injury as possible (Fig. 6), is the method of choice to reduce the extent of arterial occlusion (Holden 2008). Proximal embolization should be used only in cases in which super-selective probing of the injured vessel is difficult, time-consuming, or induces the risk of severe damage (e.g., dissection) to the vasculature. As long as portal perfusion is maintained, hepatic embolization will not lead to significant parenchymal necrosis (Holden 2008). Again, coils or vascular plugs have been widely demonstrated to achieve rapid and sufficient embolization. Unlike in splenic injuries,

recanalization and the re-bleeding of a hepatic injury are major concerns, such that a permanent arterial occlusion is preferred (Holden 2008).

2.7.2.3 Results

Success rates for the non-surgical treatment of hepatic trauma are high for hemodynamically stable patients. The frequency of surgical repair after non-surgical treatment is <15% (Meredith et al. 1994).

2.7.2.4 Complications

Open conversion is the major complication for non-surgical treatment and is mainly observed in cases of significant contrast extravasation (Fang et al. 2006). Rarely, parenchyma or gallbladder necrosis as well as bile leaks, abscesses, hemobilia, abdominal compartment, and coil migration have been described, mainly in high-grade injuries (Mohr et al. 2003). Hepatic necrosis is particularly likely to result in surgical resection, with decompressive laparotomy of the abdominal compartment (Holden 2008; Kozar et al. 2005).

2.7.3 Renal Injury

Endovascular treatment of blunt renal injuries is suitable in the majority of cases. Exceptions are hemodynamically unstable patients, major pyelo-calyceal injury, and injury to the renal vascular pedicle (Dinkel et al. 2002). However, with evolving endovascular techniques even high-grade renal injuries are treated non-surgically in an increasing number of cases (Dinkel et al. 2002).

2.7.3.1 Patient Selection

The endovascular approach is particularly appropriate for patients without either injury to the vascular pedicle or lesions involving the central collecting system (Holden 2008; Dinkel et al. 2002). Surgical repair also should be reserved for patients with bilateral renal injury or injury to a solitary functional kidney (Holden 2008).

2.7.3.2 Endovascular Procedure

Initially, a non-selective overview angiogram of the entire abdominal aorta is obtained in order to identify additional renal arteries and injury to the central renal vascular pedicle. In case of more distal vessel injury, super-selective angiography of the affected vasculature should be the next step (Fig. 7).

Dissections and occlusions of the main renal artery can be treated by stent implantation, if feasible. Otherwise, a surgical approach will be required. In case of very severe renal trauma or multiple organ injuries, complete embolization of the renal artery may be a necessary definitive treatment alternative, as it saves time and promotes hemodynamic stabilization before surgical treatment. In contrast to hepatic and splenic injuries, renal embolization should always be performed as selectively as possible (Fig. 7) (Holden 2008), as this will reduce the risk of renal infarction and conserve organ function (Sofocleous et al. 2005). Usually, coils or liquid embolic materials are used. Once renal bleeding is under control, the

interventionalist must bear in mind that a severe clot burden may be present in the urinary system, as well as severe peri-nephric hematoma, both requiring drainage (Sofocleous et al. 2005).

2.7.3.3 Results

Technical success rates can reach 90% in selected patients, with a clinical success rate >80% (Holden 2008; Sofocleous et al. 2005). Re-bleeding is mostly observed in cases in which embolization was highly super-selective in order to avoid severe renal infarction.

2.7.3.4 Complications

Complications after renal artery embolization are very rare and mostly related to re-bleeding (Holden 2008).

2.7.4 Pancreatic Injury

Injury to the pancreas is rare (<2% of abdominal injuries) and mostly observed in polytrauma patients with multiple organ injuries (Holden 2008).

2.7.4.1 Patient Selection

Non-surgical treatment is appropriate for most patients without main pancreatic duct injury (Holden 2008).

2.7.4.2 Endovascular Procedure

Selective embolization is required in cases of visible bleeding. Identification of the bleeding vessel always necessitates careful and complete angiographic evaluation of all pancreas-supplying vessels. Usually, simple coil embolization will control pancreatic bleedings.

2.7.4.3 Results

Larger series of endovascular-treated pancreatic injuries are still missing. Of primary importance in these patients is not to overlook pancreatic injuries (Holden 2008).

2.8 Acute and Chronic Gastrointestinal Ischemia

2.8.1 Gastrointestinal Ischemia

Gastrointestinal ischemia, defined as an insufficient blood flow to the intestine (Bilbao et al. 2002), can be related to many causes but especially to a

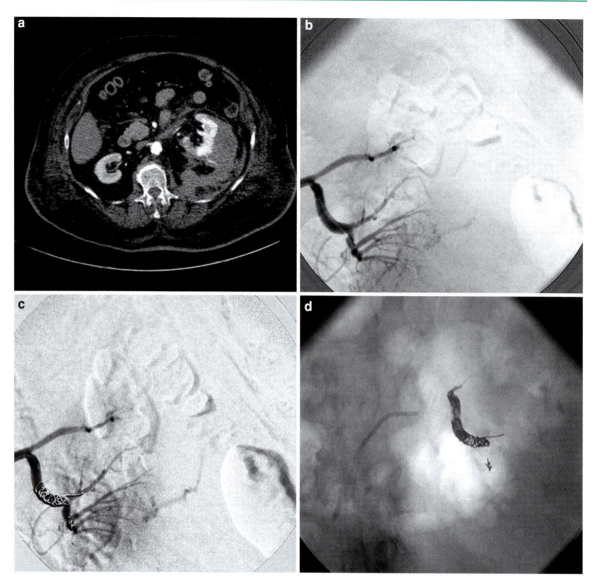

Fig. 7 Renal perforation after cardiac catheterization. **a** CT scan in the axial plane, arterial contrast phase, shows a perinephric hematoma and active contrast extravasation. **b** Superselective renal angiogram depicts active contrast extravasation, not seen on the non-selective overview angiogram due to tamponade. **c** Embolization of the lobar artery with several coils with still-active bleeding. **d** Completion of the embolization procedure by additional injection of 1 ml of Onyx-20, leading to the complete cessation of the bleeding (not shown). Renal function was conserved, with only a short, temporary increase in serum creatinine

non-occlusive decrease of intestinal blood flow, such as due to cardiac disease, infarction, hypovolemia, and arrhythmia. Other reasons for gastrointestinal ischemia are thromboembolism, bowel obstruction, inflammatory disorders, and injuries (see Table 2 for a complete list). Acute mesenteric ischemia is in most cases the result of an embolus within the superior mesenteric artery (SMA), whereas thrombosis of the SMA or the superior mesenteric vein is rare (Bilbao et al. 2002).

2.8.1.1 Diagnostic Evaluation

Gastrointestinal ischemia is preferably diagnosed with CT imaging. Doppler US may be feasible for detecting acute SMA occlusions (Bilbao et al. 2002).

Table 2 Typical causes of gastrointestinal ischemia (from Bilbao et al. 2002)

Acute mesenteric ischemia
Mesenteric vessel occlusion (mortality 90%)
Embolus (40–50%)
Thrombosis (20–40%)
Venous occlusion (<10%)
Non-occlusive mesenteric ischemia (mortality 10%)
Low-flow state
Cardiac failure
Hypotension
Bowel vasospasm
Chronic mesenteric ischemia
Atheromatous disease
Compression of celiac trunk by the median arcuate ligament

Although mesenteric angiography is still considered to be the gold standard for the diagnosis of acute mesenteric ischemia, its use is being increasingly abandoned because CT imaging is faster, in addition to demonstrating the extent of ischemia and the level and type of the vascular occlusion.

2.8.1.2 Interventional Treatment

Randomized controlled trials assessing the value of the different currently available endovascular treatment strategies are still lacking. In general, the interventionalist performing a mechanical revascularization can choose between balloons and stents and pharmacological agents (Bilbao et al. 2002).

Acute Disease

Acute disease can be caused by an embolus, thrombus, non-occlusive ischemia, or venous thrombosis. There is general agreement that SMA embolism with beginning signs of peritonism should be treated surgically, with open thrombectomy followed by the resection of necrotic bowel segments (Bilbao et al. 2002). Although there are reports of successful endovascular treatments of acute SMA embolism (Seder et al. 2009; Popovic et al. 2011), the endovascular approach should be strictly limited to special circumstances or specialized centers since time is critical in this entity (Bilbao et al. 2002). In the absence of signs of peritonism, an endovascular approach, either local fibrinolysis or mechanical thrombectomy, can be attempted (Bilbao et al. 2002).

Local fibrinolysis should always be performed using special lysis catheters, carrying several side holes that cover the entire occlusion. As a fibrinolytic agent, urokinase and rt-PA are well established. The latter has a slightly better specificity for fibrin, and thus a somewhat faster lytic action. A typical protocol for urokinase comprises a bolus injection of 100,000–300,000 IU urokinase, followed by continuous perfusion with 50,000 IU urokinase per hour, not exceeding 1.3 Mio IU within 24 h and always accompanied by systemic heparinization with a target PTT of 60–70 s. During fibrinolysis, the patient should be monitored intensively, including control of fibrinogen and lactate. In case of symptom aggravation or an increase in lactate, the patient should quickly undergo re-evaluation with abdominal CT-angiography (CTA) to decide whether surgical treatment is necessary. Control angiography should be undertaken after 12–24 h depending on the clinical state of the patient, disease severity, and signs of a thrombolytic effect. A typical protocol for rt-PA is to combine a bolus of 5 mg followed by an hourly local infusion of 5 mg, with a maximum dose of 40 mg; this maximum dose may be exceeded in selected cases depending on the patient's situation. The accompanying procedures are the same as for lysis with urokinase. Fibrinolysis also can be combined with mechanical recanalization techniques such as balloon angioplasty.

The preferred treatment of acute SMA thrombosis is likewise surgical revascularization, although successful treatment with angioplasty and stenting has been reported (Rundback et al. 2000). An important indicator for chronic mesenteric thrombosis is the late filling of SMA branches (Bilbao et al. 2002). In case of non-occlusive disease, the local infusion of vasodilators may have some benefit, potentially reducing the mortality rate (Bilbao et al. 2002). Mesenteric venous thrombosis should be treated surgically in case of urgent onset in symptomatic patients, and conservatively with oral anticoagulation in asymptomatic cases (Bilbao et al. 2002). Figure 8 provides an example of the successful fibrinolytic treatment of an embolic occlusion in a renal artery. Treatment may be the same for SMA embolus.

Chronic Disease

Intestinal angina, the typical clinical presentation of chronic mesenteric ischemia, does not require emergency treatment (Bilbao et al. 2002). It is usually

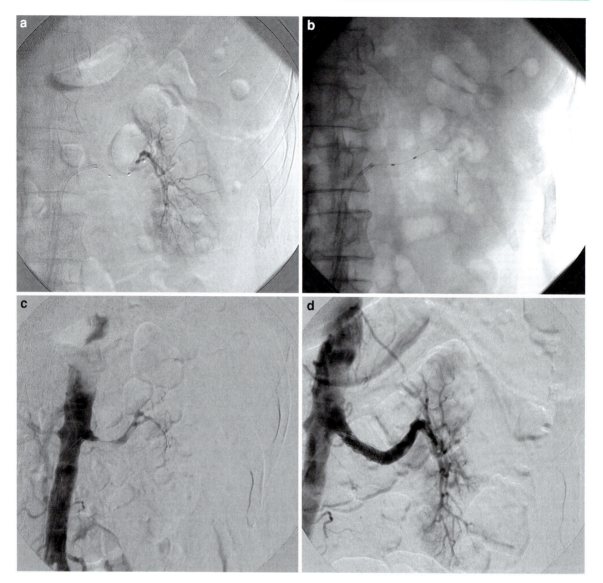

Fig. 8 Recanalization of an embolic occlusion of the left renal artery due to atrial fibrillation. The patient's serum creatinine had rapidly increased to 4.9 mg/dl and acute renal failure was imminent. **a** Recanalization of the occluded segment with a 0.014-inch guide wire, supported by a 0.014-inch support catheter (Trailblazer; ev3 Endovascular, Plymouth, MN, USA). **b** Local fibrinolysis with 20 mg rt-PA, injected using a 2.5-mm ClearWay local therapeutic infusion catheter (Atrium, Hudson, NH, USA). **c** Fibrinolysis revealed additional high-grade stenosis of the *left* renal artery. Thrombus was still present in the course of the vessel. **d** Final angiogram after stenting of the *left* renal artery and additional overnight fibrinolysis with urokinase. At 6-months follow-up, renal function was conserved albeit at a low level, with a stable serum creatinine of 2.3 mg/dl

related to atherosclerotic or stenotic disease involving the splanchnic arteries (Figs. 9, 10) or, rarely, in younger patients to an intrinsic compression of the celiac trunk by the median arcuate ligament of the diaphragm (Bilbao et al. 2002). Since many patients with isolated stenosis of a splanchnic artery are asymptomatic, careful patient selection for interventional treatment is crucial. In general, patients with typical post-prandial abdominal angina, unexplained weight loss, and stenosis in at least two of the three vessels are eligible for treatment once other types of gastrointestinal ischemia are excluded

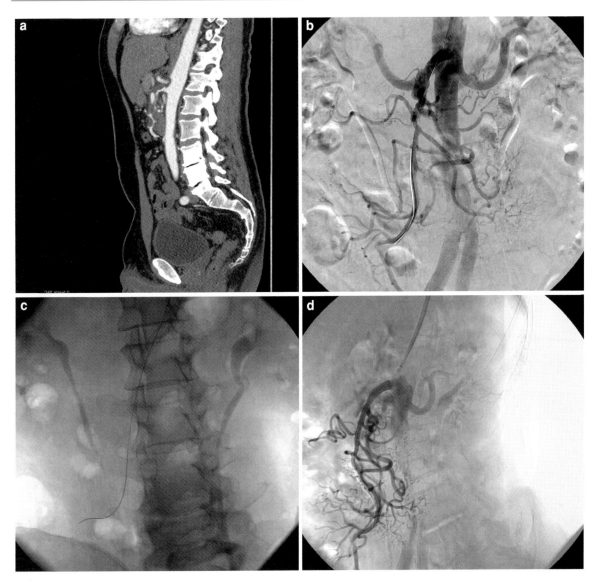

Fig. 9 Dissection of the superior mesenteric artery, treated by implantation of a multilayer aneurysm repair system (MARS). a Sagittal reconstruction of an abdominal CTA scan, demonstrating dissection and aneurysm formation involving the proximal part of the superior mesenteric artery. Side branches originating directly after the ectatic segment prevented the placement of a covered-stent graft. b Angiographic depiction of the same entity via a transbrachial access. c Delivery of a 7 × 60 mm self-expanding multilayer stent (Cardiatis SA, Isnes, Belgium) into the true lumen of the SMA, covering a major side branch. d Final angiogram after repair of the dissection and occlusion of the aneurysm. At 6 months, duplex follow-up evidenced complete repair of both the dissection and the aneurysm as well as patency of the covered side branch

(Bilbao et al. 2002). There is growing evidence that patients with 3-vessel disease, even if asymptomatic, should be treated due to the known high annual mortality rate of up to 10%. Today, endovascular treatment with balloon angioplasty and stent placement is a well-established alternative to surgical bypass of the splanchnic stenosis, although endovascular treatment has higher recurrence rates (Kasirajan et al. 2001). Ostial stenosis involving the splanchnic arteries is preferably treated by primary stenting with a balloon-expandable short stent, without covering too much of the angiographically non-diseased portion of the artery. Balloon-expandable stents are favored at this location since the plaque load in the aortic wall might compress

Fig. 10 Successful treatment of a high-grade atherosclerotic stenosis of the SMA in an 80-year-old woman with 2-vessel disease and typical abdominal angina. **a** Angiographic depiction of the ostial atherosclerotic stenosis. A 6-mm embolic protection device (Spider FX; ev3 Endovascular, Plymouth, MN, USA) was placed distally to the stenosis to avoid mesenteric embolization during balloon angioplasty. **b, c** Results after implantation of a 7 × 19-mm balloon-expandable stent. **d** Recovery of the embolic protection device revealed a relevant embolus caught within the filter

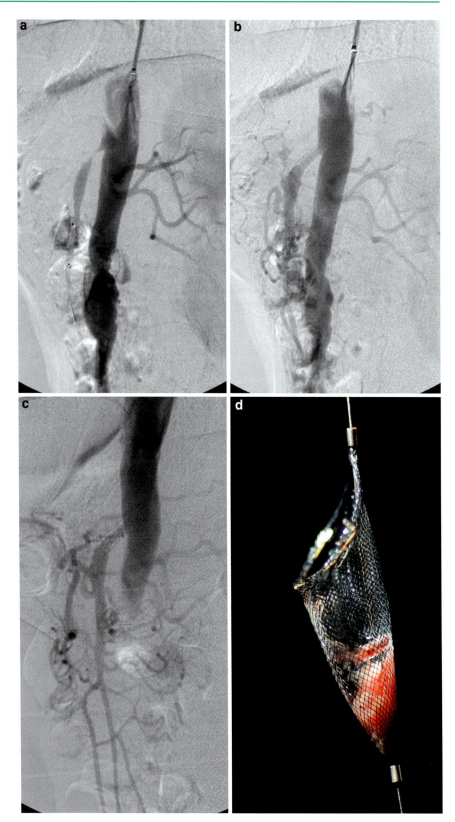

self-expanding stents. Therefore, the balloon-expandable stent should penetrate the aortic lumen for about 2 mm in order to ensure that it is stable enough to resist to aortic-plaque forces. Stenosis located more distally, on the other hand, is primarily treated by balloon angioplasty, eventually followed by placement of a self-expanding stent. This area of the vessel is acted upon by several forces, all of them related to intensive bowel movement. A balloon-expandable stent would thus be too strong, hindering vessel movement; instead, self-expanding stents are appropriate. The role of drug-eluting devices in this indication remains to be determined, but the same good results as obtained in other vascular territories can be expected.

In contrast to atherosclerotic gastrointestinal ischemia, celiac artery compression syndrome, first described by Dunbar in 1965, is still discussed controversially. It is typically seen in younger patients, mostly women, with an asthenic body habitus and presents as intermittent abdominal pain, epigastric bruits, and rapid weight loss. This syndrome does not benefit from angioplasty and stenting alone and should be treated by surgical decompression followed by arterial reconstruction (Bilbao et al. 2002; Kokotsakis et al. 2000).

2.8.2 Gastrointestinal Hemorrhage

Most (75%) gastrointestinal hemorrhages stop spontaneously (Bilbao et al. 2002). However, in all other cases imaging will be necessary if endoscopy is not able to detect the bleeding site. During the last decade, CTA and magnetic resonance angiography (MRA) have evolved enormously. Nevertheless, the detection of gastrointestinal hemorrhage requires a constant flow rate at the bleeding site, which might be too low for evaluation with either of these modalities. Therefore, early referral to DSA should be considered if there are strong indicators of gastrointestinal bleeding. DSA has the advantage of combining diagnostic evaluation and definitive treatment within one session. In contrast to all other imaging modalities, DSA detects even a minimal blood flow of 0.1 ml/min (Kruger et al. 1996) such that the majority of bleedings can be detected angiographically, especially if super-selective techniques are used. In addition, DSA detects indirect signs of bleeding, such as neovascularization, aneurysms, and arterio-venous fistulae (Bilbao et al. 2002). Provocation of the bleeding such as by the injection of fibrinolytic agents

is controversial since it might be difficult to control the results, although the procedure can be abandoned in most cases by consequent super-selective angiographic evaluation of the target vasculature. To reduce artifacts caused by bowel movement, antiperistaltic agents such as butylscopolamine should be administered, keeping in mind their contraindications.

2.8.2.1 Interventional Treatment

The bleeding site should be carefully evaluated by selective and super-selective angiography. As embolic agents, coils or liquids are employed based on their fast action, low complication and recanalization rates, and ease of use. The main problem is possible ischemia of the gut after embolization. Therefore, selecting the appropriate embolization site is crucial. If the site is too proximal to the bleeding, the vessel will still be perfused by collateral vessels. If it is distal to the vasa recta, there is a high risk of intestinal necrosis (Bilbao et al. 2002). The most appropriate method might be the direct placement of micro-coils at the bleeding site.

2.9 Other Abdominal Vascular Emergencies

2.9.1 Pelvic Injuries

Besides organ injuries and gastrointestinal hemorrhage, fracture bleedings in trauma patients are very common abdominal emergencies. The high mortality, exceeding 25%, due to abdominal fracture bleedings is associated with pelvic fractures. The bleeding derives from disrupted arteries, sheared veins, and/or oozing from bone surfaces. However, in most pelvic fractures there is also substantial bleeding from the exposed fracture margins of cancellous bone (Frevert et al. 2008). The nature of the trauma that led to the pelvic fracture defines the target vessel for bleeding complications. Anterior compression, opening the pelvic ring, may lead to rupture of the internal iliac artery. Lateral compression mostly results in rupture of the iliac vessels and retropubic veins. Vertical instability, however, causes heterogeneous patterns of vascular injury (Frevert et al. 2008).

Several treatment options are available to control bleedings deriving from pelvic fracture. In many cases, external fixation and/or pelvic compression are sufficient. If hemodynamic stability cannot be achieved, retro- or pre-peritoneal packing can be used to stop bleedings from veins and bony structures (Frevert et al. 2008). On the other hand, the endovascular repair of trauma-related pelvic bleedings has many advantages, such as less surgical stress to the patient and fast bleeding control.

2.9.1.1 Interventional Procedure

Careful selection of the appropriate access site is essential. Since pelvic bleedings mostly derive from side branches of the internal iliac artery, a contralateral access might ease probing of the target vessel. Therefore, CT scans of the trauma site should be evaluated carefully in order to define the most feasible access site. The procedure should be started by non-selective pelvic angiography, e.g., performed with a pigtail catheter placed in the infrarenal aorta. Most pelvic bleedings can be localized with this simple procedure, allowing detailed planning of the embolization procedure. Active bleedings are indicated by CM extravasation but sometimes there will be only indirect signs of vascular injuries, such as a sharp vessel cut-off, pseudoaneurysm formation, or sluggish flow.

Several endovascular treatment options are available, ranging from balloon occlusion to achieve time for treatment planning or surgical exploration, to unselective embolization of the major feeding vessel, or super-selective embolization only at the bleeding site. The ideal solution saves time and CM, in addition to avoiding severe catheter manipulations in the access vessel.

For balloon occlusion, standard PTA balloons can be used in urgent situations, although special low-pressure occlusion balloons are commercially available. For embolization, coils will achieve permanent occlusion, whereas a gelatin sponge may be used for temporary distal occlusions when it is necessary to gain time before surgical fracture repair. The gelatin sponge particles will biodegrade within several days to a few weeks, leading to reperfusion of the bleeding vessel and reducing damage to a minimum (Frevert et al. 2008). However, coils are faster, safer, and have a shorter learning curve, allowing for their use even by less-experienced interventionalists, who may be on duty during the night shift (Fig. 11). If larger arteries have to be occluded quickly and adequately but also permanently, the use of a vascular plug, consisting of

a self-expanding nitinol mesh, is advised (Frevert et al. 2008).

If the bleeding is more punctate and located in a transit vessel, sealing with covered-stent grafts offers an alternative. However, both the larger vascular access necessary for these devices, typically at least 6F or 7F, and the stiffness of these devices should be taken into account.

Embolization therapy in pelvic fractures is very safe, and complications quite unusual. The most often observed complication is caused by the embolization therapy itself is gluteal necrosis, seen in <5% of the cases. Some patients report urogenital dysfunction after pelvic fractures and embolization therapy. However, it was recently shown that urogenital dysfunction is typically related to the pelvic fracture und the accompanying damage and is not a sequela of embolization therapy (Ramirez et al. 2004).

3   CT-Guided Interventions

We now turn our discussion to CT-guided interventions. In particular, MDCT is fast, easily available, and provides high-resolution images in three dimensions. Additionally, every scanner vendor optionally recommends specific operation modes for the various CT-guided interventions. Thus, CT-guided interventional procedures have become established in cases in which guidance using standard fluoroscopy and/or US does not provide sufficient safety. The result is a minimally invasive therapeutic procedure—either alone or complementary to other treatments. Indeed, CT-guided interventional procedures may prepare or support subsequent procedures in a neo-adjuvant manner, especially in the case of fluid-type inflammatory lesions.

In the following, the typical therapeutic CT-guided intervention procedure is introduced and discussed. Daily routine work such as CT-guided biopsy is of equal importance, but is beyond the scope of this book. Similarly, the vast field of musculoskeletal interventions, including vertebro- and kypho-plasty (Hoffmann et al. 2007), CT-guided osteosyntheses (Iguchi et al. 2010; Sedat et al. 2010), and the implantation of pelvic C-clamps (Linsenmaier et al. 2003), is only touched upon herein.

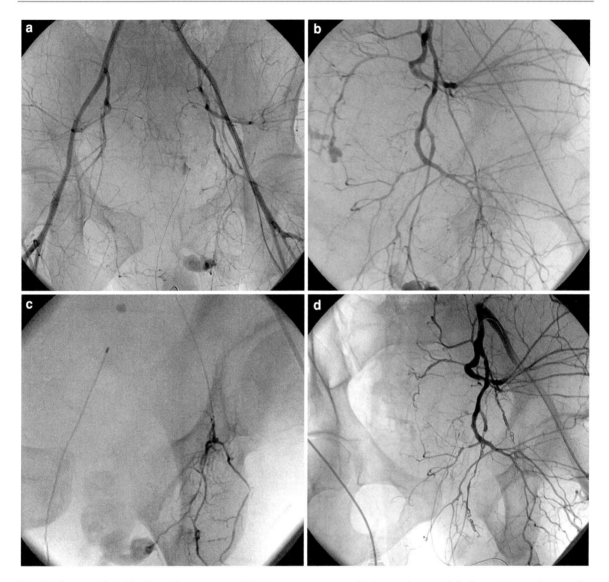

Fig. 11 Severe pelvic bleeding after trauma. **a** Pelvic overview angiogram for localization of the bleeding; **b** selective angiogram of the left internal iliac artery, depicting active bleeding and pseudoaneurysm formation after pelvic fracture; **c** super-selective angiogram; **d** final overview angiogram after super-selective embolization of several pubic side branches, which resulted in complete stoppage of the bleeding

3.1 Materials and Methods

Along with time-related effects, minimally invasive procedures can be visualized with CT in order to control the positioning of the introduced material. There are two different technical options. As each has its advantages, the combination of both is optimal. The most common is continuous CT-guidance (CT-fluoroscopy) with real-time visualization. The cardinal advantage is the complete real-time guidance of the intervention. The major disadvantage is the need for table correction to ensure continuous visualization of the tip of the introduced material. This increases the radiation dose not only to the patient, due to accumulated dose exposure time, but also to the operator, who must work either in or directly next to the beam. The alternative method is a step-by-step approach with the use of discontinuous CT-guidance. Technically, a single beam rotation is performed for every step, resulting in a defined number (usually three) of adjacent axial images. The major advantages are a reduced radiation dose to the patient, due to the reduced exposure time, and to the operator, who is able to distance to him- or herself from the beam during image acquisition. Also, as the result is essentially a mini-scan, the chance of including the tip of the working material is very high. The major weakness of discontinuous CT-guidance is that it will not include visualization of the actual material-positioning maneuvers.

3.1.1 Scan Parameters, Image Quality, and Dose Aspects

Once an initial CT has been performed for localization, the scanning parameters for CT-guidance should be modified so as to reduce the radiation dose while maintaining visualization of both the lesion and the catheter route. A protocol with fixed low-dose parameters of 100–120 kV, 10–100 mA, and 2.5- or 5-mm slice thickness is appropriate, depending on the patient's constitution and the localization (Lucey et al. 2007; Tsalafoutas et al. 2007; Yamao et al. 2010). Parameters of 120 kV, 60 mA, and a 5-mm slice thickness may serve as a useful standard for CT-guidance in the abdominal and pelvic regions. Planning- and control-scans should be limited to the region of interest. Commonly, the dose associated with the complete interventional procedure can be kept below that of a single diagnostic abdomino-pelvic scan.

3.1.2 Materials and Peri-interventional Medication

Two common techniques have been established for draining fluid collections. The first and more traditional one is to access the target using Seldinger's coaxial technique. A small needle (usually 18G) is positioned in the target and its position secured by a 0.035 guide wire. The access path is then enlarged with a dilator after which the drain is introduced using the wire as guidance. In the second technique, a completely manufactured drainage set, including a sharp stylet (mandrin) inside a coarse stabilization hollow trocar-needle, is used. This system is loaded with the hydrophilic pigtail catheter. Obviously, the two methods may be combined. Although there is no general recommendation, working with the drainage sets, on the basis of the more detailed discussion provided in the section on gastrointestinal ischemia (Sect. 2.9), is preferred by

many interventional radiologists. The drain should be size-adapted according to the viscosity of the fluid, usually resulting in ranges between 8 and 12F. The sideholes should be as large as possible. In cases of clotted material, instillation of 12,500 IU urokinase for targets of 1–3 cm or up to 100,000 IU for targets >10 cm, or repeated instillation of tissue plasminogen activator (4–6 mg tPA in 0.9% saline administered twice daily for 3 days) is likely to improve the results (Haaga et al. 2000; Beland et al. 2008). If systemic antibiosis was not previously initiated, at least a peri-interventional single-shot is recommended. According to the typical abdominal spectrum, a combination of ceftriaxone (e.g. Rocephin 500 mg) and metronidazole (e.g., Clont 400 mg) may be used. In the majority of cases, local anesthesia is sufficient although additional systemic pain relief is sometimes necessary or useful. For this, piritramide 15 mg (Dipidolor) is effective and can be administered as a 100-ml saline short-infusion. Additional information is provided in Sect. 4.1 (Peri-interventional Medication).

3.2 Patient Preparation

The operator should consider that the procedure has much in common with a surgical one. Thus, preparation is comparable and proper training of the staff accordingly is crucial. It is recommended that the team be well-rehearsed and able to provide quality assurance, especially with respect to time efforts, complications, and success rates, and to use these data for optimization purposes, with the goal of achieving best practice for the institution involved. Problems that occurred during the procedure should be subsequently discussed.

In most cases, a recent diagnostic standard contrast-enhanced CT (CECT) scan is available, which facilitates the planning of patient positioning and access route as well as recognition of the potential associated risks. However, the scan obtained prior to abscess drainage should include sufficient positive bowel contrast, which allows for sufficient differentiation between fluid-type formations and fluids within the intestine.

3.2.1 Indications and Contraindications

Typical indications include inflammatory and non-inflammatory capsulated fluid formations, e.g.,

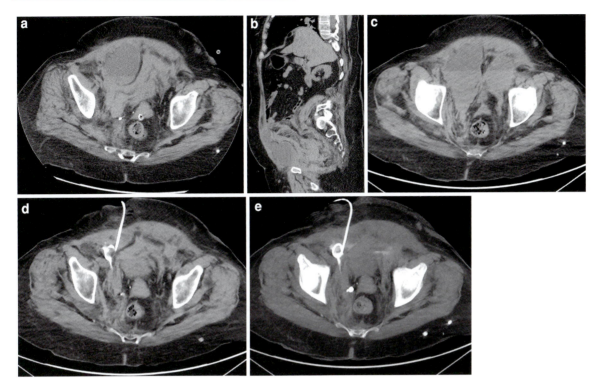

Fig. 12 Drainage of a hematoma. An 88-year-old female patient under anticoagulation therapy who complained of abdominal pain after blunt trauma (INR 4.3, pTT 66, Crea 2.4). NECT imaging revealed a large hematoma in the abdominal wall (**a, b**); 6-h control scan (**c**) with progredient hematoma followed by CT-guided draining, with immediate pain relief. The control scan (**d–e**) after injection of 20 ml 15% CM confirms both successful drainage and communication of the hematoma with the extraperitoneal space (image **e** as MIP). As the patient had renal failure, these scans were obtained without CM. The total dose-length product (DLP) was 890 mGy cm (95% location and control scan, 5% CT-guidance)

capsulated abscesses in the abdominal or pelvic region, hematoma (Fig. 12) including subcapsular hematomas of the liver and spleen, seroma, bilioma, urinoma (Fig. 13), ureteral leakage, and insufficiency of an intestinal anastomosis, as well as complications following surgical procedures such as pancreatic pseudocysts/abscesses (Fig. 14) (Gervais et al. 2004; Liu et al. 2009; Singh et al. 2006; Men et al. 2002). As material is preserved during the procedure, there is a certain degree of overlap with diagnostic procedures. Less common applications are the drainage of free fluids, the direct relaxation of gall bladder empyema, removal of fluid collections following endovascular aortic repair (EVAR) (Fig. 15), and the treatment of ano-rectal abscess formations (Fig. 16), severe prostatitis (Fig. 17), tubo-ovarian collections, and complex cases of diverticulitis (Fig. 18) (Kirat et al. 2011; Levenson et al. 2009). Percutaneous image-guided musculoskeletal drainage is also clinically useful and safe. It is highly effective for draining fluid collections involving muscle alone; however, skeletal infection is associated with a higher risk of procedural failure (Cronin et al. 2011).

Although for some indications there may be a need for immediate drainage, in most cases the indication should be discussed interdisciplinarily and finally supported by the attending physician or the respective clinician in charge.

As the risk of needle aspiration is nearly the same as that in drainage placement (exceptions are described below) but without the possibility to provide support therapy over several days, catheter drainage is recommended in nearly every case, particularly if the aspirated material is likely to be purulent or if the patient demonstrates signs of severe systemic inflammation. Needle aspiration is usually performed when it cannot be determined with certainty whether fluid formations, e.g., in the

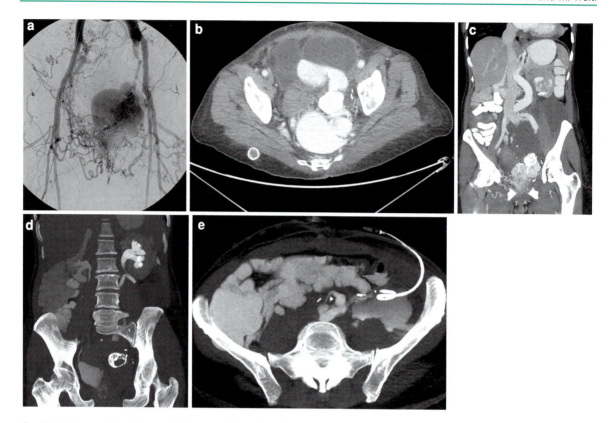

Fig. 13 Drainage of a urinoma. A 52-year-old female patient suffering from an enormous iliac arteriovenous fistula (**a**, angiography), recurrent after surgical treatment (**b, c**, diagnostic CT in portal-venous phase), developed a large urinoma (**b, c**). In urographic phase, dilatation of the left ureter and pelvis is demonstrated (**d**, MIP). Immediately after introduction of the drain, the urinoma filled with the CM administered for diagnostic scans. Communication with the left ureter is shown (**e**). The DLP was 44.5 mGy cm for the CT-guidance and 420 mGy cm for the control scan

pancreas, are infected or not (Fig. 14) and when the access route is very limited. Particularly if the patient is unable to cooperate, anesthesiologic support should be provided. Contraindications are rare but include hollow-organ perforation, acute peritonitis, and uncontrollable coagulopathy. Depending on the severity of the case, there are no further absolute contraindications.

3.2.2 Preoperative Interview

For standard procedures, the patient must provide written, informed consent after an adequate decision time. In the rare case of intervention-induced complications, legal issues may arise, particularly when documentation is incomplete.

In an emergency or in situations in which the patient is not able to provide consent, the indication and the rational basis for the intervention have to be documented in detail in the patient's record or at least in the physician's report. The typical risks of this minimally invasive intervention are to be described. These do not differ from corresponding, alternative surgical procedures but occur less commonly. It is necessary to note pre-interventional medications, especially those with effects on blood coagulation (heparin, warfarin, and thrombocyte-aggregation inhibitors). The presence of ascites may also increase the risk of bleeding. The decision for anesthesiological support should be made on the basis of clinical parameters and especially the patient interview.

3.2.3 Laboratory Values

Blood-parameter results should not be older than 24 h and the same tests are run as for comparable surgical procedures. Depending on urgency, basal TSH levels should be assessed in patients older than 40 years or

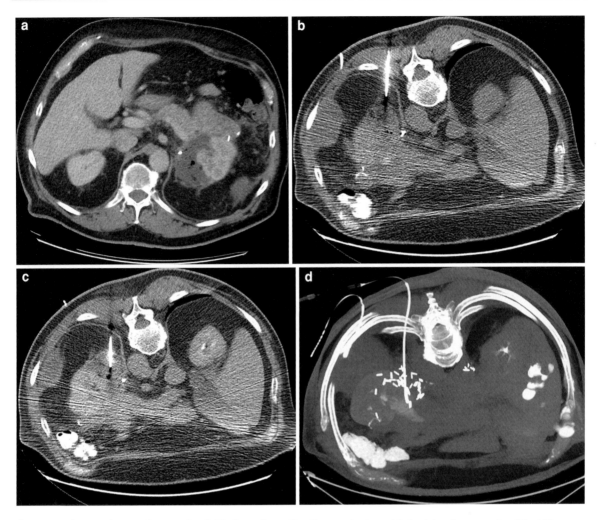

Fig. 14 Drainage of a peripancreatic fluid formation of unclear origin. A 70-year-old male patient suffering from Cushin's disease developed an inflammatory fluid formation after resection of the left adrenal gland and the pancreatic tail. The diagnostic scan showed air in the formation (**a**). Communication with the injured upper pole of the kidney was proven during CT-guided intervention (**b, c**) and the control scan (**d**). A second drain was introduced into a disjunct parasplenic abscess. Total DLP was 2430 mGy cm, including diagnostic multiphase scans, 245 mGy cm for CT-guidance

with a history of thyroid pathology. The thrombocytic count should be $>70,000/mm^3$, PTT <50 s, and the Quick value $>50\%$. Warfarin therapy should be temporarily replaced by heparin. If these conditions are not provided, appropriate additional preparations, including blood cross-matching, thrombocyte concentrates, FFP, and anesthesiological assistance, are necessary.

3.3   Interventional CT Procedure

The major points can be briefly summarized as a checklist of tips and tricks:

- Prepare optimally before the intervention; including choice of access route and patient positioning.
- Approach CT-interventions just as you would a surgical setting in the operating room.
- Ensure that the staff is well-trained.
- Protect yourself, the staff, and the patient against radiation exposure.
- Consider gravitation effects and patient comfort during and after the intervention.
- Use drainage sets whenever possible, choosing the appropriate size.
- Inject 20 ml CM i.v. 15 min prior to patient positioning if urogenital tract contrast is useful.

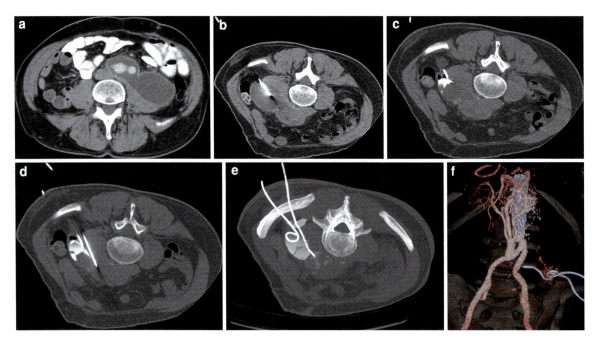

Fig. 15 Drainage of surrounding fluids, detected during a 7-year follow-up after complex EVAR. A 60-year-old male showed large fluid collections surrounding arterial iliac grafts, extending onto the psoas muscle. Diagnostic scan (**a**) reveals large fluid collections. Introduction of the first drainage set (**b**). The injection of 10 ml of 15% CM demonstrated septation of the liquids (**c**). Finally, a second drain was placed closer to the iliac prosthesis (**d**). Control scan after careful injection of 20 ml of 15% CM in the second drain (**e**, MIP). Volume-rendering of the CECT control scan shows the complex situs after EVAR and octopus-grafting (**f**). Fluoroscopy time was 35 s, DLP 203 mGy cm. Graft-versus-host reaction was identified as the underlying pathological condition

- Restrict CM administration to situations in which it is truly needed.
- Consider the patient's breathing; limit actions to identical respiratory status (mostly expiration).
- Confirm correct position before releasing the pigtail.
- Confirm samples, assure that they appear macroscopically useful
- Perform a control scan after draining the fluid by refilling with 15% CM to confirm anatomical relationships.
- Adequately secure the catheter.
- Provide quality assurance (QA).
- Provide antibiosis.

3.3.1 Standard Procedure

For most patients, a recent diagnostic abdominal and pelvic CECT-scan is available. If not, it should be performed directly before the intervention. Patient positioning depends on the best access route. As the supine position is most comfortable for the patient both during the procedure and afterwards, with the positioned catheter material, it should be given preference. If prone positioning is inevitable, the skin entry point should be located as laterally as possible since this maximizes patient comfort and prevents bending of the drain in supine position. Gravitation might influence secondary drainage effects and should be accounted for, typically by using the most caudal entry point that is safely reasonable. The patient's RR interval and pulse should be monitored. Appropriate i.v. access for medications and contrast material should be provided.

The patient and physician should be prepared according to common operating-room hygiene guidelines. An appropriate volume (approximately as much as the total volume of the fluid formation) of sterile solution containing 15% CM and 85% NaCl is prepared. In case of potential urogenital-tract crossing, 20 ml CM should be administered (if possible at least 15 min prior to intervention) for sufficient contrast during the procedure. When the procedure is not

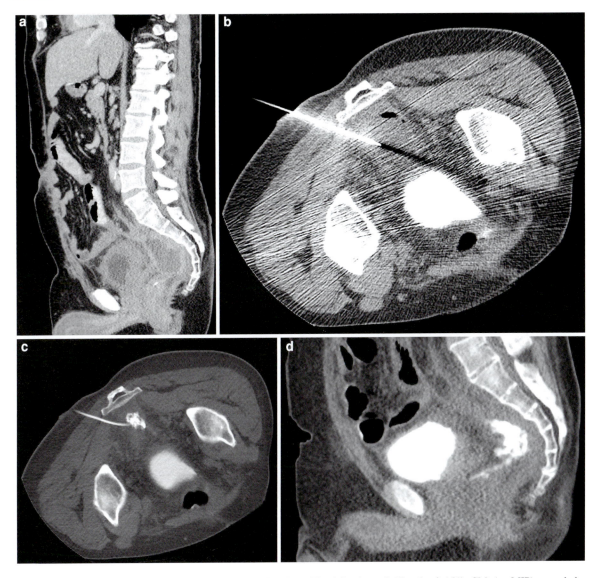

Fig. 16 Drainage of a pararectal abscess. A 51-year-old male developed a presacral abscess after resection of the rectum, resulting in a Hartmann's stump (**a**, diagnostic scan). Low-dose CTguidance (with 30 mA fixed) of drainage introduction (**b**). The injection of 20 ml of 15% CM (**c**, MIP) revealed a fistulation/insufficiency of the stump (**d**). Fluoroscopy time was 14 s, DLP 115 mGy cm

directly followed by a diagnostic scan, a location scan is required. NECT is preferable, as additional unexpected CM administration may be required. A low-dose NECT scan combined with the diagnostic scan is mostly sufficient. About half of the local anesthetic is injected at the site where the maximum pain is expected, e.g., the liver capsule and periosteum. The needle is then retracted slowly, while a quarter of the anesthetic is injected. The rest is administered sub-/intracutaneously. Skin disinfection is then repeated. If space for the accession path is very limited, sterile saline can be injected to expand the access route by shifting structures and organs. This method is commonly used when dorsally accessing the retroperitoneum between the spine and kidney in lean patients and for potential intestinal shifting.

A small incision in the skin is made and a mounted drainage catheter set is then positioned into the fluid formation under CT-guidance. The patient's breathing position is monitored visually. The drainage set

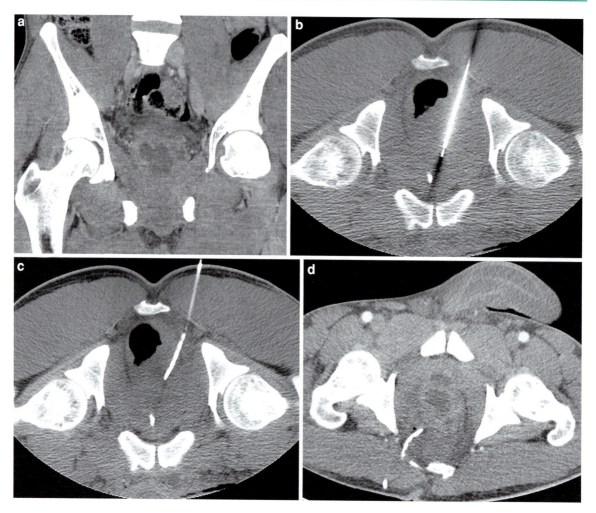

Fig. 17 Drainage of a prostatic abscess. A 35-year-old male with prostatitis presented with an extremely painful intracapsular abscess of the prostate gland (**a**, diagnostic CECT scan with 100-s delay). Introduction of the drain via the parasacral route (**b**, **c**) allowed asservation of pus (final drainage position not shown). However, a control scan one day after intervention (**d**) revealed dislocation of the drainage as the reason for unsuccessful attempts of drainage flushing on the ward

should be moved only during expiration. Additionally, make use of standardized breathing commands in order to benefit from the corresponding organ movements. If organ interfaces such as the liver capsule and pleural space are crossed, fast and confident insertion during the breath-hold is required. If critical structures, which cannot be shifted, are a potential obstacle, a minimal but safe distance has to be secured. A CECT scan adapted to the region of interest is then performed (adapt scan range, CM amount, and phase; consider use of a double-bolus injection for sufficient contrast in arterial and venous vessels). In most cases, this is sufficient for safe

adaption of a farther-removed pathway. Remove the stylet and check the proper positioning of the drain. If it is not properly secured, e.g., when the liquids are too viscous, 1 or 2 ml of the 15% CM solution should be injected. The distribution will allow assessment of the CM's position with respect to the target. If necessary, the complete drainage set has to be re-positioned after the stylet has been reintroduced. Once the target is reached, the drain is released by both sliding the pigtail forward and holding the trocar-stabilization at its position. Finally remove the stabilization, retrieve the samples, and drain the liquids. Refill the target with 15% CM up to the drained

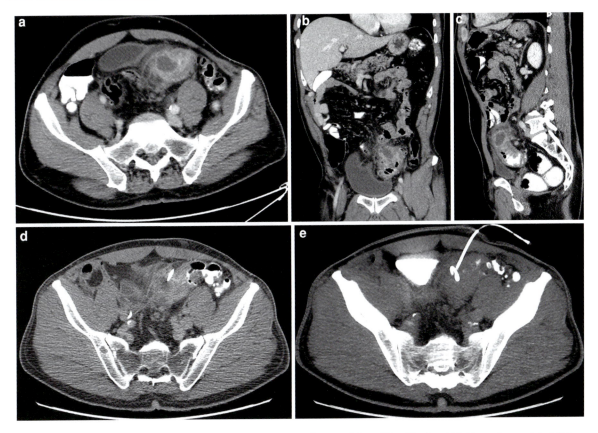

Fig. 18 Drainage of a parasigmoidal abscess caused by diverticulitis. A 56-year-old male with diverticulitis. Diagnostic scan (**a–c**), CT-guidance (**d**), and final position of the drain (**e**, MIP). After CT-intervention, the patient's leukocyte count decreased from 15 to 10 g/l and his C-reactive protein fell from 13 to 7 mg/dl in 3 days, resulting in optimized conditions for definitive surgical treatment

amount. As the intervention may be performed without bowel enhancement (unlike the diagnostic scan), this simple procedure may often yield valuable additional information, particularly regarding the communication of septated or spatially disjunct formations, exact size and position, potential fistulation to neighboring organs, or leakage of an anastomosis. After the 15% CM solution has been aspirated, repeated saline washes will almost always provide clear visualization of the target. A documentary control scan limited to the region of interest is advisable. In cases of large fluid collections, the positioning of two drains, an upper and a lower one with respect to the gravitational forces resulting from the patient's anticipated position when he or she is returned to the ward, is expedient. This strategy allows for further effective irrigation with or without additional intraluminal antibiotic treatment.

3.3.2 Complex Procedures

Sometimes, CT-intervention will be hampered by factors such as surrounding organs, difficult location, and highly viscous content, all of which render fluid collections seemingly inaccessible. In these cases, alternatives include transgluteal, transvaginal, and transrectal approaches (Maher et al. 2004; Harisinghani et al. 2003). In addition to different patient positioning or angulation of the gantry. Unfortunately, with some devices CT-guidance with tilted gantries is not possible. The most common trick is the injection of fluids to expand the access route (hydrodissection (Arellano et al. 2011)) or to initially install 15% CM through a 21G or 22G needle in order to identify alternative routes according to the distribution of the CM. If these measures are not successful, there are two options: (a) the collection or abscess is deemed unsuitable for percutaneous abscess drainage and the case is referred back to the surgeon, or (b) the intervening organ can be traversed with a catheter (Gee et al. 2010). The latter is particularly relevant for the liver and is considered to be relatively safe as a last resort. It is also appropriate for patients suffering from Crohn's disease in which there are interloop abscesses. In these cases, a 20G needle is used to aspirate the fluid, transgressing the intervening bowel in order to cleanse the surgical field prior to surgery (Maher et al. 2004). This may be combined with the subsequent injection of 15% CM as described for screening alternative access routes.

3.3.3 Postprocedure Care

The procedure is completed by adequate and comfortable but secure external fixation of the catheter. Interventional procedures must include an immediate report with information about the procedure. Relevant information must reach the referring physician and the ward in time to ensure proper handling of the drain when the patient is on the ward. Success rates of $\geq 95\%$ and a sufficient single therapeutic catheter procedure, without subsequent surgery, is achieved in 75% of the cases when established protocols are strictly followed (Gee et al. 2010).

3.4 Overlaps of Fluoroscopic- and CT-Guided Interventions

The fast-paced developments in interventional techniques have resulted in a certain degree of overlap between 2D-fluoroscopic and CT-guided procedures. Typical examples are CT-guided balloon occlusion of the aorta and other large arterial vessels in cases of severe trauma, in order to temporarily stop excessive blood loss and gain time until surgical treatment (Linsenmaier et al. 2003; Rieger et al. 1999). As with the growing acceptance of EVAR, an increasing number of institutions have adopted CT-guided occlusion of type II endoleaks and CT-controlled mounting of pelvic C-clamps (Linsenmaier et al. 2003).

Furthermore, percutaneous cholecystostomy is a minimally invasive procedure to provide gallbladder decompression, often in critically ill patient populations. Indications for this procedure include severe cholecystitis, gallbladder perforation, malignant obstruction, percutaneous biliary-stone removal, and

biliary-duct drainage. The same access may also be used for additional procedures, such as cholangiograms, gallstone dissolution, and lithotripsy. A transhepatic route is preferred in cases of large amounts of ascites and bowel interposition, offering the advantage of increased catheter stability, whereas the transperitoneal route is preferred in settings of coagulopathy and liver disease. The overall technical success rate for percutaneous cholecystostomy is >95%. Clinical improvement is achieved in 56–93% of patients. Complications occur in 3–13% and are mainly acute and minor. Of these, major complications such as bile peritonitis, significant hemorrhage, and hemo-/pneumothorax affect <5% of patients. However, sepsis and 30-day mortality rates up to 25% are usually related to underlying morbidities in critically ill patients. Catheters may be removed once the fistula track has matured (Ginat and Saad 2008).

4 Percutaneuous Transhepatic Cholangiography and Biliary Drainage

Over the past few decades, percutaneous transhepatic cholangiography with biliary drainage (PTBD) has become an established method for the effective therapy of biliary obstruction. The procedure contributes mainly by relieving patients' symptoms and restoring serum biochemistry to nearly normal constellations. Moreover, for the majority of patients with malignant causes for the obstruction, these methods improve the clinical condition thus allowing surgical resection or the administration of palliative chemotherapy or radiotherapy, resulting in improvement in the quality of life (Tapping et al. 2011). Since other important procedures such as transhepatic porto-systemic (stent) shunting (TIPS, TIPSS) are seldom indicated in emergency conditions, they are beyond the scope of this book.

4.1 Materials and Methods

4.1.1 Guidance Methods
The biliary tree is usually accessed under fluoroscopic guidance. However, especially for the left branches (Fig. 19), CT- (Kuhn et al. 2010) and US-guided (Saad 2008) access are alternative options. In particular,

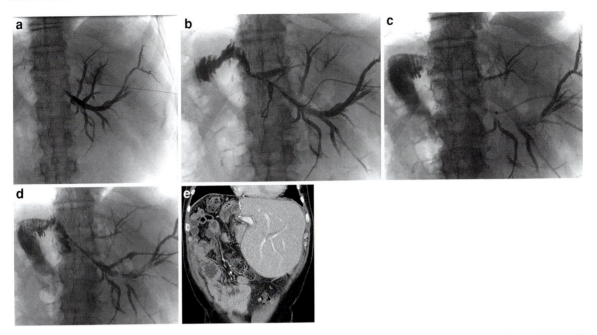

Fig. 19 Access from the left side in PTBD. A 65-year-old male with cholangiocellular carcinoma who underwent hemi-hepatectomy of the right lobe presented with recurrent cholangitis. Due to secondary hypertrophy of the left lobe, access was chosen comparable to the right side access in the 10th intercostal space after localization with US (**a**, US not shown). Further filling of the bile system shows central constriction with resulting stenosis (**b**). After dilation with a 8/40-mm balloon catheter (not shown), a 7.5F pigtail was positioned (**c, d**). CECT in portal-venous phase demonstrates the post-interventional situation after catheter removal (**e**)

these alternatives are sometimes helpful for an initial filling of the bile system followed by a more peripheral access for the proper PTBD procedure (Saad 2008).

4.1.2 Parameters, Image Quality, and Dose

The anticipated clinical benefits exceed all anticipated procedural risks, including radiation exposure. For PTBD, the mean fluoroscopy time is around 20 min (Kuhn et al. 2010). Unfortunately, this is a poor estimate of the patient's dose and the peak skin dose is usually not available as a real-time measure (Miller et al. 2010). In contrast, the kerma-area product (=dose-area product) is easily determined. Although not ideal, it has been applied for this purpose as it provides a measure of the patient entry dose. While this differs sometimes enormously depending on the clinical setting, one may consider the kerma of one fluoroscopic image shot equal to 30 s of fluoroscopy time with a pulse rate of 10/s, as a rule of thumb.

Standard recommendations (Miller et al. 2010) include:

- Collimation should be appropriate to the imaging task to limit the size of the irradiated area.
- The image receptor should be positioned as close as reasonably possible to the patient and the distance between the patient and the X-ray tube maximized.
- The patient's arms and as many bones as possible should be positioned outside the radiation field.
- Electronic magnification modes and high-dose-rate modes should be used only when necessary.
- Use the lowest fluoroscopic dose/pulse rate that is clinically acceptable.
- In many cases last image holds or fluoroscopy loops are sufficient for documentation. Additional full dose images/ series should be limited to situations with estimated relevant diagnostic gain.
- Angulation/rotation of the beam may distribute the skin dose over a larger area.
- Dose parameters must be documented.

- Anticipated clinical benefits versus radiation risk should be reconsidered during the procedure.

4.1.3 Peri-Interventional Medication

For patients, the procedure is most comfortable under conscious sedation, following slow intravenous administration of 1–5 mg midazolam (e.g., Dormicum) and with supporting systemic pain relief, in standard interventions typically through the rapid administration of half of a 15-mg piritramide (Dipidolor) short infusion at the beginning, slow infusion of another quarter during the intervention, and ongoing slow infusion of the remaining quarter in the post-interventional phase. For complex procedures, up to 1 mg alfentanil (e.g., Rapifen), administered in 0.25 mg steps, may be supportive at painful events such as the dilatation of strictures, but also more precarious.

Once the access route is planned, a local-anesthesia needle is positioned on the liver capsule. The risk of transgressing the pleural space can be minimized by assuring breath-hold conditions with a normal inspiration level, if possible. The anesthetic (e.g., 10–20 ml of 1–2% lidocaine or carbocaine without adrenaline) is injected slowly on the liver capsule in the breath-hold phase and then sub-/intracutaneously during withdrawal of the needle under normal patient breathing.

Pre-procedural broad-spectrum antibiotic prophylaxis with a combination of 2 g ceftriaxone i.v. and 400 mg metronidazole per os (e.g., Rocephin and Clont) is given to all patients undergoing biliary drainage because transient bacteremia commonly occurs during the procedure, even in the absence of signs or symptoms of infection (Covey and Brown 2008). In the case of biliary stenting, antibiotics should be continued for 48 h (Tapping et al. 2011). Alternatively oral antibiosis is also sufficient with ciprofloxacin 500 mg/day per os for 10 days (e.g., Ciprobay) (Pedicini et al. 2010).

Although there is no standard recommendation, nausea or vomiting may be suppressed with 4–8 mg ondansetron hydrochloride i.v. (e.g., Zofran) if necessary.

4.2 Preparation

Whenever possible patients should abstain from oral intake (nil per os) or be on a clear liquid diet for at least 4 h before the procedure. Patients should be well hydrated and have working venous access for sedation and antibiotic prophylaxis (Covey and Brown 2008). Constant monitoring with pulse oximetry and blood pressure measurements is an indispensable standard. Cross-sectional imaging allows for more detailed planning of the procedure, particularly the accession route(s), and is therefore recommended.

4.2.1 Indications and Contraindications

Biliary obstruction can have benign or malignant causes. Common emergencies in acute biliary conditions are acute cholecystitis, emphysematous cholecystitis, gangrenous cholecystitis, perforation, Mirizzi's syndrome, percutaneous cholecystostomy, and acute cholangitis (Menu and Vuillerme 2002). Other typical examples of benign obstruction are often iatrogenic, including during endoscopic retrograde chlangiopancreatography (ERCP), sphincterotomy, and liver or pancreatic surgery with or without bilioenteric bypass. Anastomotic strictures (Fig. 19) or postoperative bile leaks, requiring biliary drainage to divert bile from the leaking site (Fig. 20), may develop as well. Occasionally, colonized gallstones or an enteric fistula may result in cholangitis. Malignant obstruction is commonly due to pancreatic carcinoma, cholangiocarcinoma including Klatskin's cancer (Fig. 21), metastatic disease, gall bladder carcinoma, hepatocellular carcinoma, lymphoma, and advanced gastric or duodenal cancer (Covey and Brown 2008). Obstructing tumors are often not crossed, at least initially. Instead, a PTBD with external drainage is initially provided followed by an interdisciplinary decision regarding further therapy (Tapping et al. 2011). Besides these indications, PTBD may also be necessary in traumatic injury of the bile system and the post-traumatic development of bilioma (Fig. 22).

Clinical jaundice, with a serum bilirubin >3 mg%, is common. Although not necessarily in proportion to the serum bilirubin level and bile acid profile, pruritus, alteration in food taste, and anorexia are typical symptoms in these patients (Covey and Brown 2008). PTBD relieves jaundice and sepsis and decreases the risk of hepato-renal failure, providing an alternative to ERCP, which may be unsuccessful due to anatomic variations or technical difficulty, especially following surgery. In this case, PTBD sometimes allows for positioning of a stiff 0.035 guide wire for subsequent ERCP. Even when both the right and the left hepatic

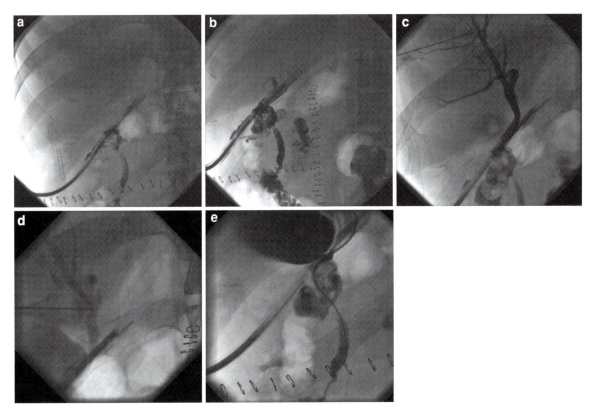

Fig. 20 Post-operative leakage of the common bile duct (CBD). A 53-year-old male patient suffering from recurrent liposarcoma after multiple surgical procedures presented with biliary leakage of the CDB. Injection of CM using the postoperative drain shows communication with the bile system (**a**, **b**). PTBD with initial filling (**c**) and secondary puncture for accessing the CBD, with the typical compression of the duct as specific proof of correct positioning (**d**). Placement of a 6F-pigtail (**e**) in the duodenum (final position not shown)

ducts are obstructed due to a hilar lesion, draining one side will relieve jaundice and pruritus in most cases. However, if this is clinically unsuccessful, the other side may also need to be drained (Tapping et al. 2011; Covey and Brown 2008).

4.2.2 Preoperative Interview

In addition to the issues discussed in Sect. 3.2.2, the interview should cover the risk of biliary rupture and leakage. For stenting in patients with a normal life expectancy, it should be emphasized that the likelihood of re-intervention is high. A specific risk stratification score, based on values for ascites, albumin, WBC count, C-reactive protein, hemoglobin, urea, bilirubin, and alanine transaminase, may be used to estimate the individual risk for a specific patient (Tapping et al. 2011).

4.2.3 Laboratory Values

In addition to the values described in Sect. 3.2.3, the pre-interventional laboratory values should include direct and indirect bilirubin, urobilinogen, γ-glutamyl transpeptidase, alanine transaminase, aspartate aminotransferase, and alkaline phosphatase.

4.3 PTBD Procedure

Biliary obstruction is divided into "low" and "high" bile duct obstruction. Low bile duct obstruction occurs below the usual insertion site of the cystic duct. In these cases, complete drainage of the entire biliary tree can be accomplished by a single, well-placed catheter or stent because the obstruction is below the confluence of the right and left bile ducts.

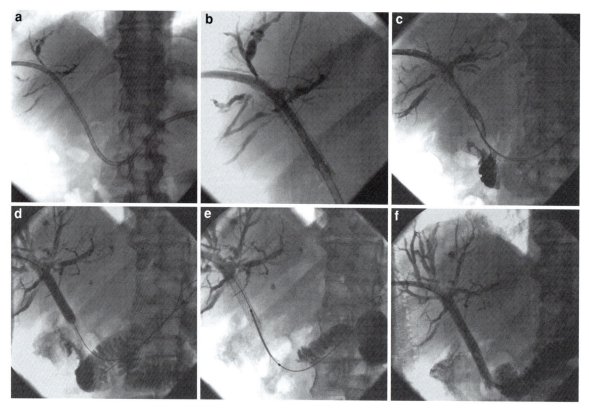

Fig. 21 Re-stenting of the CBD. A 60-year-old male patient suffering from Klatskin tumor, initially graded as Bismuth III (*right* lobe, inoperable due to metastasis and infiltration of the portal vein) with recurrent cholangitis following a prior stenting procedure of the right hepatic duct and the CBD 5 months earlier. A placed Münchner drainage was used to access the system (**a**) and for initial filling of the bile system, confirming central in-stent stenosis (**b**). A stiff 0.035 wire was positioned (**c**) followed by balloon dilatation (**d**) and the positioning of an overlapping second stent in the CBD (**e**). This restored centripetal bile flow into the duodenum (**f**)

Low bile duct obstruction is often treated endoscopically (Covey and Brown 2008).

High bile duct obstruction occurs above the cystic duct insertion. According to Bismuth and Corlette, carcinomas of the hepatic confluence are classified as type I (tumors involve the common hepatic duct, but not the confluence of the right and left hepatic ducts), type II (obstruction of the primary confluence), and type III (involves either the right or left secondary confluence). Some authors have described a type IV, in which there is involvement of the secondary confluences on the right or left sides. When bile segments are functionally isolated (e.g., missing opacification of the isolated system or ducts opacify with contrast during cholangiography but do not drain), a single drainage catheter cannot effectively drain the entire biliary tree (Covey and Brown 2008). Instead, high bile duct obstruction is best approached

percutaneously, because a specific duct can be targeted to maximize the drainage of functional parenchyma, as determined based on pre-procedure imaging. This is most commonly achieved from the right side, since it is more accessible and the volume of the right liver is usually larger. However, when there is atrophy or compromise of the portal vein on the right side, suspected segmental isolation of the right-sided ducts, and in patients with ascites, a left-sided approach is usually preferable. Cultures of bile obtained at the time of drainage should be routinely sent in patients with fever, bilioenteric anastomosis or sphincterotomy, previous ERCP, or an indwelling stent or catheter (Covey and Brown 2008).

4.3.1 Standard Procedure

The standard approach is to access the right liver lobe from the 10th or 11th intercostal space in the

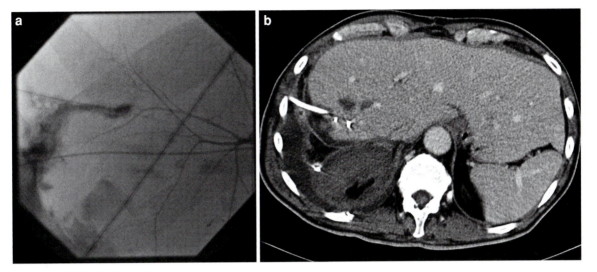

Fig. 22 Drainage of post-traumatic bilioma. A 62-year-old male polytrauma patient with biliary leakage following traumatic liver rupture of the right lobe, classified as a Moore IV lesion. Percutaneous transhepatic cholangiography (**a**) proves the biliary leak as well as undisturbed centripetal flow. CT performed after fluoroscopically controlled insertion of a 6.5F-pigtail demonstrates the cranial part of the liver rupture, pleural effusion with thoracic drainage, subhepatic bilioma, and a dorsal suprarenal hematoma in the subphrenic space (**b**)

midaxillary line or the left side from three finger breadths below the xyphoid (Kuhn et al. 2010; Covey and Brown 2008). Access from the right side usually means a lower radiation dose for the operator whereas entrance from the left side often implies a less painful procedure for the patient (Saad 2008). As modern imaging techniques allow planning of the approach based on the targeted duct, which is commonly the most dilated duct in the periphery, it is often useful to adapt the classical access routes (Covey and Brown 2008). The operator should study the course of the bile duct to determine whether it will adequately drain the biliary system and whether its course is straightforward with respect to the common hepatic duct, particularly if the access will be utilized for subsequent manipulation (stent placement, balloon dilation, stone extraction, and especially choledochoscopy) (Saad 2008; Covey and Brown 2008).

Once the site for dermatotomy is chosen, it is prepped, draped, and anesthetized. A 22G or 21G double-walled needle such as the Chiba is advanced over the cranial border of the rib into the liver parenchyma. With the stylet removed, contrast may be gingerly injected while the needle is retracted until a bile duct is opacified. During this search, diluted CM may be used to reduce the irritating contrast of paradepots. If the target duct is opacified, and the

puncture is peripheral, it may be used for drainage. Peripheral access is preferred because the risks of bleeding and inadequate drainage are higher with a central access. If, however, a central duct is opacified, undiluted contrast is injected to opacify the peripheral ducts, allowing for a more suitable access site to be punctured (Covey and Brown 2008).

For this purpose, rotation of the beam is sometimes crucial for navigation. As an example for vertical bile duct target segments, if, compared to the target, the needle moves relatively to the right in left anterior oblique projections, the duct is located anterior to it. The needle position is corrected until the tool tip again projects over the bile duct segment. If the correct position is reached, which is often clearly visible due to deformation and movement of the duct wall opposite the entry site (Fig. 20), the 0.018 wire can be introduced and directed to more central areas as far as possible (Saad 2008). If not, returning to anteroposterior projections will provide further information regarding whether the correction was insufficient or excessive. This process may be iteratively repeated. However, maximum benefit from this method is obtained when the beam rotation is perpendicular to the target. If necessary, the beam rotation axis should be adapted correspondingly. For horizontal targets, the principle may be transferred to cranio-caudal beam-tilting, with a corresponding relative movement of the needle in the cranio-caudal direction.

Following a correct final positioning, the needle is removed and replaced with an Accustick system (Boston Scientific, Natick, MA). This is a graded dilator/introducer system with an inner metal stiffener and a 2F or 3F taper to an outer dilator measuring 6.5F, allowing 0.035 guide wires (and catheters up to 4F) to be introduced and positioned in the small bowel, if possible. As the metal stiffener is designed to provide transhepatic support, its tip should be placed just before the curvature of the access wire (Saad 2008; Covey and Brown 2008).

Through the larger system, a directional catheter is inserted and advanced over a preferably hydrophilic wire beyond the obstruction and into the small bowel. The catheter can then be exchanged over a stiffer wire (e.g., Amplatz) for a multi-sidehole drainage catheter (e.g., 8F Flexima, Boston Scientific with two series of sideholes separated by a blind segment or a continuously holed 8F–12F Münchener drainage-set, Pflugbeil). These catheters are referred to as "internal–external" catheters because bile can drain externally into a bag as well as internally into the small bowel. If a catheter cannot be advanced beyond the obstruction into the small bowel, an obligatory external drainage catheter should be placed (Kuhn et al. 2010; Covey and Brown 2008; Pedicini et al. 2010).

4.3.1.1 Complex Procedure

Percutaneous drainage of a non-dilated biliary tree can be technically challenging. Usually, this is the case in the setting of an orthotopic liver transplant, postoperative bile leak, or primary sclerosing cholangitis. When a T-tube is present, one operator can inject contrast into the T-tube to opacify and distend the intrahepatic bile ducts while a second operator punctures the opacified target duct. A bile leak may result in a biloma that requires percutaneous drainage. Once the biloma resulting from a leak has been drained, injection of the catheter may result in opacification of the intrahepatic duct. In this case, the duct can be cannulated through the biloma, converting the biloma drainage catheter to a biliary drainage catheter, or the drainage catheter can at least be used to opacify the intrahepatic ducts for subsequent standard access (Covey and Brown 2008).

Especially prior to stenting, the PTBD tract may additionally provide access for biopsy forceps through a long sheath of at least 8F size (Tapping et al. 2011). When stenting is performed, self-expanding uncovered metal stents such as Wallstent (Boston Scientific) or Nitinella (Ella CS, Hradec Kralove, Czech Republic) are preferable. The distal end of the stent is placed across the ampulla (initial dilatation is usually without additional benefit (Tapping et al. 2011)), as this assures maximum biliary drainage and reduces the risk of post-procedure cholangitis. A covering 8F drain is left along the PTBD track following stent placement for 48 h, then removed (Tapping et al. 2011). Covered metal stents are also available but their use is limited due to stent migration, occlusion of side branches, including cystic or pancreatic ducts, causing cholecystitis and pancreatitis, respectively (Tapping et al. 2011). Since most metallic stents cannot be easily removed, surgeons often prefer that a metallic stent not be placed in patients who are candidates for resection (Covey and Brown 2008).

In situations in which there is already a PTBD access but a second entry is necessary because of segmental bile duct isolation, the snare-technique is a good option as it reduces additional time efforts and risks. If possible, a 4F or 5F catheter over a 0.035-inch guide wire may be used to catheterize the isolated segment transhepatically. An 8- to 10-mm diameter nitinol snare is deployed and is used as a target in gun-sight technique (that is, a strong perpendicular view to the open part of the snare). A 21G needle is then passed, which provides a view along the long axis of the needle under fluoroscopy. Once the needle has been fluoroscopically confirmed in multiple oblique views to have passed through the snare, the gooseneck snare is reduced/closed around the needle. A 0.018-inch wire is passed through the captured 21G needle, which is then withdrawn, unsheathing the wire that is then captured by the snare. The snare is pulled, which causes the wire to be pulled centrally from the peripheral duct access to the central biliary system (Saad 2008).

In cases of bile leakage, interventional treatment with an occlusion balloon, which in one study was inflated for a mean of 18 days, showed promising results with success rates of up to 100%. The technique involves the insertion of two guides into the same intrahepatic biliary duct. Over a first guide, a standard occlusion balloon catheter is inserted, positioned above the biliary leak, then inflated, and the inflation held using a high-pressure stopcock. Finally, a drainage catheter is inserted over the second guide wire and positioned above the occlusion balloon (Pedicini et al. 2010).

4.4 Post Procedure Care, Results and Complications

Typical complications particularly include pneumothorax, bleeding, infection, and bile leak. Since the hepatic artery, portal vein, and bile duct travel side by side within portal triads, it is not uncommon for blood to enter the bile duct during catheter exchanges, resulting in transient hemobilia. New or persistent hemobilia after exchange is often due to a sidehole of the catheter becoming positioned in an adjacent branch of the portal or hepatic vein and can be corrected simply by repositioning the catheter. Persistent venous bleeding from the tract may require upsizing of the catheter to tamponade the bleeding site. When a patient develops bleeding 1–2 weeks or more after biliary drainage, or pulsatile bleeding with sudden onset, particularly when there is not only hemobilia but also bleeding around the catheter, arterial injury should be suspected and the patient should undergo hepatic angiography followed by embolization of the offending arterial branch (Covey and Brown 2008).

For ERCP, the complication rate is around 5–10% and the procedure mortality rate up to 1% (Tapping et al. 2011). PTBD-related death is 0.6–5.6%, mainly due to sepsis and pneumonia. The in-hospital mortality of 13–20% is usually caused by the underlying disease (Tapping et al. 2011; van Delden and Lameris 2008). Predictors for stent failure and re-stenting are reportedly a diagnosis of cholangiocarcinoma, a lesion in the distal common bile duct, a high bilirubin, high urea and high WBC count, and postprocedure cholangitis (Tapping et al. 2011). Stents occasionally block due to either biliary sludge or tumor recurrence, resulting in recurrent jaundice. Recurrent tumor growth can be through the interstices of the stent or due to overgrowth of the proximal or distal ends. PTBD can be repeated with coaxial metal stent placement with or without balloon dilatation, as appropriate (Tapping et al. 2011). The technical success of PTBD is reported to be >90% (80% in non-dilated bile ducts (Kuhn et al. 2010)) and clinical success >75% in all major series (Tapping et al. 2011; van Delden and Lameris 2008).

PTBD and stenting with metallic stents has an overall complication rate of 8–42%, with early complications ranging from 10 to 17%. Recurrent jaundice is seen in 10–30% of patients at some point in their disease after PTBD and stenting and requires re-intervention due to tumor growth (Fig. 21) (Tapping et al. 2011). The mean stent patency of 6–9 months explains the usual restriction to patients with limited life expectancy (Covey and Brown 2008).

References

Arellano RS, Gervais DA, Mueller PR (2011) CT-guided drainage of abdominal abscesses: hydrodissection to create access routes for percutaneous drainage. AJR Am J Roentgenol 196(1):189–191

Beland MD, Gervais DA, Levis DA, Hahn PF, Arellano RS, Mueller PR (2008) Complex abdominal and pelvic abscesses: efficacy of adjunctive tissue-type plasminogen activator for drainage. Radiology 247(2):567–573

Bilbao JI, Torres E, Martinez-Cuesta A (2002) Non-traumatic abdominal emergencies: imaging and intervention in gastrointestinal hemorrhage and ischemia. Eur Radiol 12(9):2161–2171

Covey AM, Brown KT (2008) Percutaneous transhepatic biliary drainage. Tech Vasc Interv Radiol 11(1):14–20

Cronin CG, Gervais DA, Hahn PF, Arellano R, Guimaraes AR, Mueller PR (2011) Treatment of deep intramuscular and musculoskeletal abscess: experience with 99 CT-guided percutaneous catheter drainage procedures. AJR Am J Roentgenol 196(5):1182–1188

Dinkel HP, Danuser H, Triller J (2002) Blunt renal trauma: minimally invasive management with microcatheter embolization experience in nine patients. Radiology 223(3):723–730

Fang JF, Wong YC, Lin BC, Hsu YP, Chen MF (2006) The CT risk factors for the need of operative treatment in initially hemodynamically stable patients after blunt hepatic trauma. J Trauma 61(3):547–553 discussion 53-4

Frevert S, Dahl B, Lonn L (2008) Update on the roles of angiography and embolisation in pelvic fracture. Injury 39(11):1290–1294

Gee MS, Kim JY, Gervais DA, Hahn PF, Mueller PR (2010) Management of abdominal and pelvic abscesses that persist despite satisfactory percutaneous drainage catheter placement. AJR Am J Roentgenol 194(3):815–820

Gervais DA, Brown SD, Connolly SA, Brec SL, Harisinghani MG, Mueller PR (2004) Percutaneous imaging-guided abdominal and pelvic abscess drainage in children. Radiographics 24(3):737–754

Ginat D, Saad WE (2008) Cholecystostomy and transcholecystic biliary access. Tech Vasc Interv Radiol 11(1):2–13

Haaga JR, Nakamoto D, Stellato T, Novak RD, Gavant ML, Silverman SG, Bellmore M (2000) Intracavitary urokinase for enhancement of percutaneous abscess drainage: phase II trial. AJR Am J Roentgenol 174(6):1681–1685

Haan JM, Biffl W, Knudson MM, Davis KA, Oka T, Majercik S, Dicker R, Marder S, Scalea TM (2004) Splenic embolization revisited: a multicenter review. J Trauma 56(3):542–547

Haan JM, Bochicchio GV, Kramer N, Scalea TM (2005) Nonoperative management of blunt splenic injury: a 5-year experience. J Trauma 58(3):492–498

Harisinghani MG, Gervais DA, Maher MM, Cho CH, Hahn PF, Varghese J, Mueller PR (2003) Transgluteal approach for percutaneous drainage of deep pelvic abscesses: 154 cases. Radiology 228(3):701–705

Hoffmann RT, Jakobs TF, Trumm C, Weber C, Glaser C, Reiser MF (2007) Vertebroplasty in the treatment of osteoporotic vertebral body fracture. Eur Radiol 17(10):2656–2662

Holden A (2008) Abdomen—interventions for solid organ injury. Injury 39(11):1275–1289

Iguchi T, Ogawa K, Doi T, Miyasho K, Munetomo K, Hiraki T, Ozaki T, Kanazawa S (2010) Computed tomography fluoroscopy-guided placement of iliosacral screws in patients with unstable posterior pelvic fractures. Skelet Radiol 39(7):701–705

Kasirajan K, O'Hara PJ, Gray BH, Hertzer NR, Clair DG, Greenberg RK, Krajewski LP, Beven EG, Ouriel K (2001) Chronic mesenteric ischemia: open surgery versus percutaneous angioplasty and stenting. J Vasc Surg 33(1):63–71

Kirat HT, Remzi FH, Shen B, Kiran RP (2011) Pelvic abscess associated with anastomotic leak in patients with ileal pouch-anal anastomosis (IPAA): transanastomotic or CT-guided drainage? Int J Colorectal Dis [serial online]. Available at: http://www.ncbi.nlm.nih.gov/entrez/query.fcg i?cmd=Retrieve&db=PubMed&dopt=Citation&list_uids= 21773700. Accessed 20 July 2011

Kokotsakis JN, Lambidis CD, Lioulias AG, Skouteli ET, Bastounis EA, Livesay JJ (2000) Celiac artery compression syndrome. Cardiovasc Surg 8(3):219–222

Kozar RA, Moore JB, Niles SE, Holcomb JB, Moore EE, Cothren CC, Hartwell E, Moore FA (2005) Complications of nonoperative management of high-grade blunt hepatic injuries. J Trauma 59(5):1066–1071

Kruger K, Heindel W, Dolken W, Landwehr P, Lackner K (1996) Angiographic detection of gastrointestinal bleeding. An experimental comparison of conventional screen-film angiography and digital subtraction angiography. Invest Radiol 31(7):451–457

Kuhn JP, Busemann A, Lerch MM, Heidecke CD, Hosten N, Puls R (2010) Percutaneous biliary drainage in patients with nondilated intrahepatic bile ducts compared with patients with dilated intrahepatic bile ducts. AJR Am J Roentgenol 195(4):851–857

Landwehr P, Arnold S, Voshage G, Reimer P (2008) Embolotherapy: principles and indications. Radiologe 48(1): 73–95 quiz 6–7

Levenson RB, Pearson KM, Saokar A, Lee SI, Mueller PR, Hahn PF (2009) Image-guided drainage of tuboovarian abscesses of gastrointestinal or genitourinary origin: a retrospective analysis. J Vasc Interv Radiol 22(5):678–686

Linsenmaier U, Kanz KG, Rieger J, Krotz M, Mutschler W, Pfeifer KJ, Reiser M (2003) CT-guided aortic balloon occlusion in traumatic abdominal and pelvic bleeding. Rofo 175(9):1259–1263

Liu CH, Gervais DA, Hahn PF, Arellano RS, Uppot RN, Mueller PR (2009) Percutaneous hepatic abscess drainage: do multiple abscesses or multiloculated abscesses preclude drainage or affect outcome? J Vasc Interv Radiol 20(8): 1059–1065

Lucey BC, Varghese JC, Hochberg A, Blake MA, Soto JA (2007) CT-guided intervention with low radiation dose: feasibility and experience. AJR Am J Roentgenol 188(5): 1187–1194

Maher MM, Gervais DA, Kalra MK, Lucey B, Sahani DV, Arellano R, Hahn PF, Mueller PR (2004) The inaccessible or undrainable abscess: how to drain it. Radiographics 24(3): 717–735

Malhotra AK, Fabian TC, Croce MA, Gavin TJ, Kudsk KA, Minard G, Pritchard FE (2000) Blunt hepatic injury: a paradigm shift from operative to nonoperative management in the 1990s. Ann Surg 231(6):804–813

Men S, Akhan O, Koroglu M (2002) Percutaneous drainage of abdominal abscess. Eur J Radiol 43(3):204–218

Menu Y, Vuillerme MP (2002) Non-traumatic abdominal emergencies: imaging and intervention in acute biliary conditions. Eur Radiol 12(10):2397–2406

Meredith JW, Young JS, Bowling J, Roboussin D (1994) Nonoperative management of blunt hepatic trauma: the exception or the rule? J Trauma 36(4):529–534 discussion 34-5

Miller DL, Balter S, Schueler BA, Wagner LK, Strauss KJ, Vano E (2010) Clinical radiation management for fluoroscopically guided interventional procedures. Radiology 257(2):321–332

Mohr AM, Lavery RF, Barone A, Bahramipour P, Magnotti LJ, Osband AJ, Sifri Z, Livingston DH (2003) Angiographic embolization for liver injuries: low mortality, high morbidity. J Trauma 55(6):1077–1081 discussion 81-2

Nix JA, Costanza M, Daley BJ, Powell MA, Enderson BL (2001) Outcome of the current management of splenic injuries. J Trauma 50(5):835–842

Pachter HL, Guth AA, Hofstetter SR, Spencer FC (1998) Changing patterns in the management of splenic trauma: the impact of nonoperative management. Ann Surg 227(5): 708–717 discussion 17-9

Pedicini V, Poretti D, Mauri G, Trimboli M, Brambilla G, Sconfienza LM, Cornalba G, Sardanelli F (2010) Management of post-surgical biliary leakage with percutaneous transhepatic biliary drainage (PTBD) and occlusion balloon (OB) in patients without dilatation of the biliary tree: preliminary results. Eur Radiol 20(5): 1061–1068

Popovic P, Kuhelj D, Bunc M (2011) Superior mesenteric artery embolism treated with percutaneous mechanical thrombectomy. Cardiovasc Interv Radiol 34(Suppl 2):S67–S69

Ramirez JI, Velmahos GC, Best CR, Chan LS, Demetriades D (2004) Male sexual function after bilateral internal iliac artery embolization for pelvic fracture. J Trauma 56(4): 734–739 discussion 9-41

Rieger J, Linsenmaier U, Euler E, Rock C, Pfeifer KJ (1999) Temporary balloon occlusion as therapy of uncontrollable arterial hemorrhage in multiple trauma patients. Rofo 170(1): 80–83

Rundback JH, Rozenblat GN, Poplausky M, Crea G, Maddineni S, Olson C, Agrawal U (2000) Re: jejunal artery angioplasty and coronary stent placement for acute mesenteric ischemia. Cardiovasc Interv Radiol 23(5):410–412

Saad WE (2008) Transhepatic techniques for accessing the biliary tract. Tech Vasc Interv Radiol 11(1):21–42

Sedat J, Chau Y, Razafidratsiva C, Bronsard N, de Peretti F (2010) One-stage percutaneous treatment in a patient with pelvic and vertebral compression fractures. Cardiovasc Interv Radiol 33(1):219–222

Seder CW, Kramer M, Uzieblo MR, Bove P (2009) Endovascular treatment of a superior mesenteric artery embolism in a high-risk Jehovah's Witness. J Vasc Surg 49(4): 1050–1052

Singh AK, Gervais DA, Alhilali LM, Hahn PF, Mueller PR (2006) Imaging-guided catheter drainage of abdominal collections with fistulous pancreaticobiliary communication. AJR Am J Roentgenol 187(6):1591–1596

Sofocleous CT, Hinrichs C, Hubbi B, Brountzos E, Kaul S, Kannarkat G, Bahramipour P, Barone A, Contractor DG, Shah T (2005) Angiographic findings and embolotherapy in renal arterial trauma. Cardiovasc Interv Radiol 28(1):39–47

Tapping CR, Byass OR, Cast JE (2011) Percutaneous transhepatic biliary drainage (PTBD) with or without stenting-complications, re-stent rate and a new risk stratification score. Eur Radiol 21(9):1948–1955

Tsalafoutas IA, Tsapaki V, Triantopoulou C, Gorantonaki A, Papailiou J (2007) CT-guided interventional procedures without CT fluoroscopy assistance: patient effective dose and absorbed dose considerations. AJR Am J Roentgenol 188(6):1479–1484

van Delden OM, Lameris JS (2008) Percutaneous drainage and stenting for palliation of malignant bile duct obstruction. Eur Radiol 18(3):448–456

van der Vlies CH, van Delden OM, Punt BJ, Ponsen KJ, Reekers JA, Goslings JC (2010) Literature review of the role of ultrasound, computed tomography, and transcatheter arterial embolization for the treatment of traumatic splenic injuries. Cardiovasc Interv Radio 33(6):1079–1087

Velmahos GC, Toutouzas K, Radin R, Chan L, Rhee P, Tillou A, Demetriades D (2003) High success with nonoperative management of blunt hepatic trauma: the liver is a sturdy organ. Arch Surg 138(5):475–480 discussion 80-1

Yamao Y, Yamakado K, Takaki H, Yamada T, Murashima S, Uraki J, Kodama H, Nagasawa N, Takeda K (2010) Optimal scan parameters for CT fluoroscopy in lung interventional radiologic procedures: relationship between radiation dose and image quality. Radiology 255(1):233–241

Index

M. Scaglione et al. (eds.), *Emergency Radiology of the Abdomen*,
Medical Radiology. Diagnostic Imaging,
DOI: 10.1007/978-3-540-88256-5, © Springer-Verlag Berlin Heidelberg 2012

Index

277

Printing and Binding: Stürtz GmbH, Würzburg